ENDOCRINOLOGY RESEARCH AND CLINICAL DEVELOPMENTS

ESTRADIOL

SYNTHESIS, HEALTH EFFECTS AND DRUG INTERACTIONS

Endocrinology Research and Clinical Developments

Additional books in this series can be found on Nova's website
under the Series tab.

Additional e-books in this series can be found on Nova's website
under the e-book tab.

ENDOCRINOLOGY RESEARCH AND CLINICAL DEVELOPMENTS

ESTRADIOL

SYNTHESIS, HEALTH EFFECTS AND DRUG INTERACTIONS

RICCO PALMERI
AND
SAL GRIMAUDO
EDITORS

NOVA BIOMEDICAL

New York

For permission to use material from this book please contact us:
Telephone 631-231-7269; Fax 631-231-8175
Web Site: http://www.novapublishers.com

Library of Congress Cataloging-in-Publication Data

ISBN: 978-1-62808-962-2

Library of Congress Control Number: 2013947630

Published by Nova Science Publishers, Inc. † New York

Contents

Preface

Estradiol is the major steroid hormone which is involved in several organic functions, such as physiological sexual behavior, development and maintenance of male and female reproductive organs, control of visceral secretion, modulation of immune system, and tumorigenesis. In this compilation, the authors discuss the synthesis, health effects and drug interactions of estradiol. Topics include the occurrence of estradiol in environmental waters; estradiol in the central nervous system and its role in neurodegeneration; the effects of estradiol on male and female reproductive tissues and the influence of endocrine disruptors; estradiol and prostate cancer; hydroxyestradiols and methoxyestradiols as endogenous factors associated to physiological and physiopathological conditions; estrogen and functional gastrointestinal disorders; estradiol and memory; estradiol in the environment; use of combined therapy of estrogens with antidepressants; estrogen and nitric oxide as a treatment for diabetes gastroparesis; estradiol synthesis after ovarian tissue cryopreservation and transplantation; estradiol-mediated overmodulation of the neuroendocrine hormone dopamine is central to the pathophysiology of restless leg syndrome during pregnancy; and estrogen modulation on oxidative stress and synaptic plasticity in the dorsal hippocampus.

Chapter 1 - Natural estrogens are a group of steroid hormones that include the main active hormones, 17ß-estradiol (E2), estrone and estriol. Among these compounds, E2 is recognized to be the most active estrogen synthesized in female ovaries.

Environmental problems due to estrogenic compounds are mainly related to aquatic environments. Indeed, numerous studies confirmed the occurrence of these substances at concentrations of toxicological concern (e.g., the feminization of fish in large rivers and toxicological effects on wildlife). Generally, the main sources of estrogens are recognized as treated and untreated municipal and industrial effluents, as well as livestock wastes from agricultural practices, as sewage and manure often used as fertilizers. Moreover the steroid hormones found in the urine of mammals are largely present as inactive conjugates, however the behavior of these forms will deconjugate to rapidly release the free hormones in the environment. As a consequence, large quantities of estrogens are spread in environmental waters, where they may sorb to sediments and persist for relatively long periods.

Recently, the development of new analytical equipment, namely tandem mass spectrometers coupled to LC and GC systems, allowed improvements in the sensitivity, selectivity, and speed of analysis. Such improvements in sensitivity and selectivity could also be accomplished by innovative sample preparation techniques, most of them with the added benefit to be easy to execute, cost effective, and environmental friendly.

Concerning the evaluation of the biological effects of estradiol, several methods have recently been developed: on whole organisms (vitellogenine assay), cells (cell proliferation), yeast estrogen screen, ER CALUX and molecular assays.

In this chapter, various aspects of the estradiol presence in environmental waters are discussed. An overview of the current legislation related to water quality is given. The work then focuses on the health and environmental impacts and evaluation methods. Then, finally, the example case studies illustrate the health effects of estradiol and its environmental impact.

Chapter 2 - Estrogens are one of the main female sex hormones. Within this group, the most active compound with estrogenic action is estradiol. In non-pregnant women, the ovaries are the main place where estradiol is synthesized through a mechanism that depends on pituitary hormones, but there is a well-documented mechanism of estradiol synthesis independent of gonads and pituitary hormones involving the aromatase enzyme, amongst others. Not only has the presence of aromatase been found in some areas of central nervous system, but also changes in its levels after brain damage.

Estradiol is the hormone that is mainly responsible for the development of secondary sexual characteristics in females. In addition to these sexual actions, it can also have effects on the central nervous system in males. Estradiol has been found to modulate different aspects in the brain, not only in normal physiology but also in pathological conditions. It can protect against brain injury, neurodegeneration and cognitive decline, and may act as a "recovery agent" in some central nervous system disorders. In recent years, some laboratories have focused on the mechanisms of estradiol used as a neuroprotective agent in some neurodegenerative diseases, although this action is not yet fully understood. Clinical studies have shown that blood levels of estradiol are associated with decreased risk, delayed onset and progression and enhanced recovery from several traumatic or chronic neurological diseases, although there is evidence that estradiol exposure can be deleterious to some neuronal population.

This chapter will focus on the effects of estradiol in the nervous system. The authors will describe some of the recently proposed action mechanisms, summarizing some of the recent progress made on understanding the mechanisms of action of estradiol in the central nervous system including the classical and non-classical receptor-mediated and non-receptor dependent pathways, and bring together some of its putative therapeutic effects for stroke and Alzheimer's disease models. The authors' review focuses on two neurodegenerative diseases with different etiologies and evolution over time. Stroke is a trauma with a fast evolution over time, while Alzheimer's disease is chronic disease that evolves slowly. In both cases, estradiol shows neuroprotective effects in animal models.

Finally, the possibility of using estradiol as a neuroprotector and/or "recovery agent" against some neurodegenerative disorder models is discussed.

Chapter 3 - Estradiol (E2) is the major steroid hormone which is involved in several organic functions, such as physiological sexual behavior, development and maintenance of male and female reproductive organs, control of visceral secretion, modulation of immune system, tumorigenesis, and others. This hormone is essential for the acquisition of secondary sexual characteristics and hypothalamic release of gonadotropin-releasing hormone (GnRH) in mammals. In women, E2 is primarily synthesized by the granulosa cells of the ovary during aromatization of androstenedione (produced in the theca cells) to estrone, and finally to E2. An additional but not significant E2 contribution is derived from liver, adrenal and mammary glands. In both sex, testosterone can be converted into estradiol by aromatization.

In females, E2 has a key role on the functioning of reproductive organs, supporting the lining of the endometrium, cervix, uterine tubes, and vagina. Also, E2 is essential for the growth and maturation of oocytes and to orchestrate folliculogenesis. During menstrual cycle, E2 triggers the hypothalamic-pituitary events via feedback system to induce ovulation, besides participating with progesterone in the preparation of endometrium for blastocyst implantation. In males, the effect of E2 seems to be more complex. E2 is produced by the activity of aromatase mainly in leydig cells of the testis. Current researches have provided evidences that E2 is not only responsible for differentiation and function of the testes, but it may also exert actions in the epididymis, efferent ductules, prostate, seminal vesicles, and even the penis. Furthermore, excessive estrogen exposure has been postulated to be the main cause of low sperm counts which can lead to subfertility or infertility-related disorders.

E2 binds to estrogen receptors (namely ERα and ERβ subunits) at nuclear level and stimulates selective genes transcription in a tissue and cell-specific manner. The effective activation of the ERs by E2 is strongly associated with an estrogen responsive element (ERE) in the promoter region of the target genes to control its activation and/or repression. There is a variety of medications that preferentially act on one of these ER to exert such effects. Notably, endocrine-disrupting chemicals (EDCs) are synthetic or natural compounds found in the environment which interfere with hormone production and physiological functions of the reproductive organs. The most EDCs affecting reproductive function include synthetic agents used as polychlorinated biphenyls, polybrominated biphenyls, methoxychlor (MXC), phthalates, dichlorodiphenyltrichloroethane (DDT), diethylstilbestrol (DES), and other related compounds. The naturally occurring agents with estrogenic activity are originated from phytoestrogens (e.g., genistein and coumestrol). This chapter will give attention to the main actions of E2 on both male and female reproductive organs and discuss on the specific toxicity of EDCs to the reproductive function.

Chapter 4 - Although the most impressive characteristic of prostate cancer is its androgen dependence, several studies support that 17β-estradiol (E_2) also plays an important role in onset and progression of prostate cancer. Regarding the effects of E_2 in prostate carcinogenesis, the authors can highlight the carcinogenic properties of several products derived from E_2 metabolism, which play an important role on cell malignant transformation. Several polymorphisms in estrogen-related genes such as estrogen receptors (ERs) and enzymes involved in E_2 biosynthesis and metabolism have been described to favour carcinogenesis. Also, both isoforms of ERs (ERα and ERβ), which act on cells in order to maintain the normal physiology of prostate gland, are differentially expressed between neoplastic and non-neoplastic prostate cells. Therefore, this deregulation may conduct to alterations on normal gene expression in prostate cells, which may favour the progression and migration of cancer cells. On the other hand, other studies have been pointing the anti-carcinogenic activity of E_2 in prostate. These contradictory effects are based on the role of ERβ, which has been shown to exhibit anti-proliferative and anti-oxidant functions. Taking into account the scientific evidences that relate E_2 with prostate cancer, several therapeutic approaches based on ERs are being explored. This chapter summarizes the main knowledge on how E_2 may contribute to the pathophysiology of prostate gland.

In developed countries, prostate cancer (PCa) is the most frequently diagnosed malignancy in men. The aetiology of this disease is complex and remains unclear. Risk factors for a high morbidity of PCa can be classified as endogenous (family history, hormones, race, aging and oxidative stress) or exogenous (dietary factors, physical inactivity, obesity, environmental factors, occupation, smoking, sexual activity, vasectomy). However, a positive family history is the strongest epidemiological risk factor for PCa.

The relationship between hormones and the pathogenesis of PCa has been extensively studied. PCa is generally considered a paradigm of androgen-dependent tumour. However, estrogens role appears to be equally important in both normal and malignant prostate. Recent epidemiologic and experimental data have clearly pinpointed the key roles of estrogens in PCa development and progression. PCa risk in adulthood could be determined by exposure to estrogens during embryonic, perinatal/neonatal, or peripubertal development, a phenomenon referred to as ''estrogen imprinting''. Estrogens action should be considered both at a systemic endocrine level, because these steroid hormones are able to act through the pituitary gland to indirectly lower androgens, and locally within the prostate tissue . Salonia and collaborators demonstrated for the first time that the circulating 17β-estradiol (E_2, the most potent subtype of estrogens) levels are associated with a greater incidence of high grade PCa. Patients with high E_2 levels have an increased risk to develop PCa. Another study also demonstrated that E_2 exposure could neoplastically transform the rat prostatic epithelial cells *in vitro*. These results support the idea that estrogens have long been implicated in the prostate carcinogenesis. In addition, high estrogens levels and low testosterone levels induce the development of inflammation upon aging and the onset of premalignant lesions.

Understanding how estrogens are synthesized and act on prostate cells, will indubitably contribute to better understand the molecular mechanisms underlying PCa onset and progression, as well as to delineate novel strategies in diagnosis and treatment of PCa.

Chapter 5 - Estradiol (E_2) is a steroidal hormone generated by the conversion of testosterone via the p450 aromatase enzymatic complex. The E_2 physiological actions are mainly mediated by its interaction with intracellular receptors known as estrogen receptors (ERs). The E_2-ERs complex is able to alter the gene expression in its target cells binding to specific sequences in the DNA. Besides, estrogens can also activate several intracellular signal transduction cascades (e.g., cAMP-PKA, IP3-Ca^{2+}) by non-genomic mechanisms.

Following to exert its biological effects in their target tissues, E_2 must be inactivated and eliminated by the body through its conversion to soluble compounds with a insignificant or very low estrogenic activity. These reactions are accomplished by several enzymatic processes that involve reactions of oxidations and conjugations. The enzymatic modifications that a molecule of E_2 undergoes to be eliminated include sulfonations, O-methylations, hydroxylations and glucurodinations. Even though the conversion of E_2 to inactive or less active metabolites occurs mainly in the liver, it has been reported that some peripheral tissues, including breast, uterus, placenta and brain, express the enzymes required to inactive E_2.

One of the most studied enzymatic pathways that inactive estradiol in peripheral tissues consists in a C-2 hydroxylation, a reaction catalyzed by the enzyme cytochrome p450, isoform 1A1 (CYP1A1), that generates a molecule of 2-hydroxyestradiol ($2OHE_2$) and the C-4 hydroxylation, a reaction catalyzed by the enzyme CYP1B1 that generates 4-hydroxyestradiol ($4OHE_2$). Then, the hydroxyl group previously added is replaced by a methyl group through a conjugation reaction catalyzed by the enzyme Catechol-O-Methyltransferase (COMT), which originates a molecule of 2- methoxyestradiol ($2ME_2$) from $2OHE_2$ and 4-methoxyestradiol ($4ME_2$) from $4OHE_2$.

Recently, it has been demonstrated that hydroxyestradiols and methoxyestradiols are not inactive molecules since several reports have shown that these estradiol metabolites may exert physiological actions in different organs and tissues, while an unbalanced estradiol metabolization to hydroxyestradiols and methoxyestradiols could be the responsible factor of several diseases including cancer and preeclampsia. In this chapter the authors will review the available literature concerning to the physiological effects that hydroxyestradiols and methoxyestradiols exert in several organs and how an altered production of hydroxyestradiols or methoxyestradiols could have deleterious effects on several biological functions. They will specially discuss the possible physiological and physiopathological effects of $2ME_2$ in female reproductive tissues, where this estradiol metabolite is able to alter the ovum transport and change the gene expression profile. Particularly, the authors will describe a group of $2ME_2$-induced genes in the mouse uterus that could be useful as biomarkers to elucidate the role of $2ME_2$ in the female reproductive tract.

Chapter 6 - This chapter will review: 1) the pathophysiological mechanisms of functional gastrointestinal disorders (FGIDs); 2) the effects of estrogen on motor dysfunction, visceral pain, gastrointestinal (GI) symptoms and some FGIDs such as gastroesophageal reflux disease (GERD), functional dyspepsia (FD), gastroparesis, irritable bowel syndrome (IBS) and constipation.

Chapter 7 - The role of estradiol as a sex hormone is well-established. However, estradiol also exerts actions in the central nervous system that extend beyond basic sexual and reproductive functions. In this respect, estradiol exerts pronounced effects on the morphology and function of brain regions not typically considered for their contribution to reproductive function. As such, circulating levels of estradiol have been shown to produce marked effects on both reproductive and non-reproductive behaviors. The well-documented effects of estradiol on dendritic spine density in hippocampal pyramidal cells, an area critical to learning and memory, indicate an important role for estradiol in memory function. These "non-reproductive" behavioural effects remain unclear and the precise actions of estradiol on memory function are yet to be fully elucidated. The effects of estradiol on the brain throughout the lifespan are of particular interest due to the therapeutic implications which may be derived. While this is of particular interest during aging, it is also important to examine the effects of estradiol on the young adult and adolescent brain to determine the functional implications of estradiol's effects. A review of the pertinent literature concerning estradiol's morphological consequences in the brain, in particular, the hippocampus, and effects on memory function will be examined.

Chapter 8 - In last decades, increases in the occurrence of certain abnormalities in development of wildlife species brought world-wide attention to scientific community about environmental contaminants. Estradiol is a steroidal natural hormone produced by humans and animals that is excreted in urine and feces, reaching the natural environment mainly through discharge from wastewater treatment plants (WWTP). The environmental occurrence of estradiol leads to increase the frequency of appearance of reproductive disorders and cancer in wildlife and probably in humans, being nanogram-per-liter levels of this compound able to produce endocrine disruption in living organisms. Reported concentrations of estradiol in environmental matrices are usually very low and the analytical difficulties associated with the determination of this estrogen in environment have been overcome by using preconcentration and clean up steps followed by highly sensitive analytical methods and the number of analytical methods currently available for the determination of estradiol in environmental matrices is still limited.

The purpose of this chapter is to provide a general overview on estradiol occurrence and analysis in environmental matrices.

Chapter 9 - Depression is an important health problem, particularly in women around perimenopause. Controversial results exist in the efficacy of the combination of estrogens with antidepressants for depression treatment. Indeed, the use of estrogens as replacement therapy or as co-adjuvant with antidepressants has been subject of intense debate due to the possibility that estrogens may induce carcinogenic effects. However, recent reports indicate that the age of intervention -in relation with the menopause onset- is a crucial factor to explain the failure or success of the combined treatment with estrogens and antidepressants.

Other feature that contributes to the controversy is the type of compounds. Thus, the estrogenic compounds -with divergent neuropharmacological properties- differentially interact with the dissimilar kind of antidepressants: selective serotonin reuptake inhibitors, mixed reuptake inhibitors, tricyclics, atypical and monoamine-oxidase inhibitors.

The present review analyzes these two factors: age of treatment in relation to loss of ovarian function and type of estrogen/antidepressant. Thus, in the first part is presented a brief panorama of clinical and preclinical data of combining estrogenic compounds (17-β estradiol, E_2 and 17-α ethinyl-estradiol, EE_2) and antidepressants that the authors have used in basic research studies: two selective serotonin reuptake inhibitors (fluoxetine and citalopram), a mixed serotonin-noradrenaline reuptake inhibitor (venlafaxine) and a tricyclic compound preferentially with noradrenergic actions (desipramine).

Secondly, the antidepressant effects of the selective serotonin reuptake inhibitors are analyzed in relation to the subject's age and the time of loss of ovarian activity (menopause or ovariectomy) in clinical and preclinical studies. Finally, the participation of different monoaminergic and estrogen receptors as mediators of the synergism observed between estrogens and antidepressants is discussed.

Chapter 10 - Diabetic gastroparesis, defined as delayed gastric emptying, is one of the most debilitating complications of both type 1 and type 2 diabetes. Normal gastric motility/emptying requires an integrated, coordinated interplay between sympathetic, parasympathetic, and intrinsic-gut (enteric) nervous systems, interstitial cells of Cajal, and gastrointestinal smooth muscle cells. Any disturbance in their interactions has the potential to alter gastric function, and ultimately affects gastric emptying. Multiple contributing factors, including depletion of interstitial cells of Cajal, oxidative stress, excitatory and inhibitory neuropeptides, estrogen, and the nitric oxide regulator of neuronal nitric oxide synthase activity (nNOSα), have been linked to the development of gastroparesis.

Gastroparesis is far more common in women (60-70%), suggesting a possible estrogen role in gastric emptying dysfunction. Several animal and human studies have demonstrated that estradiol-17β causes delayed gastric emptying. In one study, estrogen administration in overiectomized rats, as well as postmenopausal women receieving estrogen replacement therapy, resulted in delayed gastric emptying.

Nitric oxide is a major neurotransmitter in the gut and a key physiological mediator of non-adrenergic and non-cholinergic relaxation of gastrointestinal smooth muscle cells. There is a myriad of evidence suggesting that gastroparesis is associated with changes in gastric neuronal nitric oxide synthase (nNOSα) expression and its activation state, which directly regulates the bioavailability of nitric oxide. Taken together, these evidences suggest the estrogen's role in normal gastric emptying may be via a nitric oxide regulatory pathway. The authors recently developed an animal model of diabetic gastroparesis by injecting male and female rats with streptozotocin. Male diabetic rats without gastroparesis were subsequently injected with estrogen for 3 weeks and then evaluated for the development of gastroparesis.

Although male diabetic gastroparetic (either streptozotocin- or estrogen-induced) rats exhibited similarity in disease pathology to that of females, the molecular mechanisms of development were different. The authors' results indicated that slow gastric emptying in both male diabetic groups was not associated with the level of expression and dimerization of nNOSα in gastric tissues. In contrast, females with diabetic gastroparesis demonstrated significantly impaired levels and dimerization of nNOSα in the antrum and pylorus. These results open new considerations for a potential role that estrogen may play in normal gastric emptying via a nitric oxide regulatory pathway.

Given the importance of nitric oxide in health and disease, studies on estrogen mediated regulation of nitric oxide will offer a better understanding of gastroparesis and potential development of new therapeutic interventions. In this article, the authors provide a synopsis of studies linking estrogen and nitric oxide to the development of gastroparesis. They discuss basic knowledge and their current understanding of mechanisms for gastroparesis development. Finally, perspectives on future directions of research on gastroparesis are discussed.

Chapter 11 - Fertility preservation is an effort to help cancer patients retain their fertility and an emerging discipline that now plays a central role in the care of reproductive women with cancer. An increasingly larger number of women are surviving with cancer because of improvement in diagnostic and therapeutic strategies. As a result, quality-of-life issues, including issues involving fertility preservation, have gained significant importance in cancer care. Breast cancer is the most common cancer in reproductive women in the US. Most women with breast cancer require the adjuvant chemotherapy including cyclophosphamide.

Cytotoxic treatment such as chemotherapy and/or radiotherapy can cause severe gonadal damages resulting in premature ovarian failure and infertility in female. Adjuvant chemotherapy particularly with alkylating agents such as cyclophosphamide is gonadotoxic and induces premature ovarian failure. The American Society of Clinical Oncology issued practice guideline update for fertility preservation options in cancer patients. Several well established methods for fertility preservation were introduced such as embryo and oocyte cryopreservation, gonadal shielding during radiotherapy, trachelectomy, and ovarian transposition. For fertility preservation, ovarian stimulation with gonadotropins for embryo or oocyte cryopreservation results in excessive levels of estrogen production. To reduce the estrogen exposure during ovarian stimulation in hormone dependent cancer, a novel protocol using letrozole (aromatase inhibitor) and gonadotropins was developed.

Ovarian tissue cryopreservation and transplantation is a main option to preserve their fertility in cancer patients who need cancer treatments without delay or do not want to undergo ovarian stimulation. For prepubertal girls diagnosed with cancer, ovarian tissue freezing is the only option for fertility preservation. Based on the site of transplantation of cryopreserved ovarian tissue, transplantation can be divided into two different types as orthotopic and heterotopic transplantation.

In a recent review of 60 cases of frozen-thawed ovarian transplantation, all ovarian tissue were frozen with the slow-freezing method and the restoration of ovarian activity was observed in at least 92.9%. In all cases, it took 3.5–6.5 months after transplantation before a rise in E2 and a decrease in FSH were detected (mean 4.5 months). To date, a total of 24 live births and 4 ongoing pregnancies have been reported worldwide from ovarian tissue cryopreservation and transplantation. Based on their review, the authors believe that ovarian cryopreservation and transplantation before cancer treatments is an effective option to preserve their fertility and to restore gonadal endocrine function including estradiol synthesis.

Chapter 12 - A large corpus of evidence points to an imbalance between the classical thyroid gland hormone (TH) and the neuroendocrine hormone dopamine (DA,[IMBTH/DA]) as the main derangement underpinning the pathophysiology of restless legs syndrome (RLS). DA is released by the hypothalamus into the portal blood circulation of the pituitary stalk, where it modulates the release of thyrotropin by the pituitary: DA inhibits the synthesis of the two component subunits of thyrotropin, alpha and beta. Furthermore, the dopaminergic system enhances the activity of the cytochrome P450 superfamily of enzymes via mesolimbic and tuberoinfundibular pathways. As nearly 20% of thyroid hormone is metabolized in these pathways, when DA activity increases, TH activity decreases. TH is essential for somatosensory system physiology, including the sensitivity of somatosensory receptors deep in the legs. When the thresholds of these somatic receptors are diminished, or when their signaling to the sensory cortex is too strongly transmitted, RLS may ensue. One action of TH is to positively influence the sensitivity of the receptors and the strength of their signal transmission to the sensory cortex. DA modulates this TH activity, and when DA is diminished, TH is increased, which may result in IMBTH/DA and RLS. RLS is more common in pregnant than in non-pregnant women, and during pregnancy, TH activity increases to meet the augmented metabolic necessities of pregnancy. Estradiol during pregnancy increases exponentially, and one of the effects of estradiol is the inhibition of DA release in the pituitary stalk. Furthermore, estradiol also increases thyrotropin release by increasing the sensitivity of thyrotrophic cells in the pituitary to thyrotropin-releasing hormone from the hypothalamus. It is known that estradiol levels in RLS pregnant women are higher than those in non-RLS pregnant women. In this chapter, the authors present evidence that suggests that excessive estradiol-mediated modulation of DA is central to the pathophysiology of RLS during pregnancy.

Chapter 13 - Estrogens are important for antioxidant mechanisms, maintenance of synaptic plasticity, and modulation of zinc content in the hippocampus of young and senile animals. The female brain is influenced by multiple factors including the decrease in estrogen levels, with that commonly accompanies stress and aging. However, plasticity in the hippocampus in pre- and postsynaptic sites, such as the mossy fiber system and dendritic spines, responds to the neuroprotective and antioxidant actions of hormone supplementation. Furthermore, in hippocampus, the ovariectomy produces spine pruning in pyramidal cells of CA1, a reduction of the mossy fiber area in CA3, a decrease of the zinc level in the whole hippocampus and an increase in oxidative stress. Following supplementation with a minimal dose of 17β-estradiol, these effects are reversed and these parameters have values similar to those observed during the proestrus stage of the estrous cycle, which is associated with a better performance in learning and memory in female rats. These studies confirm the roles of estrogen in protecting the hippocampus before oxidative stress and maintaining its synaptic plasticity.

In: Estradiol: Synthesis, Health Effects and Drug Interactions ISBN: 978-1-62808-962-2
Editors: Ricco Palmeri and Sal Grimaudo

Chapter 1

Occurrence of Estradiol in Environmental Waters

***Valentina F. Domingues*[1], *Virgínia C. Fernandes*[1], *Luísa Correia-Sá*[1] *and Catarina Mansilha*[2,3]**
[1]REQUIMTE, Instituto Superior de Engenharia,
Instituto Politécnico do Porto, Porto Portugal
[2]Instituto Nacional de Saúde Dr. Ricardo Jorgem Porto, Portugal
[3]REQUIMTE, Universidade do Porto, Porto, Portugal

Abstract

Natural estrogens are a group of steroid hormones that include the main active hormones, 17ß-estradiol (E2), estrone and estriol. Among these compounds, E2 is recognized to be the most active estrogen synthesized in female ovaries.

Environmental problems due to estrogenic compounds are mainly related to aquatic environments. Indeed, numerous studies confirmed the occurrence of these substances at concentrations of toxicological concern (e.g., the feminization of fish in large rivers and toxicological effects on wildlife). Generally, the main sources of estrogens are recognized as treated and untreated municipal and industrial effluents, as well as livestock wastes from agricultural practices, as sewage and manure often used as fertilizers. Moreover the steroid hormones found in the urine of mammals are largely present as inactive conjugates, however the behavior of these forms will deconjugate to rapidly release the free hormones in the environment. As a consequence, large quantities of estrogens are spread in environmental waters, where they may sorb to sediments and persist for relatively long periods.

Recently, the development of new analytical equipment, namely tandem mass spectrometers coupled to LC and GC systems, allowed improvements in the sensitivity, selectivity, and speed of analysis. Such improvements in sensitivity and selectivity could also be accomplished by innovative sample preparation techniques, most of them with the added benefit to be easy to execute, cost effective, and environmental friendly.

Concerning the evaluation of the biological effects of estradiol, several methods have recently been developed: on whole organisms (vitellogenine assay), cells (cell proliferation), yeast estrogen screen, ER CALUX and molecular assays.

In this chapter, various aspects of the estradiol presence in environmental waters are discussed. An overview of the current legislation related to water quality is given. The work then focuses on the health and environmental impacts and evaluation methods. Then, finally, the example case studies illustrate the health effects of estradiol and its environmental impact.

1. Introduction

The endocrine system is composed of different glands that control hormone metabolism. Hormones are fundamental for the regulation of a variety of biological functions including growth, metabolism, tissue function and differentiation, sexual development and behavior, and also the development of the immune system. Most hormones bind to specific membrane receptors on target cells, activating a cascade of biochemical reactions that eventually lead to the intended effect (e.g., development of a certain tissue type). However some lipophilic hormones (such as steroid and thyroid hormones) bind directly to intracellular receptors. This receptor-hormone complex interacts with transcription-control sequences of the DNA, thus modulating RNA and protein synthesis of specific genes(Leusch et al., 2006).

Natural steroids are secreted by the adrenal cortex, testis, ovary and placenta in human and animal, and include progestogens, glucocorticoids, mineralocorticoids, androgens and estrogens. Estrogens (estradiol (E2), estrone (E1) and estriol (E3)) are predominantly female hormones, which are important for maintaining the health of the reproductive tissues, breasts, skin and brain (Ying et al., 2002; Silva et al., 2012).

Steroid hormones are essential for reproduction, stress management, salt and glucose balances, as well as several other physiological processes. Due to the relatively simple chemical structure and lipophilic nature of steroids, their regulatory pathways can easily be modified by pharmacological, environmental, and/or dietary agents. Because of this, steroids or steroid-mimicking compounds are applied in many fields, making the identification of the endocrine activity of these compounds important (Sonneveld et al., 2006).

Both natural hormones (i.e. E1, 17α-estradiol and 17β-estradiol) and synthetic hormones (EE2) have the potential to behave like endocrine disrupting compounds (EDC) in the environment.

All humans, as well as animals, excrete natural and synthetic hormones in different amounts, depending on age, state of health, diet, or pregnancy (Ying et al., 2002; Silva et al., 2012). On average a menstruating female excretes 8 μg/day and a pregnant woman 600 μg/day, males also excrete E2 in a daily average of 3.9 μg/day (Johnson et al., 2000). Many of these hormones are peptides and are rapidly destroyed. However, the steroid hormones are chemically very stable and are excreted in the free form or as conjugates, which readily biotransform to the free form (Adlercreutz et al., 1987; Shore and Shemesh, 2003). One of the steroids of major concern is the E2, since it exerts physiological effects at lower concentrations than other steroids and can be found in the environment in concentrations above its lowest observable effect level (LOEL) for fish and plants (10 ng/L) (Panter et al., 1998; Irwin et al., 2001; Shore and Shemesh, 2003; Hamid and Eskicioglu, 2012).

Hormone steroids excreted by humans and animals enter the environment through the discharge of domestic sewage effluents and disposal of animal waste. Natural sources include human and animal hormones and phyto- and mycoestrogens that are intentionally or accidentally included in food and feed ingredients (Goksoyr, 2006).

These compounds could affect wildlife and human health by disrupting their normal endocrine systems. Hormone steroids have been detected in wastewater effluents and surface water as well as ground water at various levels. The behavior and fate of these hormone steroids in the environment depend on their physicochemical properties and environmental media (Yin et al., 2002).

The concern with water quality in terms of their estrogen and xenoestrogen content is an important issue when the contamination of drinking water supplies is considered. Several authors reported different analytical procedures and showed the presence of different hormones in water samples. Almost all processes operating in conventional water treatment plants (WTP) were not designed to remove such compounds leading to the occurrence of emerging contaminants in drinking, finished and/or tap waters (Jardim et al., 2012).

2. Impact of Estradiol in the Environment and Health

A growing body of scientific research indicates that some substances present in the environment may interfere with the normal function of the endocrine system of wildlife and humans (Silva et al., 2012). Since the magnitude of risks related to the presence of several EDCs (Endocrine Disrupting Chemicals), including the steroid hormones, in the environment is difficult to predict, large concern exists about these substances (Silva et al., 2012). When present in environment above a certain concentration (threshold limit value), these compounds can cause adverse health effects on wildlife (Hamid and Eskicioglu, 2012).

Among these different classes of EDCs, human and animal waste born hormones, often known as endogenous steroidal hormones, have been characterized by very high estrogenic potency (Hamid and Eskicioglu, 2012). Hormones act at extremely low levels (parts per trillion); therefore, in theory, even exposures to low levels of hormonally active agents may be of concern, particularly during sensitive periods of fetal development. Furthermore, endocrine-mediated effects may be subtle and manifest primarily in populations rather than in individuals (Solomon and Schettler, 2000). Furthermore, in the environment, chemical interactions may have profound consequences, since organisms are likely to be exposed to complex chemical mixtures of environmental pollutants (Lyssimachou and Arukwe, 2007). These complex chemical interactions have only recently become the focus of systematic investigation (Lyssimachou and Arukwe, 2007).

The presence of estrogenic compounds in the environment has become a concern because they may interfere with the reproduction of man, livestock and wildlife (Yin et al., 2002).

Natural hormones display the highest affinity for binding to nuclear estrogen receptors (ERs) and present the greatest estrogenic potency. Due to the strong estrogen affinity for ERs, the presence of low estrogen concentrations in the environment may produce endocrine disruption in a wide range of wildlife populations (Combalbert and Hernandez-Raquet, 2010).

It has now been clearly established that a number of chemical compounds and natural substances present in the aquatic environment are able to disturb the normal physiology and endocrinology of organisms (Brion et al., 2004). The natural steroid estrogens, namely the E2 have been measured in industrial and municipal sewage treatments works (STW) effluents and these discharges represent the main source of synthetic and natural estrogens into the aquatic system/environment. Nonetheless, the surface runoff is another possible source of estrogenic contamination (Brion et al., 2004). The E2 has also been detected in sewage treatment effluents. The origin of the natural steroid estrogens is predominantly from humans, and another source is from the use of conjugated estrogens for the treatment of cancer, osteoporosis, the menopause and hypogonadism. More diffuse sources come from agricultural practices (Brion et al., 2004).

In European countries, the concentrations of E2 in effluents from sewage treatment works range from low nanograms per liter up to hundreds of nanograms per liter. However, surface waters adjacent to discharges from STW effluents can receive considerable quantities of steroid estrogens (Brion et al., 2004).

E2 that is released by humans and livestock in the environment, can be considered one of the most potent endocrine disrupters even at nanogram per liter levels (Khanal et al., 2006). E2 is the main compound responsible for the estrogenic activity in sewage treatment works effluents, and given the reported concentrations in surface waters, and its estrogenic potency, E2 is now considered as an important contaminant of the aquatic systems (Brion et al., 2004). But this effect is not limited to aquatic organisms and therefore, nowadays the concern about the effect of E2, present in the environment, on human health is rising.

Indeed, estrogen hormones found in the environment appear to have physiological effects at very low concentrations, with the most supportive data being related to the effects on development, sexual differentiation, vitellogenin (VTG) production (the precursor of egg yolk protein), and reproduction of diverse fish species (Combalbert and Hernandez-Raquet, 2010) (table 1). These studies have been conducted in a variety of fish species from a number of different families but Medaka fish is the best represented. The results revealed that the major health effects (table 1) associated with exposure of different fish species to E2 included altered sexual development, presence of intersex species, changed mating behavior, decreased production and egg fertility, VTG induction, reduced male gonadosomatic index (GSI), etc.

It was showed that concentrations of E2 found in the environment could have disruptive effects on key steroidogenic enzyme pathways that control sexual development in fish (Halm et al., 2002).

The life stage of fish subjected to E2 exposure seems to have an impact in health outcome, namely in the Rare minnows. It was observed that the juvenile stage could be a critical period for the gonad development (Liao et al., 2009).

Recently Lee, Kanget et al.(Lee et al., 2012) also access the exposure effect on Medaka fish development, observing that the exposure to several EDCs including E2 significantly decreased the fluorescent intensity of the GnRH3 (Gonadotropin-releasing hormone) neurons, postponed the eye development, and retarded the growth of the embryos. Roepke et al. (Roepke et al., 2005) also mentioned that E2 and estrogenic EDCs all caused development toxicity in sea urchins through a TAM-sensitive (tamoxifen-sensitive manner) mechanism. Diotel, Nicolas et al. (Diotel et al., 2013) alos reported that E2 had an inhibitory effect on adult neurogenesis in gonad-intact adult zebrafish.

Other health effect due to E2 exposure was reported (Lerner et al., 2007) in a study conducted in an Atlantic salmon. In this experiment authors evaluated the effect of a treatment with 4-Nonylphenol (NP-L) or E2 in larvae. The authors observed a decreased gill sodium-potassium-activated adenosine triphosphatase (Na+,K+-ATPase) activity and seawater tolerance 1 year after exposure. Exposure to NP-L and E2 resulted in a latency to enter seawater and reduced preference for seawater. Both treatment groups exhibited increased plasma cortisol and decreased osmoregulatory capacity in response to a handling stressor.(Lerner et al., 2007).

The E2 genotoxicity was evaluated in *Oreochromis niloticus* using micronucleus test and the comet assay with erythrocytes, and the tested concentration of the E2 gave rise to mutagenic and genotoxic effects on the blood cells of *O. niloticus*. Therefore, the substance was considered a clastogenic chemical contaminant on both acute and chronic exposures (Sponchiado et al., 2011).

The majority of studies related to the effect of estrogens in the aquatic system were conducted on vertebrate species such as fishes. Therefore, the risk to aquatic invertebrates of exposure to estrogens is less clear although vertebrate-like sex steroids have been detected in a number of mollusks, suggesting that they may play a role in the reproductive physiology of these organisms (Peck et al., 2007). For instances, Zebra mussels rapidly bioaccumulate E2, being therefore susceptible to this compound in the environment (Peck et al., 2007).

Cubero-Leon et al. *(Cubero-Leon et al., 2010)* studied the influence of E2 and EE2 on the responses of serotonin (5-HT) receptor and COX (cyclooxygenases) mRNA expression also in mussels, *Mytilus edulis*, and the results showed that the natural estrogen, E2, as well as the synthetic estrogen, EE2, induced alterations, dependent on reproductive stage, in the mRNA expression levels of 5-HT receptor and/or COX.

The effect of E2 has also been evaluated in frogs and the results demonstrated that this exposure had animpact on the reproductive health of these animals (Hu et al., 2008).

In plants, abundant evidence exists about hormone impact on growth and seed germination (Combalbert and Hernandez-Raquet, 2010). Recent studies have reported, for example, the effect of hormones on shoot and root growth. The results of the exposure of *Medicago sativa* to E1 or E2 at 5 ng/L to 500 μg/L demonstrate that at low concentrations exposure, increased plant growth occurred, while at higher levels the opposite effect was observed (Shore et al., 1992). Similarly, exposure of alfalfa to sewage water containing between 10 to 300 ng/L of E1 and E2 induced an increase in phytoestrogen production (Shore et al., 1995).

Despite the compelling evidences on wildlife, adverse health effects of estrogenic hormones on human are still a debatable issue. Some studies have reported lower sperm count, declining male reproductive health and breast cancer as an aftermath of increased exposure to endogenous and exogenous estrogenic compounds (Ansar Ahmed, 2000; Delbès et al., 2006; McLachlan et al., 2006) while others refuted this, suggesting additional factors, namely geographic variation and cultural factors, as more important players in sperm count decline (Fisch and Goluboff, 1996; Safe, 2000). Systematic investigation of health effects on human involves many challenges, due to lag time between exposure and manifestation of clinical disorder, age and duration of exposure (Hamid and Eskicioglu, 2012).

The impact of environmental hormones in human beings is difficult to assess, in particularly on account of the presence in the environment of a wide range of endocrine-disrupting chemicals. Nevertheless, the trends in reproductive health in developed countries, which show an increase in testicular and breast cancer and a decrease in sperm quantity and quality, may result—at least partially—from exposure to estrogen hormones alone or in combination with other endocrine-disrupting compounds (Brody and Rudel, 2003; Sharpe and Irvine, 2004; Combalbert and Hernandez-Raquet, 2010).

Table 1. Heath effects in several species exposed to estradiol

Specie	Life stage	Concentration	Effects	Ref.
Oryzias latipes (Medaka fish)	Reproductive adults	29-463 ng/L	Affects reproductive capacity in the medaka fish. Both total number of produced eggs and egg fertility were significantly less in the highest E2 treatment (463 ng/L) In this study intersex gonads (testi-ova) were observed in males from a range of E2 treatments (29-463 ng/L) in water. The GSI of male medaka exposed to 463 ng/L was significantly (40%) less than that of the control fish.	(Kang Ij Fau - Yokota et al., 2002)
		1-100 nmol/L	The results indicated that exposure to E2 caused a significant decrease in the number of eggs and hatchings as compared to the negative control group at and above 3 nmol/l.	(Shioda and Wakabayashi, 2000)
		20 μg/L of 4-Nonylphenol (NP-I or NP-II) and E2	The low-level exposure resulting in the production of VTG may have subtly different biological effects on males and females. Males were more sensitive to low concentrations of NP. In samples collected following exposure to E2, the response of females was more similar to control levels following 5 d in untreated water while males continued to show heightened VTG response. It is likely that females are more metabolically equipped to cope with increased circulation and deposition of VTG and/or higher levels of estrogenic substances. These results suggest that for sampling to detect the estrogenic response of animals in the field, female tissue should be collected immediately following pulsatile exposure while male tissue should be sampled over a longer time course.	(Foran et al., 2000)
	Following hatch (5 to 8 days)	10.0, 1.0 and 0.1 μg/L	Produce exclusively female populations. E2-treated female fish had a lower fecundity in the highest concentration.	(Nimrod and Benson, 1998).
	Newly fertilized medaka embryos	0.001, 0.01, 0.1, and 1 ng/mL	The results showed that the chemicals (including E2) and the contaminated river water significantly decreased the fluorescent intensity of the GnRH3 (Gonadotropin-releasing hormone) neurons, postponed the eye development and retarded the growth of the embryos.	(Lee et al., 2012)
	Breeding medaka	0.05–1μg/L	Reproducing medaka exposed to mixtures of estrogenic compounds and equipotent treatments of E2 alone had very similar responses in mortality and reproduction (fecundity, number of spawns). However, mixtures of NP, E2, and EE2 elicited lower VTG induction than equipotent concentrations of E2 alone.	(Jukosky et al., 2008)
	Breeding pairs of medaka (≈ 5 months of age)	200 ng/L	Exposure to E2 alone resulted in significant biological changes in paired fish, including impaired reproductive capacity and plasma VTG induction.	(Sun)
	Post hatch	0.01-1μg/L	The estrogen hormones including the E2, induced intersex (i.e., testis–ova) and altered sex when the medaka fish were exposed to nanogram per liter concentrations of test compounds from hatch to approximately 100 d after hatch.	(Metcalfe Cd Fau - Metcalfe et al., 2001)
	Eggs or young varying developmental stages,	1) Varying stages, exposed to 5 mg/L for 24 h. 2) Embryo exposed to 15 mg/L	At 5 months, when exposure groups were compared to controls, significant differences were seen in reproductive success and viability of spring. Further, intersex gonads were observed in fish from all groups exposed to 15 mg/L E2. More phenotypic females than males; intersex gonads	(Koger et al., 2000)

Specie	Life stage	Concentration	Effects	Ref.
Pimephales promelas (Fathead minnow)	Reproductive adults	10, 1, and 0.1 nM (2724, 272.4, and 27.24 ng/L)	The primary effect of E2 on female is the alteration of the timing of recrudescence including VTG production. Spawning was inhibited in a way that indicated that exposure may have 'reset' the cycle of recrudescence toward the beginning of the oogenic cycle. VTG induction in male was strongly correlated with E2 exposure. An inhibition of egg production was observed.	(Kramer et al., 1998)
		1000, 100, 10, 2, 1, 0.5, 0.25, 0.125, 0.1 or 0.0625 nM	Exposure caused a reduction in size of the prominent male secondary sex characteristics, the fatpads and nuptial breeding tubercles. Females had ovaries in which most of the follicles were in the primary stage of development. There were more atretic follicles and fewer secondary and Graafian follicles. The results suggest that histological lesions could occur at ecologically-relevant exposures. Certain lesions caused by exposure of adult fathead minnows are not permanent.	(Miles-Richardson et al., 1999)
		32, 100 and 320 ng/L environmentally relevant concentrations	Exposure resulted in an oestrogenic response by a dose-dependent induction of plasma VTG and a dose-dependent inhibition of testis growth. There was an effect on P450aromB mRNA expression in the gonads; E2 up-regulated P450aromB mRNA expression in the testis and ovary in a dose-response manner after 14 d. Environmental concentrations can have disruptive effects on key steroidogenic enzyme pathways that control sexual development.	(Halm et al., 2002)
	Mature male	10, 32, 100, 320 and 1000 ng/L	The exposure to E2 lead to an increase in plasma VTG levels, which was accompanied by an inhibition of testicular growth. For the highest two concentrations of oestradiol this effect was total.	(Panter et al., 1998)
		Similar exposure to the contaminant during the 21-day; experiment 1) 17 ng /L; experiment 2)12 ng/L	All treatments responded with a rise in plasma VTG concentration when compared with the control. VTG mRNA induction, which tracked closely with plasma VTG concentrations in most treatments was not elevated in the HI treatment (in this treatment the E2 concentrations slowly decreasing through the course of the experiment), due to the lack of E2 exposure immediately prior to analysis. The ability of treatment male fish to hold nest sites in direct competition with control was sensitive to E2 exposure and did yield statistically significant differences between treatments and carrier control.	(Hyndman et al., 2010)
Gobiocypris rarus (Chinese rare minnow)	Embryo phase/ Larval/ juvenile-adult phase	E2 (1, 2.5, 5 ng/L), DES (1, 2.5, 5 ng/L), NP (0.1, 0.5, 2.0 g/L), mixtures of E2, DES and NP and control groups (0.01% DMSO).	Significant VTG induction and testis somatical index reduction were observed in adult males exposed to the mixtures. Meanwhile, the sex ratio of adult fish skewed to female was found in the fish exposed to high concentration of the mixture. These results revealed not only that the co-exposure of xenoestrogens can enhance the adverse effects on the development of fish, but that the adverse effects were induced by co-exposure of xenoestrogens below the threshold of similar detectable effects for single xenoestrogen.	(Jin et al., 2012)
	Different stages: larval, juvenile and adult.	5, 25 , 100 and 1000 ng/L	A markedly increased proportion of females and appearance of hermaphrodism were observed in the juvenile-stage group exposed to 25 ng/L. These results showed that VTG induction in the adult stage is more sensitive than in larval and juvenile stages. The juvenile stage may be the critical period of gonad development.	(Liao et al., 2009)

Table 1. (Continued)

Specie	Life stage	Concentration	Effects	Ref.
Oncorhynchus mykiss (Trout) and *Thymallus thymallus* (Grayling)	Reproductive Adults	Test 1: (0.5, 1.0, and 2.5 ng/L); Test 2: (1.0 ng/L)	At E2 ≥1 ng/L the semen volume obtained per male was significantly reduced, and after 50 days the sperm density and the sperm fertility also were reduced. When female grayling were exposed to 1.0 ng/L during the prespawning time ovulation occurred earlier than in the control group.	(Lahnsteiner et al., 2006)
Danio rerio (Zebrafish)	Embryo-larvae, juvenile and adult stages	5, 25 and 100 ng/L	The data show that the nature and level of the effects of E2 are dependent on the timing of the exposure with some effects being permanent (gonad differentiation) and others reversible (VTG induction).	(Brion et al., 2004)
	Adults	10^{-7} M	Data point to an inhibitory role of E2 on adult neurogenesis in gonad-intact adult zebrafish.	(Diotel et al., 2013)
Cyprinus carpio (Common carp)	Sexually mature male	0.1 and 1 µg/L	The mature male carp exposed failed to produce any milt and had reduced GSI. Some testis-ova occurred.	(Gimeno et al., 1998b).
	Juvenile males	9 and 23 µg/L	Immature, genetically male developed all into females.	(Gimeno et al., 1998a)
Carassius auratus (Goldfish)	Mature male	0, 1 and 10 µg/L	Regardless the exposure method, male GSI was reduced when compared to controls. In all E2 exposures fewer males had tubercles, a secondary male sex characteristic, and male sexual activity was dramatically reduced. Therefore, the exposure to E2 would result in a severe impair reproductive success.	(Bjerselius R Fau - Lundstedt-Enkel et al., 2001).
Poecilia reticulata (Guppies)	Reproductive adults	10 µg/L	Male sexual displays were dramatically inhibited. For fishes that depend on male sexual behavior to successfully reproduce, exposure to E2 could have dramatic consequences.	(Bayley et al., 1999)
		0.85 µg/L	Histological examinations revealed effects of the exposures on the gonads. Indications of blocked spermatogonial mitosis were seen in the testis structure of males after exposure to octylphenol or E2. The post-parturition ovaries of females exposed to E2 showed effects suggesting an inhibited yolk deposition.	(Kinnberg et al., 2003)
Salmo salar (Atlantic salmon)	Larvae	2 µg/L	Treatment with NP-L or E2 as yolk-sac larvae decreased gill sodium-potassium-activated adenosine triphosphatase (Na+,K+-ATPase) activity and seawater tolerance during smolt development, 1 year after exposure. Exposure to NP-L and E2 resulted in a latency to enter seawater and reduced preference for seawater approximately 2- and 5-fold, respectively. Both groups exhibited increased plasma cortisol and decreased osmoregulatory capacity in response to a handling stressor. The results suggest that early exposure to environmentally relevant concentrations of estrogenic compounds, can cause direct and delayed mortalities and that this exposure can have long term, "organizational" effects on life-history events in salmonids.	(Lerner et al., 2007)

Specie	Life stage	Concentration	Effects	Ref.
Jenynsia multidentata (Jenyns)	Adult males	0, 50, 100, and 250 ng/L E2 over 28 d	The authors' finding demonstrate that E2 exposure resulted in a very clear increase in brain aromatase transcript abundance at all assayed concentrations compared with control; however, no effects on gonadal aromatase expression were observed. Behavioral measures revealed increased sexual activity at 50 ng/L but not 100 or 250 ng/L. In contrast to the molecular and behavioral responses, the condition factor, gonadosomatic index, and sperm quality were unaltered by E2 exposure. The results suggest that E2 affects some aspects of the reproductive biology of *J. multidentata*. These modifications in the reproductive biology caused by exposure to E2 could potentially lead to long-term effects at population levels that may not always be immediately evident.	(Guyón, Roggio et al. 2012
Oreochromis niloticus (Nile tilapia)	Juvenile	6 ng/L	E2 had genotoxic potential in different periods. Differences were observed in the micronucleus frequencies of the 10 d exposure groups in relation to the control. The same was observed when comparing the nuclear abnormality frequencies of the 24 h exposure group with the negative control, and when using comet assay for 48 h evaluations. The tested concentration of the E2 gave rise to mutagenic and genotoxic effects on the blood cells, therefore the substance being considered a clastogenic chemical contaminant on both acute and chronic exposures.	(Sponchiado et al., 2011)
Strongylocentrotus purpuratus and Lytechinus anamesus) (Sea urchin embryos)	3 stages: 1) fertilization to pre-hatched blastula, 2) blastula to gastrula 3) post-gastrulation to early pluteus	The concentration ranges for each of the hormones and EDCs were centered on environmentally relevant concentrations	The stage most sensitive to E2 was the blastula stage with less overall sensitivity in the gastrula stage, regardless of concentration. Selective estrogen receptor modulators were added to the experiments individually and in combination with estrogenic EDCs to interfere with potential receptor-mediated actions. E2 and estrogenic EDCs all cause developmental toxicity in sea urchins through a TAM-sensitive.	(Roepke et al., 2005)
Dreissena polymorpha (Zebra mussel)	Adults	10 ng/L radiolabelled [14C] E2	Mussels rapidly bioconcentrated and metabolize E2 to a persistent fatty acid ester. The potential to bioaccumulate environmental estrogens suggests this mussel could be susceptible to estrogenic chemicals in the freshwater environment.	(Peck et al., 2007).
Xenopus laevis (African clawed frog)	Different developmental stages	Exp 1: 0, 1, 10, and 100 μg/L). Exp 2: 0, 1, and 100 μg/L)	E2 increased the percent of spermatocytes, spermatids, and spermatozoa compared to controls. Larval exposure did not alter hCG-induced gonadal testosterone secretion *in vitro* but significantly increased E2 secretion from ovaries of juvenile. E2 exposure during larval development appears to prevent PGC (primordial germ cell) migration to the medulla of developing gonads in a concentration-dependent manner. The degree of PGC migration to the medulla may be related to the degree of E2-induced intersex formation and feminization. Exposure during the larval period accelerates spermatogenesis and can increase ovarian E2 secretion in juveniles.	(Hu et al., 2008)

Table 1. (Continued)

Specie	Life stage	Concentration	Effects	*Ref.*
Mytilus edulis (Mussels)	Mature mussels	Exp 1: 5 and 50 ng/L Exp 2: 5 and 50 ng/L	5-HT receptor mRNA expression decreased following exposure. The opposite trend was observed at early gametogenesis stages. COX mRNA expression levels at both stages were generally decreased by E2 exposure. These results show that the E2, as well as EE2, induce alterations, dependent on reproductive stage, in the mRNA expression levels of 5-HT receptor and/or COX in this marine bivalve.	*(Cubero-Leon et al., 2010)*
Medicago sativa (Alfafa)		0.005-500 μg/L	Treatment with estrogens in the range of 0.005 to 0.5 μg/L increases both shoot and root dry weight. In contrast, estrogen in concentrations of 50 to 500 μg/L decreases plant growth. The effect of estrogen is most marked in the absence of nitrogen. Endogenous estrogen content of the plant did not increase at concentrations of 0.005-0.5 μg/L, which increased vegetative growth. Endogenous estrogen content of the plant did increase at concentrations of 50-500 μg/L, which inhibited vegetative growth and nodule weight. Estrogen in concentrations found in sewage water (0.3 μg/L) can affect the vegetative growth of alfalfa plants	(Shore et al., 1992).
		10 to 300 ng/L	The sewage water containing between 10 to 300 ng/L of E1 and E2 induced an increase in phytoestrogen production.	(Shore et al., 1995).

Estrogens affect also the functioning of several non-reproductive tissues, notably the immune system (Ansar Ahmed, 2000). Studies in several laboratories have clearly shown that natural E2 has a marked influence on the immune system. Both developmental (thymus and bone marrow) and mature (spleen and lymph nodes) lymphoid organs of normal mice are sensitive to the effects of estrogens. Therefore, estrogen affects all the major cellular players of the immune system, including T, B and antigen presenting cells (Ansar Ahmed, 2000). It is also known that clonal expansion of B lymphocyte precursors is suppressed by estrogen and that estrogen regulates the synthesis of serum and uterine IgM, IgA and IgG and augments antibody production to several non-self and self-antigens. Estrogenic hormones presumably also affect pathological conditions such as autoimmune diseases and allergies (Ansar Ahmed, 2000).

Additionally some researchers characterize certain estrogens, including the primary active endogenous estrogen E2, common pharmaceutical estrogens, and the synthetic estrogen Diethystilbestrol (DES), as carcinogens on the basis of their significant role in hormonally mediated cancers in humans and animals. Others do not consider endogenous hormones to be carcinogenic promoters because they allow neoplastically transformed cells initiated by other carcinogens to establish and grow by modifying the target tissue. In addition to acting as promoters, DES, E2, and certain metabolites of E2, including 16β- hydroxyestrone, have been shown to exhibit specific types of genotoxic activity under certain conditions. Steroidal estrogens are listed as known human carcinogens in the Report on Carcinogens, Tenth edition by the U.S. National Toxicology Program (NTP 2002) (Brody and Rudel, 2003).

Calaf et Roy (Calaf and Roy, 2008) concluded that estrogen and parathion alone, and in combination, induced malignant transformation of an immortalized human breast epithelial cell line, MCF-I0F, as indicated by anchorage independency and invasive capabilities (Calaf and Roy, 2008).

Chemical pollution of surface water presents a threat to the aquatic environment with effects such as acute and chronic toxicity to aquatic organisms, accumulation in the ecosystem and losses of habitats and biodiversity, as well as a threat to human health. As a matter of priority, causes of pollution should be identified and emissions dealt with at source, in the most economically and environmentally effective manner (Council, 2008a). The data presented raise further concerns about the effects of E2 in several species.

So, considering the high estrogenic potency of estrogenic hormones and their central role in regulating the endocrine system, the assessment of the occurrence, fate, and degradation of estrogen hormones in the environment is of particular concern (Combalbert and Hernandez-Raquet, 2010).

3. Regulation Proposals

The European Union (EU) Water Policy has as its main aims the responsibility to ensure the availability of a sufficient quantity of water of good quality throughout the EU, as well as a more efficient use of it. In 2000 the Water Framework Directive 2000/60/EC (Council, 2000) established a legal basis to protect and restore clean water across Europe and ensure its long-term, sustainable use and the prevention of deterioration. The WFD acknowledges the existence of considerable pressures on the aquatic environment, including that from chemical pollution which put in risk improvements in water quality (Commission, 2000).

Article 16 of the WFD sets out "Strategies against pollution of water" outlining the steps to be taken. The first step was the establishment of a list of priority compounds, in 2001, by Decision nº 2455/2001/EC of the European Parliament and of the Council of 20 November (Council, 2001) , that included 33 substances, or groups of substances, that were prioritized at Union level.

In 2008, and in accordance with the provisions and objectives of the WFD, the Directive 2008/105/EC (Council, 2008b) of the European Parliament and of the Council on Environmental Quality Standards in the Field of Water Policy (EQSD) layed down Environmental Quality Standards (EQS) for the 33 priority substances (PS) identified in Decision No 2455/2001/EC (Council, 2001) and 8 other pollutants that were already regulated at Union level.

The current 33 PS include a range of industrial chemicals, plant protection products and metals / metal compounds. Some PS were identified as Priority Hazardous Substances (PHS) because of their persistence, bioaccumulation and/or toxicity, or equivalent level of concern, a criteria that is consistent with the criteria for Substances of Very High Concern (SVHCs) under REACH.

Recently, the review of the list, as required by the WFD and the EQSD, involved an extensive technical analysis in identifying possible new PS and setting EQS for them.

The European Commission is now proposing to add 15 chemicals to the list of 33 pollutants that are already monitored and controlled in EU surface waters. This update will be achieved through a revision of the WFD and the EQSD. The revised list should be included in a new Directive amending the WFD. As a rule, Member States must meet environmental quality standards for new Priority Substances by 2021. The 15 substances include industrial chemicals, as well as substances used in biocides, pharmaceuticals and plant protection products. They have been selected on the basis of scientific evidence that they have a significant impact in the environment and pose a risk to human health)(Comission).

Pharmaceuticals compounds were proposed for the first time, namely: 17 alpha-ethinylestradiol (EE2), 17 beta-estradiol (E2) and diclofenac. The proposal does not put into question the medicinal value of these substances, but addresses the potential harmful effects of their presence in the aquatic environment. Concentrations above the proposed standards can affect fish health, reducing fertility, for example, and harming other living organisms (Vethaak et al., 2006).

In the United States, the Safe Drinking Water Act (SDWA) is the main federal law that ensures the quality of Americans' drinking water. Under SDWA, the United States Environmental Protection Agency (EPA) sets standards for drinking water quality having national primary drinking water regulations for more than 90 contaminants, and oversees the states, localities, and water suppliers who implement those standards.

The SDWA includes a process to identify and list new unregulated pollutants which may require a national drinking water regulation in the future. So, EPA must periodically publish a list of contaminants (called the Contaminant Candidate List or CCL) in order to prioritize research and data collection efforts to determine whether a specific contaminant should be regulated.

The final Contaminant Candidate List (CCL 3) includes 104 chemicals or chemical groups and 12 microbiological contaminants which are known or anticipated to occur in public water systems and have the potential to present health risks through drinking water exposure. The list includes chemicals used in commerce, pesticides, waterborne pathogens, disinfection byproducts, and biological toxins.

The CCL3 comprises nine hormones (17-alpha-estradiol, 17-beta estradiol, equilenin, equilin, estriol, estrone, EE2, mestranol, and norethindrone) based on new health effects and occurrence data in ambient water (EPA).

The SDWA provides for the establishment of enforceable primary maximum contaminant levels (MCLs) to regulate the concentration of microbial and chemical substances in drinking water.

With the primary purpose of the protection of public health, the World Health Organization (WHO) published the Guidelines for Drinking-water Quality that provide some recommendations for managing the risk from hazards that may compromise the safety of drinking-water. The Guidelines are addressed primarily to water and health regulators, policymakers and their advisors, to assist in the development of national standards and are also used by many others as a source of information on water quality and health and on effective management approaches. In 2011 it was published the fourth edition that in Chapter 8 introduced the pharmaceuticals as chemicals of emerging concern (WHO).

The WHO also published in 2012 a report untitled pharmaceuticals in drinking-water. This technical report aims to provide practical guidance and recommendations in managing concerns over pharmaceuticals in drinking-water, including steroid hormones and phytoestrogens, taking into consideration the available scientific knowledge and evidence. It emphasizes the importance to prioritize this emerging issue in the overall context of water safety management, which includes microbial and other chemical risks that may threaten the safety of drinking-water. (WHO, 2011b).

Natural hormones were also included in an assessment of the state of the science on endocrine disruptors prepared by a group of experts of the United Nations Environment Programme and the World Health Organization, untitled State of the Science of Endocrine Disrupting Chemicals as considerable amounts of steroid hormones used for controlling sexual development and reproduction are released daily directly to the environment in untreated sewage

The endogenous steroidal EDCs are characterized to be extremely potent when compared to other non-hormone EDCs (WHO).

In the revision of Drinking Water Quality Standards for drinking water quality analysis in Japan, E2 and EE2 were included in the list of items for further study with target values of 0.08 μg/L and 0.02 μg/L, respectively ((MHLW, 2003).

On 24 November 2007, Australian and international researchers, policy makers, regulators, water suppliers and research investors drafted the first national position paper on EDCs: The 2007 Black Mountain Declaration on Endocrine Disrupting Chemicals in Australian Waters. The paper focuses on environmental and human health implications and recommends future research objectives as well as attention to policy and public awareness.

The UK Environment Agency and the European Chemicals Bureau used the information from the UK study to draft concentrations of these chemicals that would protect aquatic life from adverse effects. They set draft guidelines for natural hormones like E1 and E2 at levels below 5 and 1 ng/L, respectively, whereas the active hormone in the contraceptive pill and hormone replacement therapy, EE2, should not exceed 0.1 ng/L (Targeting Endocrine Disruptors in Australia's Waterways. Land & Water Australia).

4. Methods of Analysis

4.1. Instrumental Methods

The entire world is paying attention to the research for finding the best method of changing the impact of E2 on human and animal health.

Estrogens have been shown to be present in the environmental waters. These compounds have been determined, by a variety of analytical procedures, in the influents and effluents of wastewater treatment plants (WWTP), fresh waters, rivers, and even drinking waters. The determination of natural and synthetic estrogens and progestogens in natural water is, however, a difficult analytical task, because of the very low detection limits required and the complexity of the matrices.

Because of the complexity of environmental and tissue matrices and the trace levels of feminizing chemicals, multi-step sample preparation is often needed to enrich analytes and reduce interferences, processes which significantly decrease throughput of the analysis. Most water samples are treated using solid-phase extraction (SPE). Disk-type adsorbents have been successfully used in SPE when analyzing feminizing chemicals in water, as they allow a flow rate up to 100 mL/min and reduce sample loading time (Chen et al., 2012) .

Thus, in general, complicated, time-consuming extraction and purification processes, usually based on the application of solid–liquid extraction, are performed before final determination by common chromatographic techniques coupled with mass spectrometry.

The first methods used primarily GC–MS or GC–ion trap-MS–MS detection at the end of the 1990s (Briciu et al., 2009). Within the last 10–15 years, the increasing use of liquid chromatography–mass spectrometry (LC–MS) has led to a revolution of environmental analysis, providing a new analytical tool that enables the identification of highly polar organic pollutants without derivatization, down to nanogram-per-liter levels in all kinds of water bodies (wastewater, surface water, groundwater, and drinking water). The major innovation that enabled this, involved the development of the appropriate ionization interfaces to couple LC with MS. Currently, electrospray ionization (ESI) and atmospheric pressure chemical ionization (APCI) are the most commonly used LC–MS interfaces. Ultra-high performance liquid chromatography (UHPLC) is an LC system that can tolerate pressures up to 19,000 psi and takes advantage of a small-particle column which possesses a very flat Van Deemter curve and increases linear velocity without significantly affecting separation. UHPLC provides rapid chromatography, increased peak capacity and better sensitivity without sacrificing LC resolution (Chen et al., 2012).

4.1.1. Extraction

Extraction of steroid sex hormones and related synthetic compounds from environmental water is usually performed by offline solid-phase extraction (SPE). Given the low analyte concentrations found in water samples, a pre-concentration by SPE is required prior to analysis.

SPE now belongs to well established methods due to the experimental simplicity, easy automation, a smaller consumption of nonaqueous solvents compared to conventional techniques, and to availability of many different sorbents. SPE is thus used in most cases as the first preconcentration technique. The procedure involves preconditioning of the sorbent, sample loading, washing of the sorbent with the sample sorbed and sample elution.

General, the procedure for preconcentration of estrogens from samples of environmental waters consists of the following steps: the samples are filtered, passed through the sorbent in the form of a disc or a cartridge, the analytes are eluted from the sorbent, the eluate is evaporated to dryness and the residue is dissolved in an organic solvent. Reverse phase sorbents are probably the best phases for estrogens (Pailler et al., 2009). Automated SPE has been reported (Zuehlke et al., 2004). Disks and, most frequently, cartridges have been employed for the SPE of these compounds. Cartridges and recently disks, have the advantage of being amenable to system automation, because specific devices are available for unattended washing, conditioning, sample loading, washing again, eventual drying, and final elution of a large number of samples (Chen et al., 2012).

Octadecyl (C18)-bonded silica gave adequate results for EDCs analysis (Noppe et al., 2007; Moreira et al., 2011) and hydrophilic lipophilic balance HLB have been the SPE adsorbents most widely employed. Although the use of styrenedivinylbenzene (SDB), packed in cartridges and SDB-XC disks, among others, has also been reported in the literature (Boyd et al., 2003; Mansilha et al., 2012).

Oasis HLB were chosen for their ability to retain a large number of compounds; basic, neutral, and acidic. It is designed, in fact, for retaining both hydrophilic and hydrophobic compounds with high capacity by means of both van der Waals and H-donor-H acceptor interactions. The Oasis HLB is one of the most important types of cartridge for the extraction of estrogenic compounds (Rocha et al., 2011b; Jardim et al., 2012). A comparison of the various types of SPE sorbents, protocols, and devices has been made by Lopez de Alda and Barcelo (Lopezde Alda and Barcelo, 2001). In this paper various procedures for the determination of several estrogens (estriol, E2, ethynyl estradiol, estrone, and diethylstilbestrol) and progestogens (progesterone, norethindrone, and levonorgestrel) in the environmental matrices, including water and river sediment, are described (Lopezde Alda and Barcelo, 2001).

A study comparing the behavior of different cartridges (C18, HLB, PLEXA, EASY) proved that the adsorbent HLB with EDTA had the best for quantitative extraction of estrogens from water. The other adsorbents were also showed acceptable recoveries for the analytes investigated. The results showed that EDTA enhanced significantly the recoveries (Pailler et al., 2009). Recently, a study compared six different cartridges (LiChrolut RP-18, LiChrolut EN/RP-18, Strata X, Strata SDB-L, GracePure C18-Fast and GracePure C18-Low) were tested. Strata SDB-L cartridges presented good performance in the extraction procedure with greater retention capacity and were chosen due to their efficiency–cost ratio (Mansilha et al., 2012).

A novel and fast, disk-type automated SPE/UHPLC methodology , which allows the quantification of the estrogens has been presented recently by Chen et al. (Chen et al., 2012). The RSD are between 6 and 12 %, while recoveries are higher than 60 %, which suggests that the method is precise and accurate. The UHPLC shortened the chromatographic time to less than 10 min, and UHPLC/MS/MS on ESI provided detection limits at sub- to few pg levels for most analytes.

To improve the stability of the compounds and also the precision and the sensitivity of the GC analysis, the derivatization is carried out in the case of compounds that have poor volatility, poor thermal stability, or that can be adsorbed in the injector will exhibit non-reproducible peak areas, heights, and shapes.

A interlaboratory procedure based on SPE followed by derivatization and GC-MS analyses was developed for the assessment of estrone, 17β-estradiol and 17α-ethinylestradiol by Mansilha et al. (Mansilha et al., 2012). This interlaboratory study was performed in two different laboratories using different equipments and chromatographic columns, in order to evaluate the robusteness of the method and increase the quality control over its application in routine analysis. The results showed that SPE/GC-MS procedure, using SDB-L cartridges, was suitable protocol for screening ultra-trace levels of the estrogens (Mansilha et al., 2012).

Table 2.Summary of analytical methodologies for estradiol determination

Sample	Sample Preparation	Method	Limits (ng/L)	Concentration found (ng/L)	Ref
Surface water	SPE: Oasis® HLB Chromabond® C-18EC, Chromabond® EASY and Bond Elut® PLEXA	HPLC-QqQ-MS	LOQ: 3	35	(Pailler et al., 2009)
	SPE: C18	HPLC-MS/MS	LOQ: 3.6	62.6	(Moreira et al., 2011)
	SPE: Oasis HLB	(LC-MS/MS)	-	<20	(Dutta et al., 2012)
	SPE: Oasis HLB cleanup: silica	HPLC-DAD	LOQ: 9.2-21.3	-	(Ribeiro et al., 2007)
River water	Disk-type automated SPE: C8 Speedisks	UHPLC/MS/MS	LOQ: 2.94	<LOD	(Chen et al., 2012)
	SPE C18	GC-MS	LOQ: 0.3	1.15-10.70	(Ra et al., 2011)
River and sea water	SPE: Oasis HLB	GC-MS	LOQ: 1.99	13.39	(Rocha et al., 2011a)
River and seacoast water	SPE: Oasis HLB	GC-MS	LOD: 0.6	>10	(Rocha et al., 2011b)
Groundwaters	SPE: HLB	GC-MS	LOD:0.75	3.18-5.17	(Li et al., 2012)
Surfacel water, groundwater	SPE: StrataX SDB	GC-MS	LOQ: 8.30-38.80	-	(Mansilha et al., 2012)
Estuary water	SPE: C18	GC-MS	LOQ: 0.25	<LOQ	(Noppe et al., 2007)
	SPE	HPLC-DAD GC-MS	LOQ: 55	<LOD	(Ribeiro et al., 2009)
Surface, ground, and drinking water	automated SPE: RP-C18	LC-MS/MS	LOQ: 0.2	-	(Zuehlke et al., 2004)
Surface water and drinking water	SDB-XC Empore disk	GC-MS/MS	LOD: 0.1	-	(Boyd et al., 2003)
	SPE: HLB Oasis	LC-MS/MS	LOQ: 0.6	nd	(Jardim et al., 2012)

4.1.2. Chromatography

Many diverse methods have been adopted for the monitoring of estrogens in environmental waters including GC-MS, LC-MS, and MS/MS detection. The use of LC-MS/MS to determining feminizing compounds is increasing because it provides good selectivity and detection sensitivity (Pacakova et al., 2009). Chemical analyses can give both quantitative and qualitative information on the chemicals in water samples. The decision to use GC or LC is usually based on the physicochemical characteristics of the target analyte. The polar functional groups and/or are thermally labile and do not lend themselves readily to GC analysis. Thus, most GC methods for estrogens must incorporate a derivatization step to overcome these limitations. LC is generally applicable to more polar compounds, in contrast to GC. The use of MS for detection in either case gives a second dimension of information, which can be used to confirm the identity of the targeted compound through its mass spectrum.

The advantages of GC involve a high separation efficiency, a high speed of analysis, the availability of highly sensitive detectors and, last but not least, environmental friendliness owing to the fact that the mobile phases are inert gases.

HPLC has some important advantages over GC techniques, namely, estrogen samples can be analysed directly, without derivatization, and aqueous samples do not require drying which is necessary in GC analyses. A number of sensitive detectors are available in an HPLC. On the other hand, a drawback of classical HPLC lies in a high consumption of solvents and, with HPLC-MS, in high cost of the instrumentation.

The HPLC separation systems for analyses of estrogens usually employ octadecyl chemically bonded stationary phases, in combination with mobile phases based on aqueous acetonitrile, eventually combined with buffers. The use of LC-MS/MS to determining feminizing compounds is increasing because it provides good selectivity and detection sensitivity (Pacakova et al., 2009). Recently, a sensitive determination of estrone, 17β-estradiol and 17α-ethinylestradiol in river waters using GC-MS/MS has been published (Rocha et al., 2013). Good sensitivity with method detection limit (MDL), obtained for E1, E2 and EE2 were 4.9, 2.5 and 3.15 ng/L. Method quantification limits (MQL) were below 25.88 ng/L. A method, which employs SPE and LC-MS/MS, using ESI in both positive and negative modes has been developed for the trace analysis of pharmaceuticals; include 3 homones (estrone, β-estradiol, and 17-α-ethinyl estradiol) in various waters. Recovery rates range from 70 to 94%, with relative standard deviations between 4 and 19% (Pailler et al., 2009).

The analysis of estrogens in the environmental waters constitutes a difficult task, because of the complexity of the matrices and their very low concentrations. The advances of the analytical chemistry are in order to achieve the best sensitivity and selectivity and simplify the sample preparation methodologies

4.2. Biological Methods

Endocrine signaling is a complex process involving synthesis, release, uptake, and the eventual degradation of hormones. The physiological response generated in the target cell due to a hormone is a composite of these processes. Thus, the effective concentration is that concentration capable of inducing a specific response in the target cell and, in the case of E2, is modified by binding to serum proteins such as albumin and sex hormone binding globulin (Arnold Sf Fau - Robinson et al., 1996).

There is currently a need to validate rapid methods to evaluate the overall androgenic and estrogenic potential of different types of environmental waters to develop risk assessment schemes. In that context, chemical analyses have limitations in that they require a priori knowledge of the nature of the biologically active chemicals present in the sample and do not take into account the different potencies of chemicals or possible interactions among the multitude of chemicals present in complex mixtures (Leusch et al., 2006). The most potent chemicals need only be present at trace concentrations to induce biological effects, and often are at or below analytical detection limits. *In vitro* bioassays can provide an assessment of the overall biological activity in an environmental sample, making them ideal for rapid and large-scale screening (Leusch et al., 2006).

Instrumental methods are reliable, but they have several potential drawbacks, such as expensive instrumentation, complex derivatization, extensive clean-up, and purification, and they also require a very high level technical expertise for operation. High cost and low throughput limit the use of these techniques (Swart and Pool, 2007). The unpredictability of the composition of environmental or field samples further hinders accurate characterization of estrogenic exposure by chemical methods. It has been demonstrated that anywhere from 15 to 50% of estrogenic chemicals, such as E2, can be bound by humic substances occurring in natural water. This suggests a potential discrepancy between the measured concentration and the biologically available concentration of contaminants (Biales et al., 2007).

The most critical issue of an *in vivo* test system is its capability to predict endocrine effects in wildlife populations. Full life-cycle or even multi-generation tests are usually regarded as the method of choice for the detection of population-relevant endpoints such as reproductive failure, but they are very time- and cost-intensive (Baumann et al., 2013). Unfortunately, analyses that focus on higher orders of biological organization, such as histopathological abnormalities, reduced fecundity, or mortality, are relatively expensive, laborious, and long-term in duration (Biales et al., 2007).

The crystal structure of the ligand binding domain of the human estrogen receptor alpha (ERα) was already elucidated. Since the gap of the ligand binding domain is much larger than E2 requires, there is space for a variety of other molecules to interact with the ERα. Thus, the recognition of estrogenic properties largely depends on empirical testing. The wide structural variety of the xenoestrogens presently known, reflecting the structure of the human ER, sets a limit to single compound chemical analysis of environmental matrices regarding time and labour. Therefore, sensitive and specific *in vitro* biotests are required for the screening of environmental samples for their content of substances with receptor-mediated estrogenic activity regardless of their chemical structure (functional analysis) (Korner W Fau - Bolz et al., 2000).

A positive result in a receptor-binding assay does not necessarily translate into receptor activation and subsequent *in vivo* effects, but rather indicates the potential for such an effect and warrants further confirmatory testing in more complex *in vitro* and particularly *in vivo* assays (Leusch et al., 2006).

Studies have also shown that different isoforms of the receptors within the same species can have different binding characteristics, and care has to be taken when comparing receptors from different tissues. Receptor binding assays also generally lack a metabolic activation step, which may cause false negatives for chemicals that are not themselves biologically active, but have metabolites that are. And while binding to the steroid receptor is the first step in a receptor-mediated response, *in vivo* responses can be mediated via other pathways and a battery of assays including *in vivo* assays should be considered in any comprehensive monitoring program on endocrine disruption (Leusch et al., 2006).

However, despite all these limitations, receptor-binding assays still provide a reliable and cost-effective platform for large-scale screening of chemicals for estrogenic or androgenic activity. Binding to the receptor is a clear indication that the chemical in question has the potential to hijack the hormonal machinery of the organism and suggests the need for further *in vivo* screening (Leusch et al., 2006).

Concerning the evaluation of the biological effects of these molecules, several methods have recently been developed: on whole organisms (Biau S Fau - Bayle et al., 2007), uterotrophic (Kanno J Fau - Onyon et al., 2001) and vitellogenine assay (Versonnen and Janssen, 2004), cells (cell proliferation)(Soto Am Fau - Fernandez et al., 1997), yeast estrogen screen (Tang X Fau - Ullah et al., 2012), ER CALUX (Brand et al., 2013) and molecular assays (Seifert, 2004). These effects are observed for a concentration range from 1 to 100 ng/L, and the experimental determination requires several hours (3 h for enzyme linked receptor assay) or days (4 days for ER CALUX and for yeast assays, 14 days for VTG assays and 21 days for uterotropic assay, for example). In most cases, the effects are evaluated via mediation of estrogen receptors (ERα and ERβ) (Habauzit et al., 2008).

Hence, in order to check if estrogenic hormones are good tracers of urban sources of contamination of EDCs in aquatic environments, it appears valuable to combine chemical analysis of estrogenic hormones with biological tests of estrogenic effects. Global biological disrupting effects are generally expressed as equivalent estrogenic quantity of E2 (EEQ) (Miège et al., 2009). These substances are able to react with an estrogen receptor, and, using this ability, they could be detected with the bioassays described previously (Miège et al., 2009).

The enzyme linked immunosorbent assay (ELISA) is a rapid, simple, and cost-effective method for quantitative analysis of estrogenic hormones. ELISA kits are commercially available for the quantification of estrogenic and androgenic hormones. Large numbers of samples can be analysed simultaneously and machines that do the readings are relatively cheap and also available in portable format that can be used in field studies (Swart and Pool, 2007).

Cellular bioassays such as the MCF-7 breast cancer cell proliferation assay (E-Screen), which measure the potency of a sample to induce cell proliferation, also provide a measure of estrogenicity (Soto et al., 1995) and complement receptor-binding assays by providing a further dimension to the estrogenicity evaluation (Leusch et al., 2006).

The yeast estrogen screen (YES) test, use a yeast strain responsive to estrogens. Yeasts do not contain sex steroid or thyroid hormone receptors, except those transfected into the strain, but they possess proteins homologous to mammalian cells that are required for activated transcription. The YES test, based on recombinant yeast cultures expressing human estrogen receptor, has been used for investigations in surface waters (Beck et al., 2006). The YES assay uses a yeast cell transformed with a human ER and a plasmid containing the estrogen-responsive element and the LacZ gene as a reporter gene coding for β-galactosidase. Activation of the receptor results in increased red coloring of the assay medium (Murk et al., 2002).

Bioluminescent yeast bioassays a *Saccharomyces cerevisiae* was used to evaluate the estrogenic activity of the water samples. Briefly, estrogenic compounds cross the yeast cell membrane and bind to human estrogen receptor protein, whose gene is located in the chromosome. The complex formed binds to estrogen response elements (ERE) activating the transcription of luxA and luxB, resulting in light emission without adding any substrates to the media. All bioassay responses were converted into E2 equivalents (ng equiv. E2 /L) by means of the ratio between the EC50 for E2 and the EC50 calculated for each compound (Jardim et al., 2012).

In the CALUX (Chemically Activated LUciferase eXpression) assay, is a measure of the ER-mediated cascade of events resulting in activation of genes. The T47D human breast adenocarcinoma cells with endogenous estrogen receptor were stably transfected with an estrogen-responsive luciferase reporter gene containing three estrogen-responsive elements. Both hydrophilic and lipophilic compounds can pass the cell membrane (Murk et al., 2002). Good correlations were found between the *in vitro* and *in vivo* studies (for the AR CALUX vs. Hershberger assay and for the ERα CALUX vs. Allen-Doisy assay) (Sonneveld et al., 2006).

The MELN test is similar to ER-CALUX test but using cells line MCF-7, stably transfected with luciferase reporter gene (Miège et al., 2009). Cell lines HELN-ERα (HELN cells transfected with ERα plasmid) (Maggioni et al., 2013) or CV-1(Hu et al., 2013) was also used to evaluate drinking water.

In these studies, biological tests were used as a global approach to give an indication of the endocrine- disruption risk for aquatic wildlife exposed in the environments studied (Miège et al., 2009). In Table 3 are described the bio testes used to evaluate the potential amount of estradiol in environmental waters.

Table 3. Bioassays used to evaluated the waters achieving results as E2 quantification

Sample	Bioassay	Achieved levels or EEQs	Ref.
Surface waters	YES test	0.02 - 4.85 ng/L	(Beck et al., 2006)I.-
River water near a sewage	ELISA (previous extraction with C-18)	0.8 – 4.7 ng/L	(Swart and Pool, 2007)
River water	MELN test	1.4 ng/L	(Pillon A Fau - Boussioux et al., 2005)
Large rivers	ER-CALUX test	0.06 - 0.46 ng/L	(Murk Aj Fau - Legler et al., 2002)
Drinking water from waterworks and from PET-bottled water	HELN-ERα cell lines	13.6 pg/L	(Maggioni et al., 2013)
Drinking water sources	CV-1 cell lines	0.12-4.8 ng/L	(Hu et al., 2013)
Drinking water	CALUX	0.008-1.074 ng/L	(Brand et al., 2013)

Vitellogenins (VTG) are the precursors of the major egg yolk proteins, vitellins (Vn), in oviparous species including teleosts fish (Tong et al., 2004). Vn provide energy reserves for embryo development in oviparous organisms. VTG are highdensity (300 to 600 kDa, according to species) glycolipophosphoproteins having Ca and Zn ligands, and are considered to have similar characteristics in vertebrates, such as fish, and invertebrates, particularly mollusks (Matozzo V Fau - Gagne et al., 2008). They are synthesized in the liver of females, in the reproductive stage (Li et al., 2005), in response to the endogenous estrogen, E2, secreted into the bloodstream and finally taken up by the developing oocytes via receptor-mediated endocytosis (Tong et al., 2004). VTG levels generally increase in sexually mature females, but are lower in juveniles and undetectable in males (Matozzo V Fau - Gagne et al., 2008). But male fish also carry the VTG gene and exposure to either natural or synthetic estrogens can trigger its expression (Li et al., 2005). In the latter case, the VTG gene is normally silent, but males may synthesize and secrete VTG in response to estrogens or estrogen mimics (Matozzo V Fau - Gagne et al., 2008).

It has been demonstrated in several fish species that exposure of male fish to E2 caused heavy induction of plasma VTG and their mRNAs (Tong et al., 2004). VTG has been focused as an ideal biomarker and widely used in fish for screening the estrogenic activity in aquatic environment (Li et al., 2006).

Fish VTG has become a major concern as a useful biomarker for estrogenic compounds in aquatic area (Li et al., 2005). A number of methods have been developed for the quantification of VTG in blood plasma, liver tissue, or whole-body homogenates from several fish species.

These methods include radioimmunoassay (RIA), ELISA, single radial immunodiffusion (Specker and Anderson, 1994) and real time polymerase chain reaction (PCR) (Celius et al., 2000). These various methods differ in sensitivity, specificity, and technical difficulty (Swart and Pool, 2009). ELISAs are widely used for quantification of VTG from such as *Cyprinus carpio* (Tyler et al., 1999), *Rhombosolea tapirina*, *Oncorhynchus mykiss* and *Salmo salar* (Watts et al., 2003; Li et al., 2005). Other studies showed that several antibodies had already been used in ELISA test against VTG of fish, e.g., *Danio rerio, Cyprinus carpio, Pimehales promelas* and *Oryzias latipes* (Nilsen Bm Fau - Berg et al., 2004), *Cyprinus carpio* and *Perca fluviatilis (Hennies M Fau - Wiesmann et al., 2003).* ELISAs are generally less expensive and easier to perform. The ELISA methods permit the use of antibodies with limited binding affinities and specificities because, in contrast to competitive assays, reagent in ELISA systems can be used in excess (Li et al., 2005).

The anti-VTG antibodies are very specific for each individual fish species and often require the production of specific antibodies for the selected species (Hansen et al., 1998) These antibody based procedures for VTG quantification may use antisera prepared against VTG from the fish species being studied. Although antisera can cross react with VTG from multiple fish species, the affinity can vary substantially (Silversand et al., 1993; Swart and Pool, 2009).

Recently, a surface plasmon resonance technique coupled with immunodetection for the determination of carp (*Cyprinus carpio*) VTG has been developed. Monoclonal antibodies were linked on the sensor surface through chemical cross-linking via a capturing antibody (Bulukin et al., 2007).

The Organization for Economic Cooperation and Development (OECD) work is ongoing to develop screening and testing programmes for endocrine disrupting effects of new chemicals, and in the focus of this development are the fish test species common carp (*Cyprinus carpio*), fathead minnow (*Pimephales promelas*), zebrafish (*Danio rerio*) and Japanese medaka (*Oryzias latipes*) (Nilsen Bm Fau - Berg et al., 2004). Although these fishes can live with polluted environments, fathead minnow, zebrafish and Japanese medaka are all small and low degree in food cycle, not suitable to reflect the food chain accumulation effect. In winter, the carp becomes torpid, retires to the bottom and stops feeding (Gwinn et al., 1992) and Japanese medaka life cycle is about one year. VTG of hardy *Carassius auratus* has the advantage to evaluate the estrogenic activity in wild environments in that the fish is omnivorous, feeding on plants, small animals and small crustaceans and other foods, and can reflect the food chain accumulation effect. In addition, it can tolerate many kinds of environments and the life cycle is about 20 years. In winter, it has not a period of dormancy (Li et al., 2005). VTG induction is usually regarded as an essential biomarker for the evaluation of EDCs affecting the sexual hormone system. However, an appropriate interpretation of VTG data is frequently only possible with information about the individual gender (Holbech et al., 2006; Baumann et al., 2013).

Table 4. Assays based on VTG or VTG mRNA measurement in several aquatic species

	Species	Method	Procedure	Detection range	Ref.
VTG protein	*Rana catesbeiana* (Bullfrog)	ELISA	Monoclonal antibodies	9.4 - 1200 ng VTG /mL	(Li et al., 2006)
		ELISA	Assay previously developed (Li et al., 2006)	100 nM – 1 μM of E2	(Lee et al., 2010)
	Oreochromis mossambicus (Tilapia)	ELISA	Polyclonal antibodies	80 ng /mL – 5.4 μg VTG /mL	(Swart and Pool, 2009)
	Moxostoma hubbsi (Copper redhorse)	Lateral flow immunoassay	VTG is captured between a particle-conjugated antibody and a capture antibody immobilized as a narrow line on a membrane strip	40 -1200 ng VTG/mL	(Maltais and Roy, 2007)
	Cyprinus carpio (Carp)	Optical immunosensor	The sensor was assembled linking the analyte specific antibodies using capturing antibodies.	0.1 – 10 ppm of VTG	(Bulukin et al., 2007)
		Optical waveguide lightmode spectroscopy biosensor	VTG bound over the sensor surface quite specifically, judging from the sensor responses according to stepwise antibody immobilization.	0.00675–67.5 nM of VTG	(Kim et al., 2008)
	Paralichthys californicus (California halibut)	ELISA	Antibody developed for another flatfish species, turbot	33–1000 ng/mL of VTG	(Palumbo et al., 2009)
mRNA	*Mugil soiuy* (mullet)	qRT-PCR	VTG and β-actin primers	0.001 – 1 μg E2/kg	(An et al., 2006)

Both mRNA and protein (levels can be detected and quantified, and both have been found to correspond to the degree of estrogenic exposure (Bowman et al., 2000; Lattier Dl Fau - Reddy et al., 2002). Vitellogenesis offers an additional advantage over other measures of estrogenic exposure in that it is considered to be directly ''downstream'' of the ligand/estrogen receptor–binding event and, thus, to exploit the specificity inherent to cellular receptors (Biales et al., 2007).

The transcription of the VTG gene takes place as a result of circulating E2 produced in the gonads of female fish during sexual maturation. The E2 enters the liver cells by diffusion and is retained in the target cells through binding to a specific receptor protein (estrogen receptor) hence inducing the activation of the VTG loci (Mommsen and Walsh, 1988; Bulukin et al., 2007)

A real-time reverse transcriptase PCR (RT-PCR) assay was developed for quantification of VTG mRNA level in both control fish and E2-treated fish. The lowest-observed-effect concentrations of E2 for the induction of VTG mRNAs were observed at 1 μg/L for zebrafish and 0.1 μg/L for medaka in a 2-day exposure experiment. Further kinetics studies of the two fish models indicated that medaka was able to respond much faster to E2 treatment than zebrafish, while the zebrafish can attain a much higher level of VTG mRNAs than medaka after a long-term E2 treatment. The implication of these observations may be that the medaka system is better in monitoring acute treatment while the zebrafish system is better in monitoring chronic exposure (Tong et al., 2004).

Quantitative real time PCR (Q-RT-PCR) is a new method for analyzing gene expression with several advantages such as speed, directness, and accuracy. Though the obtained VTG gene sequences of studied organisms are essential, methods based on degenerate primers and RT-PCR could quickly isolate a fragment of target genes, and partial sequences could be obtained in a few days (An et al., 2006) (Table 4). It have been determined VTG gene expression in Chinese sturgeon (*Acipenser sinensis* Gray) (Zhang et al., 2005), striped sea bream (Funkenstein et al., 2004), *Mugil soiuy* (mullet) (An et al., 2006) and *Elliptio complanata* (Gagné et al., 2004; Matozzo V Fau - Gagne et al., 2008) by Q-RT-PCR (An et al., 2006).

Conclusion

The excretion of steroidal hormones from human populations is a major contributor to the presence of EDCs in the aquatic environment. E2, the major estrogen in vertebrates, E1, the precursor as well as a breakdown product of E2, and EE2, the synthetic estrogen used in the birth control pill, are released in conjugated forms in urine.

The adverse effects of natural estrogens on aquatic organisms are also documented (Vos et al. 2000; Chistianshen et al. 2002). Imai et al. (2005) confirmed that exposure to E2 (>16 ng L^{-1}) affected the reproduction of marine male fishes (Desmiarti et al., 2012).

E2 is attracting attention due to its interference with the usual functioning of the endocrine system in humans and animals. When present in environment above a certain concentration, this compound can cause adverse health effects.

The awareness of the impact of some pharmaceuticals in the environment has grown considerably in recent years and has recommended future research objectives, as well as attention to policy.

Based on the literature data some public and private institutions worldwide began to define recommended maximum concentration levels for emerging contaminants, as it is E2, in order to lay down regulations to protect humans and the environment from identified chemical risks with tangible toxicological endpoints. To achieve the sensitivity and selectivity necessary for analysis of steroid sex hormones and related synthetic compounds in water, determination of these compounds currently requires the use of adequate extraction and purification steps before the final analytical determination. The use of the tandem mass spectrometry detection, coupled with GC or to LC, has improved the performance of chromatographic methods by reducing detection limits and aiding analyte identification.

In contrast to chemical analyses, biologically based indicators respond to any number of sources that activate specific, measurable intracellular events. These indicators distinguish not only xenobiotic activators mediated through prototypical receptor-binding pathways, such as estrogens, but also those that are able to stimulate intracellular events indirectly, such as metabolic breakdown products. Because the biological response of an organism to an exposure is measured, these indicators frequently have clear and immediate relevance to biological condition. Several methods have been developed: on whole organisms, uterotrophic and vitellogenine assay, cells (cell proliferation), yeast estrogen screen, ER CALUX and molecular assays. Global biological disrupting effects are generally expressed as equivalent estrogenic quantity of E2.

The evidences from laboratory (single exposure to E2 or to a mixture of EDCs) or water exposure experiments (e.g., collected river samples) link E2 with endocrine effects in several animal and plant species. The health outcomes in fishes are of such magnitude that several authors question the success of reproduction among these species. On humans the adverse health effects of E2 are still a controversial issue. Nonetheless, some studies have reported reproduction impairment and breast cancer as an outcome of increased exposure to estrogenic compounds (Ansar Ahmed, 2000; Delbès et al., 2006; McLachlan et al., 2006). Additionally, estrogens including E2 seem to affect also the functioning of several non-reproductive tissues, namely the immune system (Ansar Ahmed, 2000). Therefore, considering E2 estrogenic potency and reported health effects, the assessment of the incidence, fate, and degradation of E2 in the environment is a matter of indubitable relevance.

References

Adlercreutz, H., K. Höckerstedt, C. Bannwart, S. Bloigu, E. Hämäläinen, T. Fotsis and A. Ollus. Effect of dietary components, including lignans and phytoestrogens, on enterohepatic circulation and liver metabolism of estrogens and on sex hormone binding globulin (SHBG). *Journal of Steroid Biochemistry*, 1987 27, 4–6: 1135-1144.

An, L., J. Hu, Z. Zhang and M. Yang. Quantitative real-time RT-PCR for determination of vitellogenin mRNA in so-iuy mullet (Mugil soiuy). *Analytical and Bioanalytical Chemistry*, 2006 386, 7-8: 1995-2001.

Ansar Ahmed, S. The immune system as a potential target for environmental estrogens (endocrine disrupters): a new emerging field. *Toxicology*, 2000 150, 1–3: 191-206.

Arnold Sf Fau - Robinson, M. K., A. C. Robinson Mk Fau - Notides, L. J. Notides Ac Fau - Guillette, Jr., J. A. Guillette Lj Jr Fau - McLachlan and M. JA. - A yeast estrogen screen for examining the relative exposure of cells to natural and xenoestrogens. *Environ Health Perspect*, 1996 104, 5: 544-548.

Baumann, L., H. Holbech, S. Keiter, K. L. Kinnberg, S. Knörr, T. Nagel and T. Braunbeck. The maturity index as a tool to facilitate the interpretation of changes in vitellogenin production and sex ratio in the Fish Sexual Development Test. *Aquatic Toxicology*, 2013 128–129, 0: 34-42.

Bayley, M., J. R. Nielsen and E. Baatrup. Guppy Sexual Behavior as an Effect Biomarker of Estrogen Mimics. *Ecotoxicology and Environmental Safety*, 1999 43, 1: 68-73.

Beck, I.-C., R. Bruhn and J. Gandrass. Analysis of estrogenic activity in coastal surface waters of the Baltic Sea using the yeast estrogen screen. *Chemosphere*, 2006 63, 11: 1870-1878.

Biales, A. D., D. C. Bencic, R. W. Flick, J. Lazorchak and D. L. Lattier. Quantification and associated variability of induced vitellogenin gene transcripts in fathead minnow (Pimephales promelas) by quantitative real-time polymerase chain reaction assay. *Environmental Toxicology and Chemistry,* 2007 26, 2: 287-296.

Biau S Fau - Bayle, S., P. Bayle S Fau - de Santa Barbara, B. de Santa Barbara P Fau - Roig and R. B. - The chick embryo: an animal model for detection of the effects of hormonal compounds. *Analytical and Bioanalytical Chemistry*, 2007 387, 4: 1397-1403.

Bjerselius R Fau - Lundstedt-Enkel, K., H. Lundstedt-Enkel K Fau - Olsen, I. Olsen H Fau - Mayer, K. Mayer I Fau - Dimberg and D. K. - Male goldfish reproductive behaviour and physiology are severely affected by exogenous exposure to 17beta-estradiol. *Aquat Toxicol,* 2001 53, 2: 139-152.

Bowman, C. J., K. J. Kroll, M. J. Hemmer, L. C. Folmar and N. D. Denslow. Estrogen-induced vitellogenin mRNA and protein in sheepshead minnow (Cyprinodon variegatus). *Gen Comp Endocrinol*, 2000 120, 3: 300-313.

Boyd, G. R., H. Reemtsma, D. A. Grimm and S. Mitra. Pharmaceuticals and personal care products (PPCPs) in surface and treated waters of Louisiana, USA and Ontario, Canada. *Science of the Total Environment*, 2003 311, 1-3: 135-149.

Brand, W., C. M. de Jongh, S. C. van der Linden, W. Mennes, L. M. Puijker, C. J. van Leeuwen, A. P. van Wezel, M. Schriks and M. B. Heringa. Trigger values for investigation of hormonal activity in drinking water and its sources using CALUX bioassays. *Environment International,* 2013 55, 0: 109-118.

Briciu, R. D., A. Kot-Wasik and J. Namiesnik. Analytical Challenges and Recent Advances in the Determination of Estrogens in Water Environments. *Journal of Chromatographic Science,* 2009 47, 2: 127-139.

Brion, F., C. R. Tyler, X. Palazzi, B. Laillet, J. M. Porcher, J. Garric and P. Flammarion. Impacts of 17β-estradiol, including environmentally relevant concentrations, on reproduction after exposure during embryo-larval-, juvenile- and adult-life stages in zebrafish (Danio rerio). *Aquatic Toxicology,* 2004 68, 3: 193-217.

Brody, J. G. and R. A. Rudel. Environmental pollutants and breast cancer. *Environmental Health Perspectives*, 2003 111, 8: 1007-1019.

Bulukin, E., V. Meucci, M. Minunni, C. Pretti, L. Intorre, G. Soldani and M. Mascini. An optical immunosensor for rapid vitellogenin detection in plasma from carp (Cyprinus carpio). *Talanta*, 2007 72, 2: 785-790.

Calaf, G. M. and D. Roy. Cell adhesion proteins altered by 17 beta estradiol and parathion in breast epithelial cells. *Oncology Reports*, 2008 19, 1: 165-169.

Celius, T., J. B. Matthews, J. P. Giesy and T. R. Zacharewski. Quantification of rainbow trout (Oncorhynchus mykiss) zona radiata and vitellogenin mRNA levels using real-time PCR after in vivo treatment with estradiol-17β or α-zearalenol. *The Journal of Steroid Biochemistry and Molecular Biology*, 2000 75, 2–3: 109-119.

Chen, W.-L., G.-S. Wang, J.-C. Gwo and C.-Y. Chen. Ultra-high performance liquid chromatography/tandem mass spectrometry determination of feminizing chemicals in river water, sediment and tissue pretreated using disk-type solid-phase extraction and matrix solid-phase dispersion. *Talanta*, 2012 89, 0: 237-245.

Combalbert, S. and G. Hernandez-Raquet. Occurrence, fate, and biodegradation of estrogens in sewage and manure. *Applied Microbiology and Biotechnology*, 2010 86, 6: 1671-1692.

Comission, E., 2012. IP/12/88 -EU-Press release. Environment and Water: proposal to reduce water pollution risks. *http://europa.eu/rapid/press-release_IP-12-88_en.htm?locale=FR.*

Commission, E., 2000. Proposal for a DIRECTIVE OF THE EUROPEAN PARLIAMENT AND OF THE COUNCIL amending Directives 2000/60/EC and 2008/105/EC as regards priority substances in the field of water policy. *http://ec.europa.eu/environment/water/water-dangersub/pdf/com_2011_876.pdf.*

Council, E., 2000. Directive 2000/60/EC - establishing a framework for Community action in the field of water policy *http://eur-lex.europa.eu/LexUriServ/LexUriServ.do?uri=OJ:L:2000:327:0001:0072:EN:PDF.*

Council, E., 2001. DECISION No 2455/2001/EC -establishing the list of priority substances in the field of water policy and amending Directive 2000/60/EC. *http://eur-lex.europa.eu/LexUriServ/LexUriServ.do?uri=OJ:L:2001:331:0001:0005:EN:PDF.*

Council, E., 2008a. Directive 2008/105/EC *http://eur-lex.europa.eu/LexUriServ/LexUriServ.do?uri=OJ:L:2008:348:0084:0097:EN:PDF.*

Council, E., 2008b. DIRECTIVE 2008/105/EC - on environmental quality standards in the field of water policy, amending and subsequently repealing Council Directives 82/176/EEC, 83/513/EEC, 84/156/EEC, 84/491/EEC, 86/280/EEC and amending Directive 2000/60/EC of the European Parliament and of the Council. *http://eur-lex.europa.eu/LexUriServ/LexUriServ.do?uri=OJ:L:2008:348:0084:0097:EN:PDF.*

Cubero-Leon, E., C. M. Ciocan, E. M. Hill, M. Osada, M. Kishida, N. Itoh, R. Kondo, C. Minier and J. M. Rotchell. Estrogens disrupt serotonin receptor and cyclooxygenase mRNA expression in the gonads of mussels (Mytilus edulis). *Aquatic Toxicology*, 2010 98, 2: 178-187.

Delbès, G., C. Levacher and R. Habert. Estrogen effects on fetal and neonatal testicular development. *Reproduction*, 2006 132, 4: 527-538.

Desmiarti, R., J. Li and F. Li. Behavior of Natural Estrogens in Reservoir: Investigations Based on Continuous Flow Experiments and Model Analysis. *Water, Air, & Soil Pollution,* 2012 223, 6: 3307-3320.

Diotel, N., C. Vaillant, C. Gabbero, S. Mironov, A. Fostier, M.-M. Gueguen, I. Anglade, O. Kah and E. Pellegrini. Effects of estradiol in adult neurogenesis and brain repair in zebrafish. *Hormones and Behavior,* 2013 63, 2: 193-207.

Dutta, S. K., S. P. Inamdar, J. Tso and D. S. Aga. Concentrations of free and conjugated estrogens at different landscape positions in an agricultural watershed receiving poultry litter. *Water, Air, and Soil Pollution,* 2012 223, 5: 2821-2836.

EPA, 2009. Contaminant Candidate List 3 - CCL -Final Third Drinking Water Contaminant Candidate List *http://water.*

Fisch, H. and E. T. Goluboff. Geographic variations in sperm counts: a potential cause of bias in studies of semen quality. *Fertility and sterility,* 1996 65, 5: 1044-1046.

Foran, C. M., E. R. Bennett and W. H. Benson. Exposure to environmentally relevant concentrations of different nonylphenol formulations in Japanese medaka. *Marine Environmental Research,* 2000 50, 1-5: 135-139.

Funkenstein, B., A. Dyman, B. Levavi-Sivan and M. Tom. Application of real-time PCR for quantitative determination of hepatic vitellogenin transcript levels in the striped sea bream, Lithognathus mormyrus. *Marine Environmental Research,* 2004 58, 2–5: 659-663.

Gagné, F., C. Blaise and J. Hellou. Endocrine disruption and health effects of caged mussels, Elliptio complanata, placed downstream from a primary-treated municipal effluent plume for 1 year. *Comparative Biochemistry and Physiology Part C: Toxicology & Pharmacology,* 2004 138, 1: 33-44.

Gimeno, S., H. Komen, A. G. M. Gerritsen and T. Bowmer. Feminisation of young males of the common carp, Cyprinus carpio, exposed to 4-tert-pentylphenol during sexual differentiation. *Aquatic Toxicology,* 1998a 43, 2–3: 77-92.

Gimeno, S., H. Komen, S. Jobling, J. Sumpter and T. Bowmer. Demasculinisation of sexually mature male common carp, Cyprinus carpio, exposed to 4-tert-pentylphenol during spermatogenesis. *Aquatic Toxicology*, 1998b 43, 2–3: 93-109.

Goksoyr, A. Endocrine disruptors in the marine environment: Mechanisms of toxicity and their influence on reproductive processes in fish. *Journal of Toxicology and Environmental Health-Part a-Current Issues*, 2006 69, 1-2: 175-184.

Gwinn, R. P., P. B. Norton and P. W. Geotz 1992. *The New Encyclopedia Britannica.* Chicago, Encyclopedia Britannica Inc.

Habauzit, D., J. Armengaud, B. Roig and J. Chopineau. Determination of estrogen presence in water by SPR using estrogen receptor dimerization. *Analytical and Bioanalytical Chemistry*, 2008 390, 3: 873-883.

Halm, S., N. Pounds, S. Maddix, M. Rand-Weaver, J. P. Sumpter, T. H. Hutchinson and C. R. Tyler. Exposure to exogenous 17 beta-oestradiol disrupts P450aromB mRNA expression in the brain and gonad of adult fathead minnows (Pimephales promelas). *Aquatic Toxicology*, 2002 60, 3-4: 285-299.

Hamid, H. and C. Eskicioglu. Fate of estrogenic hormones in wastewater and sludge treatment: A review of properties and analytical detection techniques in sludge matrix. *Water Research,* 2012 46, 18: 5813-5833.

Hansen, P. D., H. Dizer, B. Hock, A. Marx, J. Sherry, M. McMaster and C. Blaise. Vitellogenin – a biomarker for endocrine disruptors. *TrAC Trends in Analytical Chemistry,* 1998 17, 7: 448-451.

Hennies M Fau - Wiesmann, M., B. Wiesmann M Fau - Allner, H. Allner B Fau - Sauerwein and S. H. - Vitellogenin in carp (Cyprinus carpio) and perch (Perca fluviatilis): purification, characterization and development of an ELISA for the detection of estrogenic effects. *Sci Total Environ*, 2003 309, 1-3: 93-103.

Holbech, H., K. Kinnberg, G. I. Petersen, P. Jackson, K. Hylland, L. Norrgren and P. Bjerregaard. Detection of endocrine disrupters: Evaluation of a Fish Sexual Development Test (FSDT). *Comparative Biochemistry and Physiology Part C: Toxicology & Pharmacology*, 2006 144, 1: 57-66.

Hu, F., E. E. Smith and J. A. Carr. Effects of larval exposure to estradiol on spermatogenesis and in vitro gonadal steroid secretion in African clawed frogs, Xenopus laevis. *General and Comparative Endocrinology*, 2008 155, 1: 190-200.

Hu, X., W. Shi, F. Cao, G. Hu, Y. Hao, S. Wei, X. Wang and H. Yu. Bioanalytical and instrumental analysis of estrogenic activities in drinking water sources from Yangtze River Delta. *Chemosphere*, 2013 90, 7: 2123-2128.

Hyndman, K. M., A. Biales, S. E. Bartell and H. L. Schoenfuss. Assessing the effects of exposure timing on biomarker expression using 17β-estradiol. *Aquatic Toxicology*, 2010 96, 4: 264-272.

Irwin, L. K., S. Gray and E. Oberdörster. Vitellogenin induction in painted turtle, Chrysemys picta, as a biomarker of exposure to environmental levels of estradiol. *Aquatic Toxicology,* 2001 55, 1–2: 49-60.

Jardim, W. F., C. C. Montagner, I. C. Pescara, G. A. Umbuzeiro, A. M. Di Dea Bergamasco, M. L. Eldridge and F. F. Sodré. An integrated approach to evaluate emerging contaminants in drinking water. *Separation and Purification Technology*, 2012 84, 0: 3-8.

Jin, S., F. Yang, T. Liao, Y. Hui, S. Wen and Y. Xu. Enhanced effects by mixtures of three estrogenic compounds at environmentally relevant levels on development of Chinese rare minnow (Gobiocypris rarus). *Environmental Toxicology and Pharmacology,* 2012 33, 2: 277-283.

Johnson, A. C., A. Belfroid and A. Di Corcia. Estimating steroid oestrogen inputs into activated sludge treatment works and observations on their removal from the effluent. *Science of The Total Environment*, 2000 256, 2–3: 163-173.

Jukosky, J. A., M. C. Watzin and J. C. Leiter. The effects of environmentally relevant mixtures of estrogens on Japanese medaka (Oryzias latipes) reproduction. *Aquatic Toxicology*, 2008 86, 2: 323-331.

Kang Ij Fau - Yokota, H., Y. Yokota H Fau - Oshima, Y. Oshima Y Fau - Tsuruda, T. Tsuruda Y Fau - Yamaguchi, M. Yamaguchi T Fau - Maeda, N. Maeda M Fau - Imada, H. Imada N Fau - Tadokoro, T. Tadokoro H Fau - Honjo and H. T. - Effect of 17beta-estradiol on the reproduction of Japanese medaka (Oryzias latipes). *Chemosphere*, 2002 47, 1: 71-80.

Kanno J Fau - Onyon, L., J. Onyon L Fau - Haseman, P. Haseman J Fau - Fenner-Crisp, J. Fenner-Crisp P Fau - Ashby, W. Ashby J Fau - Owens and O. W. - The OECD program to validate the rat uterotrophic bioassay to screen compounds for in vivo estrogenic responses: phase 1. *Environ Health Perspect,* 2001 109, 8: 785-794.

Khanal, S. K., B. Xie, M. L. Thompson, S. Sung, S.-K. Ong and J. van Leeuwen. Fate, Transport, and Biodegradation of Natural Estrogens in the Environment and Engineered Systems. *Environmental Science & Technology,* 2006 40, 21: 6537-6546.

Kim, N., D.-K. Kim, Y.-J. Cho, D.-K. Moon and W.-Y. Kim. Carp vitellogenin detection by an optical waveguide lightmode spectroscopy biosensor. *Biosensors and Bioelectronics,* 2008 24, 3: 391-396.

Kinnberg, K., B. Korsgaard and P. Bjerregaard. Effects of octylphenol and 17 beta-estradiol on the gonads of guppies (Poecilia reticulata) exposed as adults via the water or as embryos via the mother. *Comparative Biochemistry and Physiology C-Toxicology & Pharmacology*, 2003 134, 1: 45-55.

Koger, C. S., S. J. Teh and D. E. Hinton. Determining the sensitive developmental stages of intersex induction in medaka (Oryzias latipes) exposed to 17β-estradiol or testosterone. *Marine Environmental Research*, 2000 50, 1–5: 201-206.

Korner W Fau - Bolz, U., W. Bolz U Fau - Sussmuth, G. Sussmuth W Fau - Hiller, W. Hiller G Fau - Schuller, V. Schuller W Fau - Hanf, H. Hanf V Fau - Hagenmaier and H. H. - Input/output balance of estrogenic active compounds in a major municipal sewage plant in Germany. *Chemosphere*, 2000 40, 9-11: 1131-1142.

Kramer, V. J., S. Miles-Richardson, S. L. Pierens and J. P. Giesy. Reproductive impairment and induction of alkaline-labile phosphate, a biomarker of estrogen exposure, in fathead minnows (Pimephales promelas) exposed to waterborne 17β-estradiol. *Aquatic Toxicology,* 1998 40, 4: 335-360.

Lahnsteiner, F., B. Berger, A. Kletzl and T. Weismann. Effect of 17 beta-estradiol on gamete quality and maturation in two salmonid species. *Aquatic Toxicology*, 2006 79, 2: 124-131.

Lattier Dl Fau - Reddy, T. V., D. A. Reddy Tv Fau - Gordon, J. M. Gordon Da Fau - Lazorchak, M. E. Lazorchak Jm Fau - Smith, D. E. Smith Me Fau - Williams, B. Williams De Fau - Wiechman, R. W. Wiechman B Fau - Flick, A. L. Flick Rw Fau - Miracle, G. P. Miracle Al Fau - Toth and T. GP. - 17alpha-ethynylestradiol-induced vitellogenin gene transcription quantified in livers of adult males, larvae, and gills of fathead minnows (Pimephales promelas). *Environ Toxicol Chem,* 2002 21, 11: 2385-2393.

Lee, K., Z. Chang, B.-S. Oh, M. Lu and J.-S. Park. Estrogenic Response in Male Bullfrog (Rana catesbeiana) Hepatocytes After Single or Combined Exposure to Cadmium (Cd) and 17beta-Estradiol (E2). *Bulletin of Environmental Contamination and Toxicology,* 2010 85, 5: 452-456.

Lee, W., C.-W. Kang, C.-K. Su, K. Okubo and Y. Nagahama. Screening estrogenic activity of environmental contaminants and water samples using a transgenic medaka embryo bioassay. *Chemosphere*, 2012 88, 8: 945-952.

Lerner, D. T., B. T. Bjornsson and S. D. McCormick. Larval exposure to 4-nonylphenol and 17 beta-estradiol affects physiological and behavioral development of seawater adaptation in atlantic salmon smolts. *Environmental Science & Technology*, 2007 41, 12: 4479-4485.

Leusch, F. D. L., M. R. van den Heuvel, H. F. Chapman, S. R. Gooneratne, A. M. E. Eriksson and L. A. Tremblay. Development of methods for extraction and in vitro quantification of estrogenic and androgenic activity of wastewater samples. *Comparative Biochemistry and Physiology Part C: Toxicology & Pharmacology*, 2006 143, 1: 117-126.

Li, C.-R., K.-S. Jung, S.-H. Lee, A. Kim and J.-S. Park. Development of a sandwich enzyme-linked immunosorbant assay for the quantification of vitellogeinin in Bullfrog (Rana catesbeiana). *Chemosphere*, 2006 63, 9: 1485-1490.

Li, C.-R., K.-T. Kim, Y.-J. Kang, A. Kim, S.-W. Kang and J.-S. Park. A novel enzyme-linked immunosorbent assay system for the quantitative analysis of Carassius auratus vitellogenin. *Chemosphere*, 2005 59, 7: 997-1003.

Li, Y. X., W. Han, M. Yang, C. H. Feng, X. F. Lu and F. S. Zhang. Migration of natural estrogens around a concentrated dairy-feeding operation. *Environmental Monitoring and Assessment*, 2012 184, 8: 5035-5041.

Liao, T., Q. L. Guo, S. W. Jin, W. Cheng and Y. Xu. Comparative responses in rare minnow exposed to 17 beta-estradiol during different life stages. *Fish Physiology and Biochemistry,* 2009 35, 3: 341-349.

Lopezde Alda, M. J. and D. Barcelo. Use of solid-phase extraction in various of its modalities for sample preparation in the determination of estrogens and progestogens in sediment and water. *Journal of chromatography. A*, 2001 938, 1-2: 145-153.

Lyssimachou, A. and A. Arukwe. Alteration of brain and interrenal StAR protein, P450scc, and Cyp11 beta mRNA levels in Atlantic salmon after nominal waterborne exposure to the synthetic pharmaceutical estrogen ethynylestradiol. *Journal of Toxicology and Environmental Health-Part a-Current Issues,* 2007 70, 7: 606-613.

Maggioni, S., P. Balaguer, C. Chiozzotto and E. Benfenati. Screening of endocrine-disrupting phenols, herbicides, steroid estrogens, and estrogenicity in drinking water from the waterworks of 35 Italian cities and from PET-bottled mineral water. *Environmental Science and Pollution Research*, 2013 20, 3: 1649-1660.

Maltais, D. and R. L. Roy. A lateral flow immunoassay for rapid evaluation of vitellogenin levels in plasma and surface mucus of the copper redhorse (Moxostoma hubbsi). *Environmental Toxicology and Chemistry*, 2007 26, 8: 1672-1676.

Mansilha, C., S. Rocha, P. Gameiro, C. Pinho, I. M. P. L. V. O. Ferreira, P. Silva and V. Domingues. Interlaboratory validation of an environmental monitoring method for trace analysis of endocrine disrupting compounds. *Analytical Methods,* 2012 4, 11: 3724-3732.

Matozzo V Fau - Gagne, F., M. G. Gagne F Fau - Marin, F. Marin Mg Fau - Ricciardi, C. Ricciardi F Fau - Blaise and B. C. - Vitellogenin as a biomarker of exposure to estrogenic compounds in aquatic invertebrates: a review. *Environ Int*, 2008 34, 4: 531-545.

McLachlan, J. A., E. Simpson and M. Martin. Endocrine disrupters and female reproductive health. *Best Pract Res Clin Endocrinol Metab*, 2006 20, 1: 63-75.

Metcalfe Cd Fau - Metcalfe, T. L., Y. Metcalfe Tl Fau - Kiparissis, B. G. Kiparissis Y Fau - Koenig, C. Koenig Bg Fau - Khan, R. J. Khan C Fau - Hughes, T. R. Hughes Rj Fau - Croley, R. E. Croley Tr Fau - March, T. March Re Fau - Potter and P. T. - Estrogenic potency of chemicals detected in sewage treatment plant effluents as determined by in vivo assays with Japanese medaka (Oryzias latipes). *Environ Toxicol Chem*, 2001 20, 2: 297-308.

MHLW, 2003. Revision of Drinking Water quality standards and QA/QC for drinking water quality analysis in Japan. *http://www.nilim.go.jp/lab/bcg/siryou/tnn/tnn0264pdf/ks0264011.pdf.*

Miège, C., V. Gabet, M. Coquery, S. Karolak N, M. L. Jugan, L. Oziol, Y. Levi and M. Chevreuil. Evaluation of estrogenic disrupting potency in aquatic environments and urban wastewaters by combining chemical and biological analysis. T*rAC Trends in Analytical Chemistry,* 2009 28, 2: 186-195.

Miles-Richardson, S. R., V. J. Kramer, S. D. Fitzgerald, J. A. Render, B. Yamini, S. J. Barbee and J. P. Giesy. Effects of waterborne exposure of 17 β-estradiol on secondary sex characteristics and gonads of fathead minnows (Pimephales promelas). *Aquatic Toxicology,* 1999 47, 2: 129-145.

Mommsen, T. P. and P. J. Walsh (1988). 5 Vitellogenesis and Oocyte Assembly. *Fish Physiology.* W. S. Hoar and D. J. Randall, Academic Press. Volume 11, Part A: 347-406.

Moreira, M., S. Aquino, M. Coutrim, J. Silva and R. Afonso. Determination of endocrine-disrupting compounds in waters from Rio das Velhas, Brazil, by liquid chromatography/high resolution mass spectrometry (ESI-LC-IT-TOF/MS). *Environmental Technology*, 2011 32, 12: 1409-1417.

Murk Aj Fau - Legler, J., M. M. H. Legler J Fau - van Lipzig, J. H. N. van Lipzig Mm Fau - Meerman, A. C. Meerman Jh Fau - Belfroid, A. Belfroid Ac Fau - Spenkelink, B. Spenkelink A Fau - van der Burg, G. B. J. van der Burg B Fau - Rijs, D. Rijs Gb Fau - Vethaak and V. D. - Detection of estrogenic potency in wastewater and surface water with three in vitro bioassays. *Environ Toxicol Chem*, 2002 21, 1: 16-23.

Murk, A. J., J. Legler, M. M. H. van Lipzig, J. H. N. Meerman, A. C. Belfroid, A. Spenkelink, B. van der Burg, G. B. J. Rijs and D. Vethaak. Detection of estrogenic potency in wastewater and surface water with three in vitro bioassays. *Environmental Toxicology and Chemistry*, 2002 21, 1: 16-23.

Nilsen Bm Fau - Berg, K., J. K. Berg K Fau - Eidem, S.-I. Eidem Jk Fau - Kristiansen, F. Kristiansen Si Fau - Brion, J.-M. Brion F Fau - Porcher, A. Porcher Jm Fau - Goksoyr and G. A. - Development of quantitative vitellogenin-ELISAs for fish test species used in endocrine disruptor screening. *Analytical and Bioanalytical Chemistry*, 2004 378, 3: 621-633.

Nimrod, A. C. and W. H. Benson. Reproduction and development of Japanese medaka following an early life stage exposure to xenoestrogens. *Aquatic Toxicology,* 1998 44, 1–2: 141-156.

Noppe, H., T. Verslycke, E. De Wulf, K. Verheyden, E. Monteyne, P. Van Caeter, C. R. Janssen and H. F. De brabander. Occurrence of estrogens in the Scheldt estuary: A 2-year survey. *Ecotoxicology and Environmental Safety*, 2007 66, 1: 1-8.

Pacakova, V., L. Loukotkova, Z. Bosakova and K. Stulik. Analysis for estrogens as environmental pollutants - A review. *Journal of Separation Science*, 2009 32, 5-6: 867-882.

Pailler, J. Y., A. Krein, L. Pfister, L. Hoffmann and C. Guignard. Solid phase extraction coupled to liquid chromatography-tandem mass spectrometry analysis of sulfonamides, tetracyclines, analgesics and hormones in surface water and wastewater in Luxembourg. *Science of the Total Environment*, 2009 407, 16: 4736-4743.

Palumbo, A. J., M. Koivunen and R. S. Tjeerdema. Optimization and validation of a California halibut environmental estrogen bioassay using a heterologous ELISA. *Science of The Total Environment,* 2009 407, 2: 953-961.

Panter, G. H., R. S. Thompson and J. P. Sumpter. Adverse reproductive effects in male fathead minnows (Pimephales promelas) exposed to environmentally relevant concentrations of the natural oestrogens, oestradiol and oestrone. *Aquatic Toxicology,* 1998 42, 4: 243-253.

Peck, M. R., P. Labadie, C. Minier and E. M. Hill. Profiles of environmental and endogenous estrogens in the zebra mussel Dreissena polymorpha. *Chemosphere*, 2007 69, 1: 1-8.

Pillon A Fau - Boussioux, A.-M., A. Boussioux Am Fau - Escande, S. Escande A Fau - Ait-Aissa, E. Ait-Aissa S Fau - Gomez, H. Gomez E Fau - Fenet, M. Fenet H Fau - Ruff, D. Ruff M Fau - Moras, F. Moras D Fau - Vignon, M.-J. Vignon F Fau - Duchesne, C. Duchesne Mj Fau - Casellas, J.-C. Casellas C Fau - Nicolas, P. Nicolas Jc Fau - Balaguer and B. P. - Binding of estrogenic compounds to recombinant estrogen receptor-alpha: application to environmental analysis. *Environ Health Perspect*, 2005 113, 3: 278-284.

Ra, J.-S., S.-H. Lee, J. Lee, H. Y. Kim, B. J. Lim, S. H. Kim and S. D. Kim. Occurrence of estrogenic chemicals in South Korean surface waters and municipal wastewaters. *Journal of Environmental Monitoring*, 2011 13, 1: 101-109.

Ribeiro, C., M. A. Pardal, M. E. Tiritan, E. Rocha, R. M. Margalho and M. J. Rocha. Spatial distribution and quantification of endocrine-disrupting chemicals in Sado River estuary, Portugal. *Environmental Monitoring and Assessment,* 2009 159, 1-4: 415-427.

Ribeiro, C., M. E. Tiritan, E. Rocha and M. J. Rocha. Development and validation of a HPLC-DAD method for determination of several endocrine disrupting compounds in estuarine water. *Journal of Liquid Chromatography & Related Technologies,* 2007 30, 18: 2729-2746.

Rocha, M. J., C. Ribeiro and M. Ribeiro. Development and optimisation of a GC-MS method for the evaluation of oestrogens and persistent pollutants in river and seawater samples. *International Journal of Environmental Analytical Chemistry*, 2011a 91, 12: 1191-1205.

Rocha, M. J., M. Ribeiro, C. Ribeiro, C. Couto, C. Cruzeiro and E. Rocha. Endocrine disruptors in the Leça River and nearby Porto Coast (NW Portugal): presence of estrogenic compounds and hypoxic conditions. *Toxicological & Environmental Chemistry*, 2011b 94, 2: 262-274.

Rocha, S., V. Domingues, C. Pinho, V. Fernandes, C. Delerue-Matos, P. Gameiro and C. Mansilha. Occurrence of Bisphenol A, Estrone, 17β-Estradiol and 17α-Ethinylestradiol in Portuguese Rivers. *Bulletin of Environmental Contamination and Toxicology*, 2013 90, 1: 73-78.

Roepke, T. A., M. J. Snyder and G. N. Cherr. Estradiol and endocrine disrupting compounds adversely affect development of sea urchin embryos at environmentally relevant concentrations. *Aquatic Toxicology*, 2005 71, 2: 155-173.

Safe, S. H. Endocrine disruptors and human health--is there a problem? An update. *Environ Health Perspect,* 2000 108, 6: 487-493.

Seifert, M. Luminescent enzyme-linked receptor assay for estrogenic compounds. *Analytical and Bioanalytical Chemistry*, 2004 378, 3: 684-687.

Sharpe, R. M. and D. S. Irvine. How strong is the evidence of a link between environmental chemicals and adverse effects on human reproductive health? *Bmj*, 2004 328, 7437: 447-451.

Shioda, T. and M. Wakabayashi. Effect of certain chemicals on the reproduction of medaka (Oryzias latipes). *Chemosphere*, 2000 40, 3: 239-243.

Shore, L. S., Y. Kapulnik, B. Ben-Dor, Y. Fridman, S. Wininger and M. Shemesh. Effects of estrone and 17 β-estradiol on vegetative growth of Medicago sativa. *Physiologia Plantarum,* 1992 84, 2: 217-222.

Shore, L. S., Y. Kapulnik, M. Gurevich, S. Wininger, H. Badamy and M. Shemesh. Induction of phytoestrogen production in Medicago sativa leaves by irrigation with sewage water. *Environmental and Experimental Botany*, 1995 35, 3: 363-369.

Shore, L. S. and M. Shemesh. Naturally produced steroid hormones and their release into the environment. *Pure and Applied Chemistry*, 2003 75, 11-12: 1859-1871.

Silva, C. P., M. Otero and V. Esteves. Processes for the elimination of estrogenic steroid hormones from water: A review. *Environmental Pollution,* 2012 165: 38-58.

Silversand, C., S. J. Hyllner and C. Haux. Isolation, immunochemical detection, and observations of the instability of vitellogenin from four teleosts. *Journal of Experimental Zoology,* 1993 267, 6: 587-597.

Solomon, G. M. and T. Schettler. Environment and health: 6. Endocrine disruption and potential human health implications. *Canadian Medical Association Journal*, 2000 163, 11: 1471-1476.

Sonneveld, E., J. A. C. Riteco, H. J. Jansen, B. Pieterse, A. Brouwer, W. G. Schoonen and B. van der Burg. Comparison of In Vitro and In Vivo Screening Models for Androgenic and Estrogenic Activities. *Toxicological Sciences*, 2006 89, 1: 173-187.

Soto Am Fau - Fernandez, M. F., M. F. Fernandez Mf Fau - Luizzi, A. S. Luizzi Mf Fau - Oles Karasko, C. Oles Karasko As Fau - Sonnenschein and S. C. - Developing a marker of exposure to xenoestrogen mixtures in human serum. *Environ Health Perspect,* 1997 3: 647-654.

Soto, A. M., C. Sonnenschein, K. L. Chung, M. F. Fernandez, N. Olea and F. O. Serrano. THE E-SCREEN ASSAY AS A TOOL TO IDENTIFY ESTROGENS - AN UPDATE ON ESTROGENIC ENVIRONMENTAL-POLLUTANTS. *Environmental Health Perspectives,* 1995 103: 113-122.

Specker, L. L. and T. R. Anderson (1994). Developing an ELISA for a model proteinvitellogenin. In *Biochemistry and Molecular Biology of Fishes: Analytical Techniques,*. P. W. Hochanchka and T. P. Mommsen. Amsterdam, Elsevier: 567–578.

Sponchiado, G., E. M. Fortunato de Lucena Reynaldo, A. C. B. de Andrade, E. C. de Vasconcelos, M. L. Adam and C. M. Ribas de Oliveira. Genotoxic Effects in Erythrocytes of Oreochromis niloticus Exposed to Nanograms-per-Liter Concentration of 17 beta-Estradiol (E-2): An Assessment Using Micronucleus Test and Comet Assay. *Water Air and Soil Pollution,* 2011 218, 1-4: 353-360.

Sun, L., J. Zha and Z. Wang. Effects of binary mixtures of estrogen and antiestrogens on Japanese medaka (Oryzias latipes). *Aquatic Toxicology*, 2009 93, 1: 83-89.

Swart, J. C. and E. J. Pool. The Development and Validation of a Quantitative ELISA for in vivo and in vitro Synthesized Vitellogenin from Mossambicus tilapia (Oreochromis mossambicus). *Journal of Immunoassay and Immunochemistry*, 2009 30, 2: 208-223.

Swart, N. and E. Pool. Rapid Detection of Selected Steroid Hormones from Sewage Effluents using an ELISA in the Kuils River Water Catchment Area, South Africa. *Journal of Immunoassay and Immunochemistry*, 2007 28, 4: 395-408.

Tang X Fau - Ullah, N., C. Ullah N Fau - Yu, Z. Yu C Fau - Qin, R. Qin Z Fau - Huang, X. Huang R Fau - Zhu, C. Zhu X Fau - Shen, Y. Shen C Fau - Chen and C. Y. - Chemical and bioassay analysis of estrogen pollution in the surface water of the Tiaoxi River, the source river for Taihu Lake. *Bull Environ Contam Toxicol*, 2012 89, 4: 816-819.

Tong, Y., T. Shan, Y. K. Poh, T. Yan, H. Wang, S. H. Lam and Z. Gong. Molecular cloning of zebrafish and medaka vitellogenin genes and comparison of their expression in response to 17β-estradiol. *Gene*, 2004 328, 0: 25-36.

Tyler, C. R., R. van Aerle, T. H. Hutchinson, S. Maddix and H. Trip. An in vivo testing system for endocrine disruptors in fish early life stages using induction of vitellogenin. *Environmental Toxicology and Chemistry,* 1999 18, 2: 337-347.

Versonnen, B. J. and C. R. Janssen. Xenoestrogenic effects of ethinylestradiol in zebrafish (Danio rerio). *Environmental Toxicology,* 2004 19, 3: 198-206.

Vethaak, A. D., S. M. Schrap and P. de Voogt 2006. *Estrogens and Xenoestrogens in the Aquatic Environment: An Integrated Approach for Field Monitoring and Effect Assessment*, Society of Environmental Toxicology and Chemistry.

Watts, M., N. W. Pankhurst, A. Pryce and B. Sun. Vitellogenin isolation, purification and antigenic cross-reactivity in three teleost species. *Comparative Biochemistry and Physiology Part B: Biochemistry and Molecular Biology,* 2003 134, 3: 467-476.

WHO, 2011a. Guidelines for Drinking-water Quality. *http://whqlibdoc.who.int/publications/ 2011/9789241548151_eng.pdf.*

WHO 2011b. Pharmaceuticals in drinking-water.

WHO 2012. *State of the science of endocrine disrupting chemicals 2012,* United Nations Environment Programme and the World Health Organization.

Yin, G.-G., R. S. Kookana and Y.-J. Ru. Occurrence and fate of hormone steroids in the environment. *Environment International,* 2002 28, 6: 545-551.

Ying, G.-G., R. S. Kookana and Y.-J. Ru. Occurrence and fate of hormone steroids in the environment. *Environment International,* 2002 28, 6: 545-551.

Zhang, Z., J. Hu, W. A. F. Jin, L. An, S. Tao and J. Chen. Induction of vitellogenin mRNA in juvenile chinese sturgeon (acipenser sinensis gray) treated with 17β-estradiol and 4-nonylphenol. *Environmental Toxicology and Chemistry*, 2005 24, 8: 1944-1950.

Zuehlke, S., U. Duennbier, T. Heberer and B. Fritz. Analysis of endocrine disrupting steroids: Investigation of their release into the environment and their behavior during bank filtration. *Ground Water Monitoring and Remediation,* 2004 24, 2: 78-85.

In: Estradiol: Synthesis, Health Effects and Drug Interactions ISBN: 978-1-62808-962-2
Editors: Ricco Palmeri and Sal Grimaudo

Chapter 2

Estradiol in CNS: Role in Neurodegeneration

***M. J. Pérez-Álvarez*[1,2] *and F. Wandosell*[2,3*]**
[1]Departamento de Biología (Fisiología Animal), Univ. Autónoma de Madrid, Madrid, Spain
[2]Centro de Biología Molecular "Severo Ochoa", CSIC-UAM, Univ. Autónoma de Madrid, Madrid, Spain
[3]Centro de Investigación Biomédica en Red sobre Enfermedades Neurodegenerativas (CIBERNED), Spain

Abstract

Estrogens are one of the main female sex hormones. Within this group, the most active compound with estrogenic action is estradiol. In non-pregnant women, the ovaries are the main place where estradiol is synthesized through a mechanism that depends on pituitary hormones, but there is a well-documented mechanism of estradiol synthesis independent of gonads and pituitary hormones involving the aromatase enzyme, amongst others. Not only has the presence of aromatase been found in some areas of central nervous system, but also changes in its levels after brain damage.

Estradiol is the hormone that is mainly responsible for the development of secondary sexual characteristics in females. In addition to these sexual actions, it can also have effects on the central nervous system in males. Estradiol has been found to modulate different aspects in the brain, not only in normal physiology but also in pathological conditions. It can protect against brain injury, neurodegeneration and cognitive decline, and may act as a "recovery agent" in some central nervous system disorders. In recent years, some laboratories have focused on the mechanisms of estradiol used as a neuroprotective agent in some neurodegenerative diseases, although this action is not yet fully understood. Clinical studies have shown that blood levels of estradiol are associated with decreased risk, delayed onset and progression and enhanced recovery from several

* Corresponding Author address: Departamento de Biología (Fisiología Animal), Univ. Autónoma de Madrid, 28049 Madrid, Spain. Email: mj.perez@uam.es.

traumatic or chronic neurological diseases, although there is evidence that estradiol exposure can be deleterious to some neuronal population.

This chapter will focus on the effects of estradiol in the nervous system. We will describe some of the recently proposed action mechanisms, summarizing some of the recent progress made on understanding the mechanisms of action of estradiol in the central nervous system including the classical and non-classical receptor-mediated and non-receptor dependent pathways, and bring together some of its putative therapeutic effects for stroke and Alzheimer's disease models. Our review focuses on two neurodegenerative diseases with different etiologies and evolution over time. Stroke is a trauma with a fast evolution over time, while Alzheimer's disease is chronic disease that evolves slowly. In both cases, estradiol shows neuroprotective effects in animal models.

Finally, the possibility of using estradiol as a neuroprotector and/or "recovery agent" against some neurodegenerative disorder models is discussed.

Keywords: Neuroesteroids, Estradiol, Brain Damage, Neurodegeneration, Ischemia, Alzheimer, Stroke, MCAO

Introduction

Estradiol is one of the female sexual hormones in the steroid hormone family. There are two main groups of female sexual hormones: estrogens and progestins. All of them derive from cholesterol and are mainly produced by the ovaries under pituitary control in females. The importance of the organs/places involved in the production of estrogens varies with female reproductive physiology. In a non-pregnant woman, only the ovaries produce significant amounts of estrogens and secrete them to the blood, while the adrenal cortex secretes to a lesser extent. During pregnancy, the placenta secretes large amounts of estrogen. In males, only the adrenal glands synthesize and release estrogens into general circulation.

The three major estrogens detected in plasma are: β-estradiol (hereafter estradiol), estrone and estriol (structures in Figure 1). The main estrogen produced and secreted by the ovaries and adrenal glands is estradiol, although they also secrete small amounts of estrone. Most estrone is also synthesized in peripheral tissues from androgens produced by the adrenal cortex, theca cells and ovarian stroma. Estriol is an oxidation product derivative, as both estradiol and estrone and produced by the liver. The estrogenic action of estradiol, estrone and estriol shows different power. Estradiol is 12 times more powerful than estrone and 80 times more than estriol. Estradiol is therefore considered to be the principal estrogen.

The main function of estrogens is related to the development of secondary sexual characteristics in women acting on the uterus, external genitals, Fallopian tubes and breasts. They also have others effects on the skeleton (increased osteoblastic activity, deposition of bone matrix and calcium/phosphate on the bones), skin, metabolism, lipid deposition etc. They also influence the development, growth, differentiation, maturation and function of the peripheral and central nervous system [1].

All estrogens are derived from blood cholesterol. In the synthesis pathway, the first molecule formed is pregnenolone, which is subsequently transformed to testosterone and afterwards to estradiol. The last step in this pathway, the conversion of androgens to estrogens, is catalyzed by aromatase. Figure 1 shows the major intermediates and enzymes involved in the synthesis pathway of steroid sex hormones. In most vertebrates aromatase is expressed in the gonads [2], placenta [3], adipose tissue [4] and brain [2]. This expression pattern suggests that circulating androgens can be converted into active estrogenic metabolites in specific target tissue.

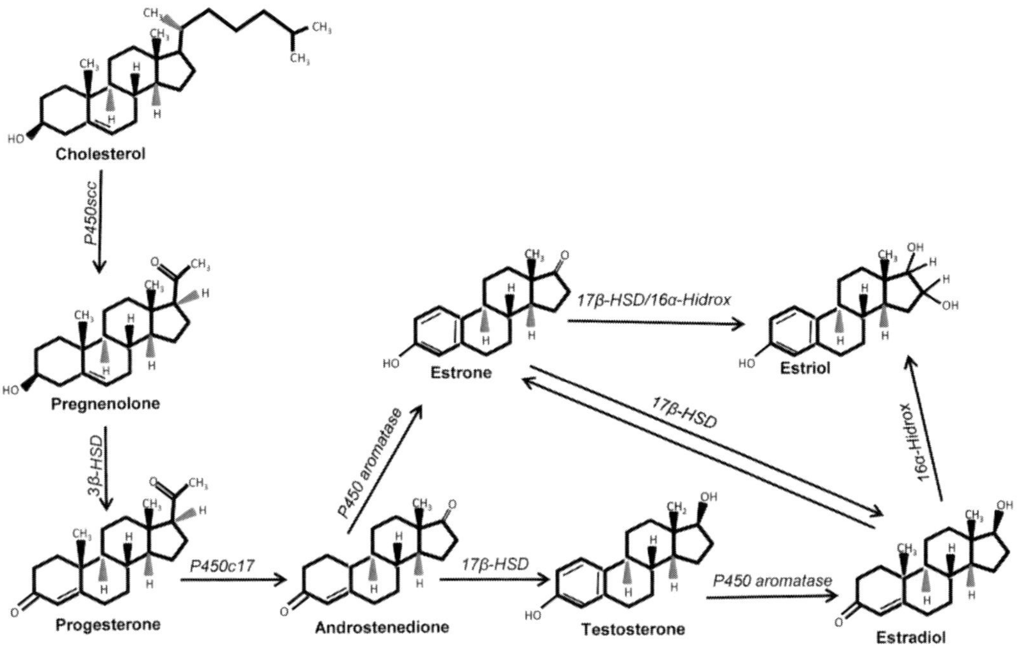

Nomenclature: P450 scc: cytochrome P450 side-chain cleavage; P450 c17: 17α-hydroxylase/C17–20-lyase; 3βHSD: 3β-hydroxysteroid dehydrogenase; 17βHSD: 17β-hydroxysteroid dehydrogenase; 16α-Hidox: 16α-hidoxilase; P450 Aromatase: cytochrome P450 aromatase.

Figure 1. A schematic view of the steroidogenic pathway. The figure includes the enzymes implicated in the synthesis pathway of esteroids hormones, and some of the main intermediary products.

The brain is an important site of estrogens synthesis in vertebrates derived from cholesterol, pregnenolone or androgens. This fact was first demonstrated in mammals by Naftolin et al. in 1971 [5], who found direct evidence that some regions of the central nervous system like limbic system, diencephalon and hypothalamus were able to convert androgens into estrogens [5]. Some laboratories have proven that the central nervous system can synthetize estrogens such as estradiol from cholesterol *de novo* [6-8]. These brain-derived estrogens may play a role in neuronal and/or glial signaling, which are different from sexual action. Cerebral aromatase can thus act by converting circulating metabolites, like circulating androgens, into active estrogenic compounds in some central nervous system regions, or act as part of the endogenous neuroesteroid mechanism to specific regions of the brain. Aromatase is highly expressed in hypothalamus and limbic system regions of the brain involved in physiological and behavioral aspects of reproduction, but there are other sites of aromatase expression in the brain that are not involved in reproduction, such as hippocampus, cerebral cortex, amongst others. Some neuroanatomical studies using both immunohistochemistry and *in situ* hybridization have confirmed the distribution pattern of aromatase in both central and peripheral nervous system including: hypothalamus, amygdala (where it is highly expressed), hippocampus [6], cerebral cortex [9, 10], midbrain [11], sensory peripheral neurons [12] and spinal cord [13]. This suggests that brain-derived estrogens are involved in physiological and behavioral aspects of reproduction and other neuronal function such a cognition, memory, pain and sensory perception [14]. Aromatase is expressed by neurons under normal condition. This neuronal aromatase has been located in different compartments of neurons such as somas, processes and synaptic terminals. Aromatase is also expressed in astrocytes isolated from the cerebral cortex of neonatal rats and maintained under culture conditions [7, 15, 16]. This expression is enhanced *in vitro* by different stress situations such as addition of glutamate or serum deprivation [17]. Similar results have been obtained in reactive astrocytes of mammals and birds after brain injury and ischemia [18-20]. Sexual differences have been found in the expression of aromatase mRNA, indicating that local estrogen levels may be gender-related. A higher aromatase expression has been found in the bed nucleus of the *stria terminalis* of male rats than females [21, 22].

A. Estradiol and Its Receptors

The brain is a target of circulating estrogens from peripheral tissues and also estrogens produced locally by the brain itself. Most biological actions are initiated by the estrogen binding with specific intracellular receptors. Two different types of ER have been identified, to date:

- First, a group known as the "classical ERs" which function as nuclear transcription factors, belonging to the nuclear receptor superfamily [23].
- Second, receptors known as "ER-membrane associated", such as G-protein-coupled-receptor 30 (GPR30). However alternative ER-membrane associated effects have been reported to be not necessary linked to GRP30 [24, 25].

With respect to the first group, two "classical" estrogen receptors (ERs) have been identified alpha (ERα) [26] and beta (ERβ) [27]. Studies using histochemical techniques and *in situ* hybridization have described the presence of both *classical* estradiol receptors in mammal nervous system [28]. In recent years, six splice variants for ERβ (ERβ1, ERβ2, ERβ1δ3, ERβ2δ3, ERβ1δ4, ERβ2δ4) have been reported in rodents and humans, all of them also located in the brain [29, 30]. In general, the β2 variants are less abundantly expressed that their β1 counterparts. ERβ1 is the most abundant variant expressed in brain and ERβ2δ3 the least [29], adding greater complexity to the genomic regulation of the cell by estradiol.

Both subtypes of receptors show similar domain organization and substantial sequence homology. ERα and ERβ share similar DNA-binding domains (96% homology) and similar ligand-binding-domains (56% homology) and bind to the same hormone response element in DNA [27]. *In vitro* studies have shown that ERα and ERβ can exist as hetero- or homodimers, and that these forms may interact differentially with response elements on genes [31]. Nonetheless, they have differences in their affinities for ligands [32] and in their function [29], suggesting distinct roles in estrogen-mediated actions. Studies with ERα (Estr $1^{-/-}$) and ERβ (Estr $2^{-/-}$) knockout mice (ERα-KO and ERβ-KO respectively) showed that ERα-KO mice manifest severely impaired reproductive function leading to infertility [29], whereas ERβ-KO are fertile [33], indicating different roles for these two receptors in such functions. Behavioral studies with ERβ-KO and ERα-KO mice have been performed to test for their possible brain functions. Results using ERβ-KO mice indicate that ERβ may be involved in controlling anxiety-like behavior [34, 35], cognitive functions and memory [28], feeding behavior [36], whereas ERα is essential for neuroendocrine function related to reproduction, since it is involved in regulating the secretion of female sexual hormones by anterior pituitary [29]. *In situ* hybridization techniques [37] have shown that both ERα and ERβ are present in the rat central nervous system but are differentially expressed. Some regions only have ERα or ERβ mRNA, whereas other regions express both. mRNA of ERβ was present in the anterior olfactory nuclei, cerebral and piriform cortex, supraoptic and paraventricular nuclei of the hypothalamus, ventral tegmental area, substancia nigra, pontine nuclei, cerebellum, anterior horn of the spinal cord, pineal gland, areas in which ERα was absent or sparse. ERα mRNA but not ERβ was detected in the ventromedial hypothalamic nucleus, subfornical organ, ventrolateral thalamic nucleus, lateral and basolateral amigdaloid nucleus, and dorsal endopiriform nucleus. The distribution of ERα and ERβ mRNAs overlap in some regions such as the preoptic area, the bed nucleus of the stria terminalis, lower brainstem, arcuate nucleus, hippocampus and dorsal horn of the spinal cord. For a long time, the presence of protein for ERs could not be definitively confirmed in certain regions of the brain, where estradiol was known to act due to the lack of good ER antibodies. Later, the development of better antibodies allowed most investigations to definitively confirm the expression of the protein for ERs within the mammalian brain in both tissue obtained from adults [38-40] and postnatal rat brain [41].

Specifically in the adult rat brain, ERα and ERβ containing structures have been found throughout the adult brain and spinal cord with an analogous pattern observed using hybridization probes. Evaluation of the distribution of ERα and ERβ immunoreactive cerebral nuclei did not reveal great gender differences except in some regions. There is greater expression of ER in males than females in the medial septum, the bed nucleus of the stria terminalis, medial preoptic area and locus subceruleus, while there are higher levels in the female hippocampus than in male [40].

Regarding the cell type expressed ERα and ERβ, some researchers have found that both neurons and glial cells express the two receptors, and while several effects caused by the activation of these receptors upon neuronal functions have been described, the function on glial cells is not fully understand.

There is less information about GRP30 [42-45], but some of the signaling reported to be initiated by estradiol such as the activation of mitogen activated protein kinase (MAPK) [46], or phosphoinositide 3-kinase (PI3K) [47], or protein kinase C (PKC) [48] could be legitimately attributed to this type of receptor.

However the exact contribution of GRP30 to the neuronal and/or glia physiology is yet to be illustrated.

B. Mechanisms of Action in the Central Nervous System: Classical and Non-Classical Receptor-Mediated and Non-Receptor Dependent Pathways

Sex hormones are all cholesterol-derived steroid compounds. Females and males synthesize both estrogens and androgens, which are widely distributed in many mammalian tissues, included in the brain. In addition to the circulating levels many data suggested that sex hormones such as estradiol or testosterone may by synthetized inside the brain [for review see: [49]].

In the case of estrogens, different type of actions have been reported [for review see [5]]. Many data have indicated that estradiol carries out a plethora of functions based on its capacity to simply diffuse through the lipid bilayer of the membrane because it is a lipid, and associated with its receptors (ERs). Many of these actions could be classified as follows:

- ER-independent mechanisms, such as the antioxidant effects reported by estradiol [51].
- ER-dependent mechanism by "classical ERs".
- ER-dependent mechanisms by non-classical ERs, such as those mediated by G-protein-coupled-receptor 30 (GPR30). Alternative ER-membrane associated effects have been reported [24, 25], but we will focused on the GRP30 in this review.

Many data have indicated that at least in mammalian brain, neurons and glia presented specific response to estradiol which implicates ERs [37], although the exact contribution of ERα, ERβ and GRP30 in each neural cell type is not fully established.

The second open issue is the determination and characterization of level and variations of the estradiol locally generated in the brain, in either neuron or glia.

Most of the data from the different actions are from the "classical ERs" and their transcriptional activity. This activity is triggered by dimerization of receptors in the presence of the hormone, using two different classes of ER, denoted as ERα and ERβ [26, 27]. After that, they translocate to the nucleus and may trigger transcription, using either the estrogen responsive element sequences (ERE), (for review see: [52, 53]) dispersed through the genome, or complexes with other transcription factors, such as AP1 [54].

Besides the nuclear actions of estradiol in the cells, the mechanism of action involving binding of estrogen to nuclear estrogen receptors and subsequent regulation of transcription, rapid estrogen effects have been described that occur within minutes and thus cannot be attributed to a genomic mechanism of action. These rapid effects have thus been designated as "non-genomic" effects of estrogen. The existence of non-genomic ERs mediating rapid cell signaling has been proposed in a number of studies [55, 56].

More recently, different ERs have been proposed as a membrane bound protein, and at least one has been fully characterized, the G-protein-coupled-receptor 30 (GPR30), a "non-classical ER" transmembrane receptor coupled to the G-protein [43-45].

This type of ER would be responsible of some of the cytoplasmic effect described for many laboratories, which suggest that in addition to the transcriptional effect orchestrated by classical ER's, rapid cytoplasmic action of estradiol may be reported in some systems.

In fact, diversified data suggest that estradiol may activate MAPK/Erk [46], or PI3K [47], or PKC [48], as mentioned above.

We recently demonstrated that ER is linked to PI3K associated "cytoplasmic signaling" in the brain and in primary neurons. However, some of these data indicated that the signaling is associated with the classical ER, either α and/or β. Indeed the ER α/β is associated with the PI3K regulatory subunit, p85 [57, 58]. We inferred from the phosphorylation level of some Akt substrates, or by the increase of phosphorylation in the residues 308 and 473, that estradiol activates Akt, at short time [59].

Using embryonic neurons or brain tissue samples we detected and described a novel multiprotein complex in which ER, GSK3 and β-catenin were associated. In this complex the estradiol transiently stabilized β-catenin, which is disassociated from this ER–complex, in a clear correlation with the inhibition of GSK3 [58].

Also, in breast cancer cells, a similar interaction has been reported between ERα with p85 subunit of PI3K and Src which is mediated by ERα methylation on the residue Arg260. In this complex, FAK is recruited to this complex, modulating migration process. Using human tissue these authors demonstrated that ERα is methylated in normal epithelial breast cells, and is hypermethylated in some breast cancers. They propose that this methylation is necessary for cytoplasmic functions of ERα, to propagate downstream transduction cascades that coordinate cell proliferation and survival events [60, 61].

We demonstrated in both neuronal cell lineage and primary culture neurons that estradiol transiently leads to activation of Akt and the subsequent inhibition of GSK3. This may be confirmed by the inhibitor of PI3K, LY 290024, which prevented the activation of Akt and the inhibition of GSK3. These cooperative -and in some way reciprocal- effects from estradiol signaling and IGF-1/PI3K pathway have been reported not only in neural tissue, but also in other cellular systems such as breast cancer cells.[47, 57, 58].

We must point out that the estradiol-mediated stabilization of β-catenin would be an important secondary effect of this hormone, bearing in mind the dual role of this protein in cell adhesion as well as nuclear transcription. β-catenin is a key component on the Wnt signaling pathway [62, 63], and an important element of the cell adhesion system (*i.e.*: cadherins, and integrins) [64, 65]. It has been established in many cellular system that the presence of Wnts triggers different pathways. One of them regulates a multi-protein complex that inhibits the GSK3 activity and promotes β-catenin stabilization. Next this β-catenin cooperates in a transcriptional response mediated by its nuclear partner, the TCF-Lef family protein [66-68]. We therefore studied whether the stabilization of β-catenin, estradiol-mediated can generate a similar response in neurons, and detected increased β-catenin-mediated transcription upon estradiol addition in a time and concentration-dependent manner. Our data indicated that this transcription is TCF-mediated. We subsequently generated an established neuronal cell line containing a dominant negative version of LEF-1. The differential expression analysis using these cells treated with either, estradiol or Wnt3a, and control solvents, permitted the identification of the mRNA response and subsequently the early response genes to this hormone. Our analysis focused on genes with a differential respond to estradiol or Wnt. Accordingly, we discarded genes with a similar response after estradiol (either positive or negative) but which were insensitive to the presence of dominant negative LEF-1, and thus removed all genes that were directly ERE-dependent. The comparative analysis of the LEF-1-sensitive genes led a major conclusion. We found that some genes are regulated similarly by estradiol and Wnt3a. However, a significant fraction of genes were expressed differentially, which strongly suggested that the expression pattern of estradiol and Wnt3a, sensitive to LEF-1, was different [69, 70].

These results permit the proposal of a novel mechanism by which the estrogen receptor can modulate gene expression using the β-catenin/TCFs/DNA complex in neurons sharing some elements with Wnt signaling [66, 71, 72].

However, our findings to date strongly support that the estradiol-induced transcriptional activation differs from Wnt, revealing new roles for estrogens in the neurons.

It's tempting to hypothesize that some of these estradiol-mediated signals may represent a general mechanism. This hypothesis should be revised, at least in two major fields. Firstly, considering the role of GSK3 in survival, neurodegeneration [73-79] and Alzheimer disease [80], our data suggest that part of the neuroprotective effect of estrogen may be due to the control of GSK3 activity and some GSK3-dowstream pathways. Secondly, in view of the possible role of estradiol in the initiation or maintenance of some hormone-dependent tumors, estradiol behaves, at least in part, like Wnts, modulating important proteins such as β-catenin [81], Cyclin D [82-84], c-myc [85], implicated in tumor progression [63].

In conclusion, this new estradiol signaling pathway merits further analysis. The figure 2 shows a schematic outline of the principal mechanisms of action of estradiol described until now, including the *classical* and *non-clasical* receptor-mediated pathways.

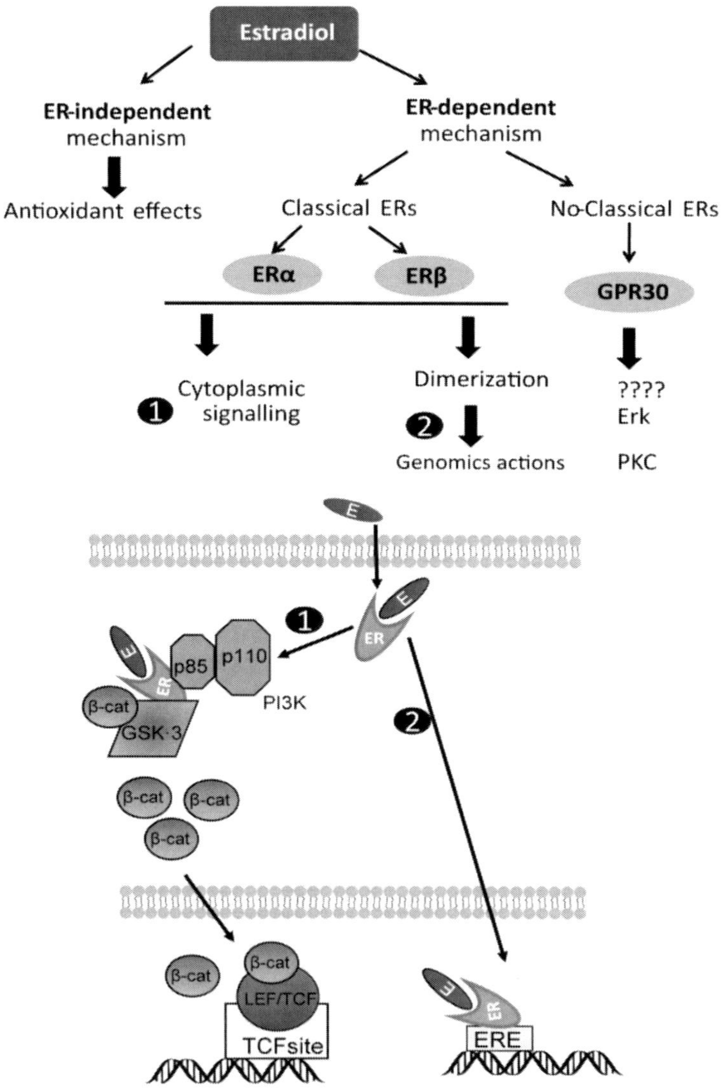

Figure 2. Mechanism of action of estradiol. Summary of the mechanisms proposed for the actions of estradiol and some estrogenic derivatives. ER-independent and ER-dependent mechanism mediated by *classical* and *non- classical* receptors.

C. Physiological Action of Estradiol in the Brain

Estradiol is an important hormone that regulates the physiology of multiple body tissues and functions. Estradiol also acts on the nervous system, modulating certain brain functions. Here we shall present a summary of the main physiological effects of estradiol in the central nervous system. Brain functions can be broadly divided into three different main categories: sensory, motor and "superior or higher" functions. Within the superior functions, subcategories such as mood or emotion, behavior, cognition (learning and memory) can be defined. Estradiol has a strong influence over all three and also sensorial perception of nociception.

CNS Development

Estradiol regulates the differentiation of neurons and glial cells in the central nervous system. These developmental action of estradiol have been characterized in hypothalamus [86, 87], where sex differences are generated in neuronal circuits controlling neuroendocrine events, reproduction, growth; the midbrain [88], cerebellum [89, 90], hippocampus [91] and neocortex [92]. Estradiol regulates at least four aspects of neuronal development: the growth of axons, the growth of dendrites; the growth of dendritic spines and the formation of synapses [93]. Different mechanisms may be implicated in each of these developmental actions of estradiol, and it is also possible that the mechanisms differ between the neuronal type and the brain region under consideration. These developmental actions of estradiol do not always correspond to a hormonal effect, since estradiol, synthesized locally by neurons or astrocytes, also participates in the regulation of neuronal development by paracrine or autocrine mechanism [92, 94-96].

Cognition and Memory

ERα and ERβ are both expressed in the hippocampus, a region of the brain involved in cognitive function and memory.

The importance of estradiol in cognitive function has been highlighted by examining cognition in relation to phases of the menstrual cycle, menopausal symptoms, circulating hormones levels and aging in women [97-99].

In rodents, estradiol has been reported to enhance learning in some rodent memory tasks including Morris water maze [100], a function mediated by the ERβ receptor. ERβ-KO mice treated with estradiol show impairments in acquisition of spatial reference memory [101], deficits in hippocampal neuronal activity [102]. In addition, the use of a ERβ selective agonist enhances spatial memory in ovariectomized rats in Morris water maze tests, while a ERα selective agonist does not [103].

At cellular level, estrogens have been reported to promote the formation of new dendritic spines and alter spine density in the hippocampus in both granule and pyramidal cells in young adult and aging female rats [104, 105], as well as increasing the expression of the NMDA receptor subunit NR2B and enhanced NMDAR-mediated synaptic activity and long-term potentiation [93, 106].

Estradiol has also been shown to increase phosphorylation of cyclic AMP response element-binding protein (CREB), a process which has been strongly implicated in the formation of long-term memory [28].

Hypothalamic-Pituitary-Adrenal Axis

Estradiol and gonadal steroids hormones play a vital role in modulating hypothalamic-pituitary-adrenal (HPA) axis function. It has now been established that basal and stress-induced adrenal steroid secretion is greater in females than in males [107, 108], and that the activating effects of gonadal steroids play an integral role in this sex difference [109]. But there is evidence that estrogen can increase or reduce stress.

In females, ovariectomy reduces stress-induced cortisol and ACTH, and this is reversed by estrogen treatment [108]. However, several groups have reported that estrogen can inhibit responses to stress [110-112].

Again, this effect can be explained by the different role of estradiol receptors in the HPA axis. The treatment of ovariectomized females with an ERβ-selective agonist causes a significant decrease, while treatment with an ERα selective agonist causes a significant increase in stress-induced ACTH and cortisol [113].

Stress-Anxiety-Related Behaviors

Several studies have reported that Major Depressive Disorder episodes, one of the most common psychiatric disorders, are twice as common in women as compare to men [114]. A link between the inherent sex differences in this disorder could be explained by the action of estradiol. Estrogens are a well-known mood regulator, with reported effects of estradiol treatment ranging from depressant to antidepressant [115]. These opposing effects of estradiol on emotion have been associated with the activation of different receptors. There is increasing evidences that ERα activation is anxiogenic [29, 116, 117], whereas ERβ activation is anxiolytic [113, 118]. Behavioral actions of ERβ activation may be explained by direct effects on regulation of neuropeptides or hormones that are involved in the stress response such as adenocorticotropin hormone, corticosterone, oxytocine, serotonin [29]. In fact ERβ has been implicated in serotonin reuptake dynamics [119, 120].

In studies of aggressive behavior, ERα and ERβ show opposing effects. Based on the behavior of ERα-KO and ERβ-KO mice, it has been suggested that ERα enhances aggressive behavior and ERβ reduces aggression [121-123].

Pain

Estradiol is involved in pain modulation. Some studies show that treatment using estradiol reduces endogenous pain caused by increased nociceptive neuronal activity [124], an effect mediated by ERβ. Treatment with ERβ agonist alleviated chronic but not acute inflammatory pain states [125]. These and others results show the potential interest of ERβ as a target drug for of pain treatment.

D. Neuroprotective Effect of Estradiol

Estradiol is considered to be a neuroprotective hormone for several reasons. First, because analysis of human populations has provided evidence that the normal age-related depletion of sex steroid hormones is a major risk factor for some diseases such as cardiovascular and neurodegenerative disorders. Second, because sex differences in the onset and severity of neurodegenerative disease and mental disorders have been described.

The losses of estrogen hormonal control at menopause in women and the more gradual decrease in testosterone in aging men is risk factors for neurodegenerative diseases such stroke [77], Alzheimer (AD) [80] and some type of Parkinson [126-128]. Thus, the hypothesis is that the depletion of sex hormones along normal aging is associated with brain vulnerability to these diseases. In fact, following menopause, women quickly lose the circulating levels of ovarian hormones, estradiol and progesterone, increasing the prevalence of several neurodegenerative diseases. However the concept of neuroprotective effects of estrogen in women following menopause remains controversial because these effects may vary with the timing of treatment [129, 130] (see section E).

Estradiol directly promotes survival, synaptic plasticity and prevents axonal and dendritic pruning [1, 131]. It can also prevent the loss of neuronal functions by modifying the levels of neurotransmitters, receptors, second messengers, and signaling pathways activity. Moreover, estradiol may have indirect neuroprotective effects through its action on other body organs or systems such as reducing cholesterol levels or altering the immune function.

There are three main areas of support for the estrogen protection hypothesis: epidemiological findings, clinical evidence and animal studies exploring the effects of estrogens on different models that imitate neurodegenerative diseases. In this chapter we focus on the effects of estradiol as a neuroprotective agent in two such diseases with different etiologies and evolution over time: stroke and Alzheimer disease. We will also present some of the experimental evidence on the neuroprotective effect of estradiol in others disorders.

Parkinson's Disease

Parkinson's disease (PD) is a chronic neurodegenerative disorder of unknown etiology, although it probably arises from the interplay of environmental and genetic factors. PD is characterized by destruction of dopaminergic neurons in the *susbtantia nigra pars compacta* and their terminals in the *dorsal striatum*. This destruction leads to disturbances in sensorimotor control (primary manifestations), often associated with depression and dementia (secondary symptoms) [132]. Some studies suggested there may be sex differences in the risk of PD, the severity of symptoms, and treatment outcome.

A higher incidence of PD in men than women has been reported [133-135]. They are also sex differences in symptom severity and response to antiparkinsonism medication between male and female patients [136]. The reason for sex differences in PD remains unclear, but there is growing evidence that estrogen may play a neuroprotective role in this disease, despite the sparse expression of estradiol receptors in striatum and *substantia nigra*, at least in rodents.

Thus, both animal and human studies suggest a beneficial regulatory effect of estrogen on the nigroestriatal dopaminergic system, which may underlie putative protective effects of estrogen in PD. [137-139]

Multiple Sclerosis

Multiple sclerosis is an autoimmune disease that affects the nervous system with flare-ups that are initially intermittent. Patients can show complete recovery between recurring episodes, and eventually irreversible neurological deficits leading to cumulative disability. Some characteristics of this disease are axonal damage and demyelinated plaques. Neuronal loss as a consequence of such damage has been proposed [140]. This disease show sexual dimorphism that reflects multiple factors including gender-specific hormonal effects on immune responsiveness, genetic susceptibility, and modulation of target cell activity. Estrogen in particular is thought to be beneficial in multiple sclerosis, based on the fact that estrogen levels inversely correlate with the incidence of exacerbations, and that the disease is ameliorated during pregnancy and then is increased in the post-partum period [141, 142]. This could be explained by the ability of estradiol to influence cytokine expression that may impact several different aspects of this inflammatory disease (see below).

Inflammatory Response of Glial Cell

Most neurodegenerative disorders such as strokes, Parkinson's and Alzheimer's diseases are often accompanied by inflammation events within the nervous system (neuroinflammation). The response of neural tissue to injury comprises a sequence of events leading to the activation of glial cells (microglia and astrocytes) and the release of inflammatory mediators. These include pro-inflammatory cytokines, prostaglandins, free radicals and complements, which in turn induces chemokines and adhesion molecules expression and the recruitment of immune cells [122]. This response is aimed at protecting the neural tissue, but the excessive and chronic activation of glial cells may lead to neurotoxicity and hence be injurious for nervous tissue. The inflammatory response that occurs in the nervous system after damage can be divided into two phases: acute and chronic. The acute phase comprises a rapid activation of glial cells (microglia and astrocytes). The glial cells undergo changes in their morphology and begin to proliferate. They then start to release a set of growth factors and pro-inflammatory molecules to the extracellular compartment in the damaged regions and the surrounding tissue. These molecules partially restore the stability and function of the surrounding areas in a paracrine way, a defensive response aimed at repairing or preventing the spread of the damage. Over time, however, the situation becomes a chronic response. Pro-inflammatory cytokines and chemokines attract macrophages, more microglia, lymphocytes (especially T cells) to the inflammation focus [143, 144], which promotes additional injury and propagates a feed-forward inflammatory response, resulting in a progressive neurodegeneration.

At least part of the neuroprotective actions of estradiol after injury in the brain are mediated by effects of the hormone in this inflammatory process, through its effects on the glial cells. Estradiol has shown to be anti-inflammatory agent and the reduction of inflammation by this hormone in the central nervous system has been well documented on animal models of neurodegenerative diseases [129, 145, 146] and in vitro [147-149]. This estrogen anti-inflammatory activity in brain could be a therapeutic opportunity for neurodegenerative diseases.

All these observations suggest that estrogen exerts a beneficial effect by limiting damage to the central nervous system. However, one aspect that is still not completely clear is the molecular mechanism responsible for estradiol neuroprotection. Studies of many model systems such as amyloide toxicity and glutamate excitotoxicity suggest that specific pathways such as PI3K-Akt may be implicated [78, 80, 129]. However, in many cases nuclear transcription-activity associated with classical ERs happens at the same time, and cannot be dissociated from the "cytoplasmic" signaling triggered by estradiol.

E. Putative Therapeutic Effect in Stroke Models

Cerebrovascular accident (CVA) or stroke is a complex neurodegenerative disease with a high incidence in the population. Furthermore, CVA is the leading cause of disability and the second causes of death in the world. Men have a higher incidence of strokes than women until menopause, when this pattern is inverted [150]. In Spain, strokes are the second cause of death in the entire population and the leading cause of mortality in post-menopausal women. Women also experience several physiological periods of higher stroke risk such pregnancy, childbirth, peri-menopause (45-55 years) and old age (over 85), all of which correspond with a depletion of sexual hormones. These statistical data in humans suggest that sexual hormones, including estradiol, play a role in the incidence and progression of stroke. Stroke is considered to be a neurodegenerative disease, since either subtype of stroke can cause neuronal cell death and result in profound disability.

Approximately 87% of CVA are ischemic, where a brain region suffers a decrease or interruption of the oxygenated blood flow for a significant period of time and 13% are hemorrhagic (10% intracerebral hemorrhage and 3% subarachnoid hemorrhage), during which a blood vessel bursts inside the brain [150, 151]. Some animal models have mimicked ischemic CVA, which can be divided into two main groups. One is global ischemia (four vessel occlusion) that mimics the effects on the brain of a cardiac arrest, and the other is focal ischemia (middle cerebral artery occlusion, MCAO) that mimics a focal occlusion of a cerebral artery either by an embolus or by local thrombosis [152, 153]. The MCAO models can be subdivided into two groups: transient MCAO (tMCAO) and permanent MCAO (pMCAO). tMCAO is when the artery occlusion is sustained for a short period of time (30-120 minutes) and after, injured tissue reperfusion is allowed, and pMCAO is when the artery occlusion is maintained until the animal's sacrifice. tMCAO mimics a therapeutic intervention on patients who have suffered a stroke, while pMCAO imitates no therapeutic intervention. Estradiol has profound protective actions on all stroke models. There are some evidences that support this fact. Female animals sustain less brain tissue injury from MCAO than do age-matched males, and this advantage is abolished by ovariectomy (OVX) [154, 155]. In ovary intact females, circulating estradiol levels are inversely correlated with MCAO-induced infarct size [156], and when exogenous estradiol is administered before [154, 157] or after [129, 158] the onset of MCAO the brain is protected during experimental stroke in both males and females. In addition physiological levels of estradiol administered chronically prior to tMCAO in OVX female rats show dose-dependent amelioration of ischemia-induce injury [155, 159]. Pretreatment using an antagonist of ERs (ICI 182,780 a competitive antagonist of both estrogen receptor isoforms, ERα and ERβ) prior to stroke induction has been found to enhance the size of the infarct [160].

There is also evidence that brain-derived estrogens may act as a natural neuroprotection factor. The extent of the infarct volume increased in aromatase knockout females compared with wild-type and pre-treatment with aromatase inhibitors, exacerbating ischemic injury in rodent brains [151, 161]. Likewise, induction of expression of aromatase after brain stroke has been described. Increased expression was found in the peri-infarct region where injured cells have survived the initial ischemic insult, but could later become incorporated into the irreversibly damaged infarct core [18].

Ischemic brain injury results from a complex sequence of pathophysiological events that evolve over time and space. The major pathogenic mechanisms of this ischemic cascade include excitotoxicity, peri-infarct depolarizations, inflammation and programmed cell death (apoptosis) [152, 153]. In some of them, estradiol has shown protective effects. A schematic view of the principal pathophysiological mechanisms triggered after ischemia and the main processes where estradiol may have neuroprotective effects, is presented in Figure 3.

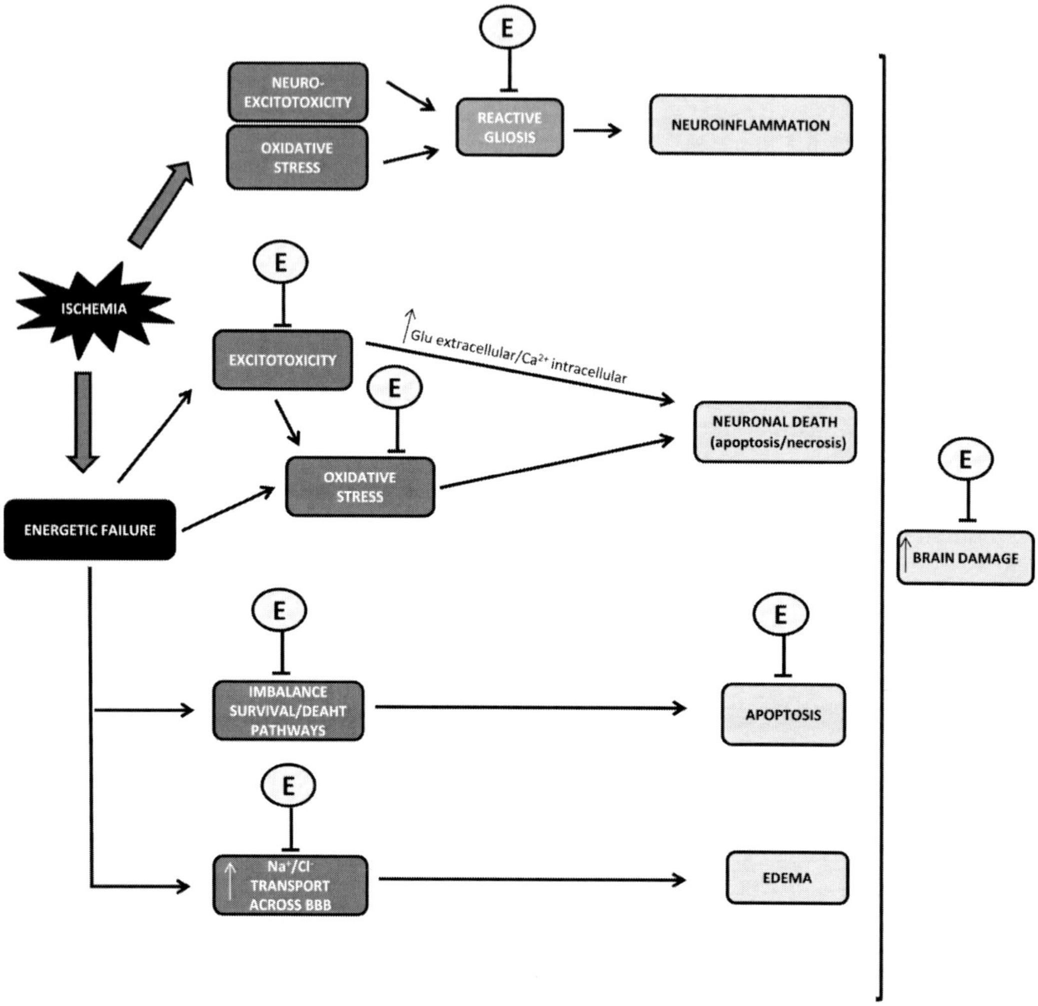

Figure 3. A basic scheme of the main pathophysiological mechanisms triggered after an ischemic insult. The illustration represents some of the best reported dysfunctions generated after ischemia. E-Represent the possible localization/routes that may influence estradiol reducing brain injury.

It seems clear that excitotoxicity is an early mechanism in cerebral ischemia. Due to a lack or dramatic reduction of cerebral blood flow, the delivery of oxygen and glucose to the brain is restricted and neurons become to be unable to maintain ionic gradients. Consequently, presynaptic voltage-dependent calcium channels become activated and excitatory amino acids (glutamate) are released into the extracellular space. At the same time, reuptake of excitatory amino acids is impeded because of the energy failure, which further increases the accumulation of glutamate in the synaptic clef. Activation of NMDA and metabotropic glutamate receptors contributes to cell death. Estradiol has also been shown to interact with and inhibit the activation of NMDA receptors to attenuate *in vitro* glutamate-mediated excitotoxicity using cultured cortical or hippocampal neurons [162, 163]. *In vivo* experiments using the pMCAO model suggest that estradiol-mediated neuroprotection involves a reduction of ischemia induced excitotoxicity primarily through interaction with NMDA receptors [164].

An increase in the intracellular levels of Ca^{2+} as a result of glutamate mediated over-activation after ischemic damage is thought to initiate a series of cytoplasmatic and nuclear events that profoundly impact the development of tissue damage. Events such as the activation of proteolytic enzymes, which degrade cytoskeletal proteins, and the activation of phospholipase A2 and cyclooxygenase, which generate free-radical species, produce lipid peroxidation and membrane damage. This oxidative stress, together with mitochondrial dysfunction, has been found to play a role in promoting neuronal damage and death in cerebral ischemia [165, 166].

Although estradiol is an antioxidant molecule when administered at high dosage [167, 168], low dosage of estradiol has been found to attenuate NADPH oxidase activation and O_2^- production in the hippocampal CA1 region following reperfusion, and this effect is blocked by ER antagonist ICI180.782, in a model of global cerebral ischemia [151]. Estradiol treatment thus attenuates oxidative damage induced by ischemia, at least in hippocampal CA1 cells.

Oxygen free radicals also serve as important molecules that trigger inflammation and apoptosis. Following ischemic injury, brain cells that are compromised by excessive glutamate-receptor activation, Ca^{2+} excess, oxygen radicals and/or by mitochondrial and DNA damage, can die from necrosis or apoptosis. Necrosis is the predominant mechanism that follows acute vascular occlusion, and occurs mainly in the core area after a stroke. In low-grade injury regions, cell suicide develops and death occurred by apoptosis, particularly within the ischemic penumbra. This region is a brain area that surrounds the core, with low blood perfusion, in which cells have lost their membrane potential. The core and penumbra are dynamic areas in space and time, and if the artery occlusion persists, the penumbra can become a core region and hence increase the infarct area and aggravate the symptoms and the prognosis of the disease [152]. Because cells mainly die from preventable apoptosis in the penumbra, several studies have focused on the role of estradiol as an anti-apoptotic or pro-survival agent.

Classical ER receptors are ligand-activated transcription factors and play a crucial role in mediating neuroprotective actions, since they are involved in the regulation of the transcription of various pro and anti-apoptotic genes [138]. These receptors are also implicated in the activation of multiple signaling cascades such ERK/MAPK [169, 170] and PI3K/Akt [129, 171] to promote neuron survival.

In vivo studies in a pMCAO model have shown that estradiol administered before the onset of ischemia increases transcription of pro-survival *bcl2* after injury and prevents transcription of pro-apoptotic *bad* in OVX female rats [172]. Estradiol also prevents the translocation of cytochrome c, activation of caspase-3, and DNA fragmentation, both of which occur during apoptosis [173]. Ischemia also induces and increases the levels of Fas (CD95/Apo1) and Fas-associated Death Domain (FADD), and enhances the activity of caspase-3 and caspase-8 (components of Fas mediated apoptosis). Estradiol significantly reduces the ischemia induction of this apoptosis pathway [174]. Results from a model of global ischemia show that estradiol strongly enhances the expression of the anti-apoptotic prosurvival factor surviving in the CA1 hippocampal region [175] and reduces ischemia-increased mRNA levels of *c-fos* [173].

A large body of evidence supports a role for estradiol in the rapid activation of neuronal signaling pathways (MAPK family and PI3K-Akt) related to the survival/death balance.

The MAPK family is involved in cerebral ischemia. JNK and p38 appear to be detrimental after stroke, and their inhibition blocks apoptosis. However, the role of ERK in ischemia models is questionable because its activity is involved in both neuroprotection and exacerbation of damage (for review see [176]). ERK phosphorylation has been found to decrease during focal and global ischemia [176]. In a model of pMCAO estradiol administration prior to ischemia prevented the ischemia reduction of MEK1/2 and ERK1/2 phosphorylation and decreased the volume of the infarct [170]. In a model of global ischemia, estradiol exerted a prolonged attenuation of phosphorylation of JNK at Thr183/Tyr185 (phosphorylation sites critical for JNK activation) in the CA1 region of the hippocampus. Work in our laboratory on the PI3K-Akt survival pathway found that cerebral ischemia induced in male rats produced a profound down-regulation of this pathway. Treatment with estradiol after 6 hours of the onset of pMCAO, caused a rescue of the activity on this pathway [129].

The intracellular signaling pathways activated during excitotoxicity trigger the expression of genes that initiate post-ischemic inflammation, another pathogenic process that contributes the worsening of ischemic injury. Few data are available in literature about the effects of estradiol in the inflammatory processes following strokes. The nuclear factor-kappa B (NFkB) plays an essential role in the regulation of post-ischemic inflammation, which is detrimental to recovery after an ischemic stroke. During the first 24 hours after tMCAO, there is a rapid increase in the inflammatory response, including: IkB phosphorylation, NF-kB activation, iNOS over-expression [177], and tumor necrosis factor-alpha, interleukin 6, and interleukin 1beta mRNA over-expression [178]. Estradiol treatment before tMCAO produced protective effects by reducing inflammatory responses, decreasing the activation or over-expression of the above factors [177, 178].

When damage occurs in the nervous system, glial cells, mainly astrocytes and microglia, respond through a complex phenomenon called *reactive gliosis*. This process involves proliferation and migration of these glial cells towards the injury sites. In addition, the activation of microglia and astrocytes during *reactive gliosis* is accompanied by a local increased release of chemokines and cytokines, which regulate the inflammatory process [179]. Astrocytes can also release the transforming growth factor-β (TGF-β), which can protect neurons from death. Estradiol has been found to stimulate the expression and release of TGF-β in culture [180]. This would be another form of neuroprotection to promote neuronal survival TGF-β-mediated from astrocytes that should be explored in greater depth. However, recently we have reported an increase in the amount of microglia and astrocytes 54 hours after of the onset of pMCAO. Post-ischemia treatment with estradiol reduced the number of glial cells to control levels. [129].

During a stroke, cerebral edema can form as increased transport of Na^+ and Cl^- from blood into the brain occurs across the blood-brain barrier (BBB). Estradiol significantly decreased brain swelling and lesion volume during pMCAO. Estradiol also abolished activity and decreased the levels of Na-K-Cl co-transporter of cerebral microvascular endothelial cells stimulated by chemical hypoxia. These findings support the hypothesis that estrogen also attenuates the stimulation of BBB Na-K-Cl co-transporter activity, reducing edema formation during stroke [181].

All of the above evidence indicates that estradiol acts as a neuroprotective agent in ischemic stroke, interfering in several pathophysiological mechanisms triggered after an ischemic insult, such as excitoxicity, survival pathways, inflammation and edema. The mechanisms of action of estradiol as a neuroprotective agent after cerebral ischemia are not fully understood and could involve the complementary activation of both "classical" and "non-classical" receptors.

To date, the question about which receptor subtype plays a predominant role in estradiol-mediated neuroprotection in stroke models has not been resolved. It has been described that the expression of receptor ERα and ERβ are differentially modulated after the evolution of cerebral ischemia, in fact the induction of expression of ERα in both males and females, takes place earlier than ERβ modulation. ERα is dramatically increased in neuronal population of cerebral cortex after stroke and pretreatment using estradiol accelerates and amplifies this event, while after ischemic injury ERβ is down-regulated. Estradiol administered before pMCAO, prevent this down-regulation in the late stages of brain injury [182]. Experimental evidence suggests that ERβ is not essential to neuroprotection after stroke. Estradiol continues to protect the brain against ischemia in the absence of ERβ in knockout mice [183]. The use of a selective agonist of ERβ (diarylpropiolnitrile, DNP) in a rat model of stroke revealed no significant differences in hemispheric lesion volumes or in sensorimotor function between vehicle- and DPN-treated groups [184]. However, activation of ERβ has been shown to promote neuroprotection against glutamate excitotoxicity in cultured hippocampal neurons [185]. Selective activation of ERβ, administering DNP before the onset of ischemia, provided neuroprotection within cerebral cortex against tMCAO in male rats [186] but not in pMCAO males. Elsewhere, pre-treatment with G-1, a selective agonist for GPR30, has been reported to exert neuroprotection against cerebral ischemia induced by tMCAO in females [187] and in a model of cardiac arrest and cardiopulmonary resuscitation (CA/CPR) in males [188]. This evidence suggests that estrogen receptor subtypes play different roles in protecting against injury associated with ischemia, which are probably complementary.

F. Putative Therapeutic Effect in Alzheimer's Disease Models

Alzheimer's disease (AD) is one of the most prevalent neurodegenerative disorders, in which age is the most significant risk factor. It is generally sporadic, with a small percentage of affected individuals presenting autosomal dominant mutations, however even in such cases; it develops during middle and old age. As mentioned previously, the loss of estrogen hormonal control at menopause in women and the more gradual decrease in testosterone in aging men increases the prevalence of several neurodegenerative diseases, not only AD.

Final estradiol levels in the brain can be notably different from circulating levels due to either the presence of brain steroid converting enzymes (e.g., Aromatase), the local synthesis of neurosteroid, or even sequestration by sex hormone binding globulin [189, 190]. Similarly, it has been found that testosterone levels in men decline in the brain during aging, with low levels by the age of 80, while the potent androgenic metabolite dihydrotestosterone (DHT) is not reduced with age. These differences would explain the differential prevalence of age-related AD between men and women.

AD is characterized by two histopathological hallmarks, the accumulation of β–amyloid peptide, known as *senile plaques* (for review see: [191, 192]) and by the accumulation of phosphorylated tau, *tangle*s composed of PHFs [193]. In several animal models, although many of them are only part of this complex pathology, the accumulation of amyloid and/or several neurodegenerative markers present sex differences. For instance in some reports indicated that in Tg2576, APPswe/PS1 and 3xTgAD transgenic mice, the accumulation of Aβ is different in males and females [194-197].

In addition, some data show that estradiol may regulate either APP metabolism and/or β–amyloid generation/accumulation [80, 198-200].

These data and recent studies in animal models confirm the beneficial effects of hormone therapy (HT), which may be a helpful brain protection therapy against AD [80, 201]. However, HT data from female Alzheimer´s patients have been controversial [130] with some showing a reduced risk of AD in women who's HT started at the time of menopause and an increased risk of AD in those who began therapy 10–15 years after menopause [202-206].

Changes in hormone and/or receptor responsiveness with age may help to partially explain this controversial timing effect. During the menopause transition, neural sensitivity to estrogens may decline, suggesting that there is a "critical period" around the time of menopause during which HT may protect cognitive functions [206] and allow the body to maintain hormone responsiveness before the irreversible, age-related hormone fluctuations begin.

Indeed, our information on the behaviour of ERs (stability, presence, localization, affinity, etc.) present in neurons and glia, in the female brain after menopause, is by no means clear. Thus, more information is needed to understand why estradiol is still a successful therapy in some animal models and not in humans.

Conclusion

In animal models at least, estradiol exerts a powerful neuroprotective effect against neurodegenerative diseases such as PD, Alzheimer's disease, stroke and multiple sclerosis, caused by different insults. This hormone also presents anti-inflammatory action. Inflammation is a common mechanism triggered by neurodegeneration that implies the activation of glial cells (astrocytes and microglia). In some cases this activation may exacerbate the brain damage. At the cell level, numerous studies have shown that estradiol promotes different neurothropic actions on neurons and glial cells, including neuronal survival, synaptic plasticity, and prevents axonal and dendritic pruning. For all these reasons, it was initially considered a good candidate as a neuroprotective molecule against neurodegenerative illness until 2003, when a study by Women's Health Initiative (WHI) was published. This study showed that the HT in postmenopausal women not only did not prevent mild cognitive impairment, but moreover promoted an increased risk of dementia and stroke in women over 65 years of age who received HT compared to those who received placebo. These findings questioned the evidence of neurodegenerative diseases from animal models, and highlighted the lack of knowledge about the complex estradiol action.

However, we must not forget that estradiol acts at systemic level, and is also the main hormone that determines secondary sexual characteristics in females. The discovery in 1996 of a new ER receptor (ERβ) [27], and that only ERα is the isoform implicated in reproduction, in rodents at least [29, 33], opened up new possibilities for the use of estradiol as a neuroprotective agent. Subsequent studies have shown that the estradiol-mediated actions may be contradictory, depending on the ER isoform (see section C). Moreover some of the neuroprotective actions of estradiol were too fast to involve, at least exclusively, transcriptional-mediated mechanisms. A rapid cytoplasmic signaling associated with the application of the hormone began to suggest the existence of a new estradiol receptor apart from the already known ERs (see section A). We now know that these fast actions of estradiol can be mediated by both: the ER-membrane associated receptor (GPR30 or others) and by the association of ER (α and/or β) with the p85 subunit of PI3K (see section B). The latter could be an important mechanism in neuroprotection, but it has also been found to promote/enhance cell division in breast cancer, once again calling into question the use of estradiol as a neuroprotective agent. It has also been shown that the selective agonist of GPR30 reduces ischemia-induced damage.

On the other hand, it seems that ERβ is not essential to neuroprotection after stroke (see section E), while a different expression of ERα and ERβ after cerebral ischemia has been described which can be modulated by estradiol administered after the insult (see section E). All this information suggests that the estradiol-mediated neuroprotection is a complex phenomenon that is not yet fully understood. Estradiol-mediated neuroprotection probably requires a complex interaction between all subtype receptors. This leads us to think that the level of expression and the location of estradiol subtypes receptors is probably an important factor to be considered.

Most studies of ischemia models have involved young animals and the results show that estradiol protects against ischemic injury when administered before, after or even during the damage (see section E). However, it has also been reported that estradiol administered chronically at physiological levels (experimentally mimicking HT) in long-term OVX female rodents provides little or no benefit in focal or global ischemia.

The average age of the women who enrolled in WHI clinical trials was 63.3, the majority postmenopausal for 13 years on average prior to the start of HT. The quantity and distribution of estradiol receptors is probably not the same in young females, who are physiologically exposed at high blood estradiol levels, as in older females who have suffered a dramatic reduction in sexual hormones levels.

Therefore, the effect of exogenous administration of estradiol does not have to be the same, hence the proposal of the "critical period hypothesis" to explain these controversial results [159], which suggests that there is an appropriate time window for estradiol to maintain its beneficial action following ovarian hormone removal. If HT is not begun within this time window, estradiol may no longer protect the brain against neurodegenerative insults. On other hand, in male rats we have found that estradiol protects against ischemic insults when administered 6 hours after the onset of the damage [129]. More research is needed to accurately determine the therapeutic window of estradiol in different neurodegenerative disease models.

Estradiol dosage is another important issue. Estradiol pellets that maintain high physiological hormone levels exacerbate focal ischemia-induced infarcts in reproductively senescent, middle-aged female rats [207]. In contrast, pretreatment with intermediate levels of estradiol protects the brain from ischemic cell death in middle-aged female rats OVX for 8 weeks [208, 209] and also in reproductively senescent females. Low physiological levels of estradiol (10–25 pg/ml) protect young mice following focal ischemia, and young and middle-aged rats after global ischemia when initiated immediately (within hours), but not when initiated 10 weeks after ovariectomy [210, 211]. The dose is thus an important factor to take into account, as it can reduce or exacerbate damage.

Estradiol dosage and also the timing of treatment are thus major factors that define the effectiveness of estradiol as a neuroprotective agent. Further studies are also needed to determine the mechanism of action of estradiol as a neuroprotective agent, and also the impact of each of the receptors involved in these actions in different stages of neurodegenerative diseases.

This knowledge could provide an opportunity to design drugs that enhance the neuroprotective effects of estradiol and avoid the undesirable effects of this hormone at both the systemic level and also in the central nervous system.

Participants

- Maria Jose Pérez-Álvarez
Departamento de Biología (Fisiologia Animal), UAM. & Centro de Biología Molecular "Severo Ochoa", CSIC-UAM
Universidad Autónoma de Madrid, Cantoblanco,
C/Darwin nº2
28049 Madrid, Spain
Phone: 34 914972819
e-mail: mj.perez@uam.es

-Francisco Wandosell
Centro de Biología Molecular "Severo Ochoa", CSIC-UAM, Univ. Autónoma de Madrid, & Centro de Investigación Biomédica en Red sobre Enfermedades Neurodegenerativas (CIBERNED),
Universidad Autónoma de Madrid, Cantoblanco,
C/ Nicolás Cabrera nº 1,
28049 Madrid, Spain.
Phone: 34 91 1964561
e-mail: fwandosell@cbm.uam.es,

Acknowledgment and Funding

This work was supported by grants from CIBERNED (which was an initiative of ISCIII), and DGCYT [DGCYT, SAF2012-39148-C03-01]; and by an Institutional grant from the "Fundación Areces". In addition some aspects of this work were partially supported by a grant form EU-FP7-2009-CT222887 and by CAM S2010/BMD-231-(2010-14)."NEURODEGMODELS".

The funders had no role in study design, data collection and analysis, decision to publish, or preparation of the manuscript.

References

[1] Hoffman G, Merchenthaler I, Zup S. Neuroprotection by ovarian hormones in animal models of neurological disease. *Endocrine*. 2006;29(2):217-31.

[2] Simpson ER. Sources of estrogen and their importance. *The Journal of Steroid Biochemistry and Molecular Biology*. 2003;86:225-30.

[3] Ryan KJ. Biological Aromatization of Steroids. *Journal of Biological Chemistry*. 1959;234:268-272.

[4] Grodin JM, Siiteri PK, Macdonald PC. Source of Estrogen Production in Postmenopausal Women. *Journal of Clinical Endocrinology and Metabolism*.1973;36: 207-14.

[5] Naftolin F, Ryan KJ, Petro Z. Aromatization of androstenedione by limbic system tissue from human foetuses. *Journal of Endocrinology. 1*971; 71:795-796.

[6] Hojo Y, Hattori T-A, Enami T, Furukawa A, Suzuki K, Ishii H-t, et al. Adult male rat hippocampus synthesizes estradiol from pregnenolone by cytochromes P450α and P450 aromatase localized in neurons. *Proceedings of the National Academy of Sciences*. 2004;101:865-70.

[7] Zwain IH, Yen SSC. Neurosteroidogenesis in Astrocytes, Oligodendrocytes, and Neurons of Cerebral Cortex of Rat Brain. *Endocrinology*. 1999;140:3843-52.

[8] Holloway CC, Clayton DF. Estrogen synthesis in the male brain triggers development of the avian song control pathway in vitro. *Nature Neuroscience*. 2001;4(2):170-5.

[9] MacLusky NJ, Walters MJ, Clark AS, Toran-Allerand CD. Aromatase in the Cerebral Cortex, Hippocampus, and Mid-Brain: Ontogeny and Developmental *Implications. Molecular and Cellular Neuroscience*. 1994;5(6):691-8.

[10] Yague JG, Muñoz A, de Monasterio-Schrader P, DeFelipe J, Garcia-Segura LM, Azcoitia I. Aromatase expression in the human temporal cortex. *Neuroscience*. 2006;138(2):389-401.

[11] MacLusky NJ, Walters MJ, Clark AS, Toran-Allerand CD. Aromatase in the cerebral cortex, hippocampus, and mid-brain: ontogeny and developmental implications. *Mol. Cell Neurosci.* 1994;5(6):691-8.

[12] Horvath TL, Wikler KC. Aromatase in developing sensory systems of the rat brain. J. *Neuroendocrinol*. 1999;11(2):77-84.

[13] Evrard HC. Estrogen synthesis in the spinal dorsal horn: a new central mechanism for the hormonal regulation of pain. American Journal of Physiology - Regulatory, *Integrative and Comparative Physiology*. 2006;291(2):R291-9.

[14] Roselli CF. Brain aromatase: Roles in reproduction and neuroprotection. *The Journal of Steroid Biochemistry and Molecular Biology*. 2007;106:143-50.

[15] Zwain IH, Yen SSC, Cheng CY. Astrocytes cultured in vitro produce estradiol-17β and express aromatase cytochrome P-450 (P-450 AROM) mRNA. *Biochimica et Biophysica Acta* 1997;140(8):3843-52.

[16] Liu M, Hurn PD, Roselli CE, Alkayed NJ. Role of P450 aromatase in sex-specific astrocytic cell death. *Journal of Cerebral Blood Flow and Metabolism*. 2006;27(1):135-41.

[17] Azcoitia I, Sierra A, Veiga S, Garcia-Segura LM. Aromatase Expression by Reactive Astroglia Is Neuroprotective. *Annals of the New York Academy of Sciences.* 2003;1007(1):298-305.

[18] Carswell HVO, Dominiczak AF, Garcia-Segura LM, Harada N, Hutchison JB, Macrae IM. Brain aromatase expression after experimental stroke: Topography and time course. *The Journal of Steroid Biochemistry and Molecular Biology.* 2005;96(1):89-91.

[19] Garcia-Segura LM, Veiga S, Sierra A, Melcangi RC, Azcoitia Ii. Aromatase: a neuroprotective enzyme. *Progress in Neurobiology.* 2003;71(1):31-41.

[20] Peterson RS, Saldanha CJ, Schlinger BA. Rapid Upregulation of Aromatase mRNA and Protein Following Neural Injury in the Zebra Finch (Taeniopygia guttata). *Journal of Neuroendocrinology.* 2001;13(4):317-23.

[21] Lauber ME, Sarasin A, Lichtensteiger W. Transient Sex Differences of Aromatase (CYP19) mRNA Expression in the Developing Rat Brain. *Neuroendocrinology.* 1997;66:173-80.

[22] Wagner CK, Morrell JI. Neuroanatomical distribution of aromatase mRNA in the rat brain: indications of regional regulation. *The Journal of Steroid Biochemistry and Molecular Biology.* 1997;61:307-14.

[23] Hewitt SC, Li Y, Li L, Korach KS. Estrogen-mediated regulation of Igf1 transcription and uterine growth involves direct binding of estrogen receptor alpha to estrogen-responsive elements. *Journal of Biological Chemistry.* 2010;285(4):2676-85.

[24] Bulayeva NN, Wozniak AL, Lash LL, Watson CS. Mechanisms of membrane estrogen receptor-alpha-mediated rapid stimulation of Ca2+ levels and prolactin release in a pituitary cell line. *American Journal of Physiology and Endocrinolology Metabolism* 2005;288(2):E388-97.

[25] Revankar CM, Cimino DF, Sklar LA, Arterburn JB, Prossnitz ER. A transmembrane intracellular estrogen receptor mediates rapid cell signaling. *Science.* 2005;307(5715):1625-30.

[26] Koike S, Sakai M, Muramatsu M. Molecular cloning and charcterization of rat estrogen receptor cDNA. *Nucleic Acids Research.* 1987; 15:2499-513.

[27] Kuiper GG, Enmark E, Pelto-Huikko M, Nilsson S, Gustafsson JA. Cloning of a novel receptor expressed in rat prostate and ovary. *Proceedings of the National Academy of Sciences.*1996;93:5925-30.

[28] Liu F, Day M, Muniz LC, Bitran D, Arias R, Revilla-Sanchez R, et al. Activation of estrogen receptor-[beta] regulates hippocampal synaptic plasticity and improves memory. *Nature Neuroscience.* 2008;11(3):334-43.

[29] Weiser MJ, Foradori CD, Handa RJ. Estrogen receptor beta in the brain: From form to function. *Brain Research Reviews.* 2008;57(2):309-20.

[30] Handa RJ, Ogawa S, Wang JM, Herbison AE. Roles for Oestrogen Receptor β in Adult Brain Function. *Journal of Neuroendocrinology.* 2011;24(1):160-73.

[31] Saunders PT. Oestrogen receptor beta (ER beta). *Reviews of Reproduction.*1998;3:164-71.

[32] Gruber CJ, Tschugguel W, Schneeberger C, Huber JC. Production and Actions of Estrogens. *The New England Journal of Medicine* 2002;346:340-52.

[33] Krege JH, Hodgin JB, Couse JF, Enmark E, Warner M, Mahler JF, et al. Generation and reproductive phenotypes of mice lacking estrogen receptor β. *Proceedings of the National Academy of Sciences* 1998;95:15677-82.

[34] Krezel W, Dupont S, Krust A, Chambon P, Chapman PF. Increased anxiety and synaptic plasticity in estrogen receptor β-deficient mice. *Proceedings of the National Academy of Sciences* 2001;98:12278-82.

[35] Imwalle DB, Gustafsson J-A, Rissman EF. Lack of functional estrogen receptor β influences anxiety behavior and serotonin content in female mice. *Physiology & Behavior.* 2005;84(1):157-63.

[36] Liang Y-Q, Akishita M, Kim S, Ako J, Hashimoto M, Iijima K, et al. Estrogen receptor ß is involved in the anorectic action of estrogen. *International Journal of Obesity.* 2002;26:1103-1109.

[37] Shughrue P, Scrimo P, Lane M, Askew R, Merchenthaler I. The Distribution of Estrogen Receptor- β mRNA in Forebrain Regions of the Estrogen Receptor-α Knockout Mouse. *Endocrinology* 1997;138:5649-52.

[38] Laflamme N, Nappi RE, Drolet G, Labrie C, Rivest S. Expression and neuropeptidergic characterization of estrogen receptors (ERα and ERβ) throughout the rat brain: Anatomical evidence of distinct roles of each subtype. *Journal of Neurobiology.* 1998;36(3):357-78.

[39] Shughrue PJ, Merchenthaler I. Distribution of estrogen receptor β immunoreactivity in the rat central nervous system. *The Journal of Comparative Neurology.* 2001;436(1):64-81.

[40] Zhang J-Q, Cai W-Q, Zhou D-S, Su B-Y. Distribution and differences of estrogen receptor beta immunoreactivity in the brain of adult male and female rats. *Brain Research.* 2002;935:73-80.

[41] Perez SE, Chen EY, Mufson EJ. Distribution of estrogen receptor alpha and beta immunoreactive profiles in the postnatal rat brain. *Developmental Brain Research.* 2003;145(1):117-39.

[42] Filardo EJ, Quinn JA, Frackelton AR, Jr., Bland KI. Estrogen action via the G protein-coupled receptor, GPR30: stimulation of adenylyl cyclase and cAMP-mediated attenuation of the epidermal growth factor receptor-to-MAPK signaling axis. *Mol. Endocrinol.* 2002;16(1):70-84.

[43] Filardo EJ, Thomas P. GPR30: a seven-transmembrane-spanning estrogen receptor that triggers EGF release. *Trends in Endocrinology & Metabolism.* 2005;16(8):362-7.

[44] Prossnitz ER, Arterburn JB, Sklar LA. GPR30: A G protein-coupled receptor for estrogen. *Molecular and Cellular Endocrinology.* 2007;265-266:138-42.

[45] Prossnitz ER, Arterburn JB, Smith HO, Oprea TI, Sklar LA, Hathaway HJ. Estrogen signaling through the transmembrane G protein-coupled receptor GPR30. *Annual Reviews of Physiology.* 2008;70:165-90.

[46] Singh M, Setalo G, Jr., Guan X, Warren M, Toran-Allerand CD. Estrogen-induced activation of mitogen-activated protein kinase in cerebral cortical explants: convergence of estrogen and neurotrophin signaling pathways. *Journal of Neurosciences* 1999;19(4):1179-88.

[47] Honda K, Sawada H, Kihara T, Urushitani M, Nakamizo T, Akaike A, et al. Phosphatidylinositol 3-kinase mediates neuroprotection by estrogen in cultured cortical neurons. *Journal of Neurosciences Research.* 2000;60(3):321-327.

[48] Cordey M, Gundimeda U, Gopalakrishna R, Pike CJ. Estrogen activates protein kinase C in neurons: role in neuroprotection. *Journal of Neurochemistry.* 2003;84(6):1340-1348.

[49] Toran-Allerand CD. Estrogen and the brain: beyond ER-alpha, ER-beta, and 17beta-estradiol. *Annals of New York. Academy of Sciences.* 2005;1052:136-44.

[50] Levin ER. Cell localization, physiology, and nongenomic actions of estrogen receptors. *Journal of Applied Physioogyl.* 2001;91(4):1860-7.

[51] Mann V, Huber C, Kogianni G, Collins F, Noble B. The antioxidant effect of estrogen and Selective Estrogen Receptor Modulators in the inhibition of osteocyte apoptosis in vitro. *Bone.* 2007;40(3):674-84.

[52] He J, Cheng Q, Xie W. Minireview: Nuclear receptor-controlled steroid hormone synthesis and metabolism. *Molecular Endocrinology.* 2010;24(1):11-21.

[53] Huang P, Chandra V, Rastinejad F. Structural overview of the nuclear receptor superfamily: insights into physiology and therapeutics. *Annuals Reviews of Physiology.* 2010;72:247-272.

[54] Vivar OI, Zhao X, Saunier EF, Griffin C, Mayba OS, Tagliaferri M, et al. Estrogen receptor beta binds to and regulates three distinct classes of target genes. *Journal of Biologycal Chemistry.* 2010;285(29):22059-22066.

[55] Raz L, Khan MM, Mahesh VB, Vadlamudi RK, Brann DW. Rapid Estrogen Signaling in the Brain. *Neurosignals.* 2008;16(2-3):140-153.

[56] Toran-Allerand CD, Guan X, MacLusky NJ, Horvath TL, Diano S, Singh M, et al. ER-X: A Novel, Plasma Membrane-Associated, Putative Estrogen Receptor That Is Regulated during Development and after Ischemic Brain Injury. *The Journal of Neuroscience.*2002;22:8391-401.

[57] Mendez P, Azcoitia I, Garcia-Segura LM. Estrogen receptor alpha forms estrogen-dependent multimolecular complexes with insulin-like growth factor receptor and phosphatidylinositol 3-kinase in the adult rat brain. *Brain Research Molecular Brain Researc.* 2003;112(1-2):170-176.

[58] Cardona-Gomez P, Perez M, Avila J, Garcia-Segura LM, Wandosell F. Estradiol inhibits GSK3 and regulates interaction of estrogen receptors, GSK3, and beta-catenin in the hippocampus. *Molecular and Cellular Neuroscience.* 2004;25(3):363-373.

[59] Varea O, Escoll M, Diez H, Garrido JJ, Wandosell F. Oestradiol signalling through the Akt-mTORC1-S6K1. *Biochimica et Biophysica Acta.* 2013;1833(5):1052-1064.

[60] Le Romancer M, Treilleux I, Bouchekioua-Bouzaghou K, Sentis S, Corbo L. Methylation, a key step for nongenomic estrogen signaling in breast tumors. *Steroids.* 2010;75(8–9):560-4.

[61] Le Romancer M, Treilleux I, Leconte N, Robin-Lespinasse Y, Sentis S, Bouchekioua-Bouzaghou K, et al. Regulation of estrogen rapid signaling through arginine methylation by PRMT1. *Molecular Cell.* 2008;31(2):212-221.

[62] Moon RT, Kohn AD, De Ferrari GV, Kaykas A. WNT and beta-catenin signalling: diseases and therapies. *Nature Reviews Genetics.* 2004;5(9):691-701.

[63] Bienz M, Clevers H. Linking colorectal cancer to Wnt signaling. *Cell.* 2000;103(2):311-20.

[64] Moon RT, DeMarais A, Olson DJ. Responses to Wnt signals in vertebrate embryos may involve changes in cell adhesion and cell movement. *J. Cell. Sci. Suppl.* 1993;17:183-8.

[65] Bienz M. beta-Catenin: a pivot between cell adhesion and Wnt signalling. *Current. Bio*logy. 2005;15(2):R64-7.

[66] Mulholland DJ, Dedhar S, Coetzee GA, Nelson CC. Interaction of Nuclear Receptors with Wnt/{beta}-catenin/Tcf Signalling: Wnt you like to know?. *Endocrine Reviews*. 2005;26(7):898-915.
[67] Arce L, Yokoyama NN, Waterman ML. Diversity of LEF/TCF action in development and disease. *Oncogene*. 2006;25(57):7492-504.
[68] Barolo S. Transgenic Wnt/TCF pathway reporters: all you need is Lef? *Oncogene*. 2006;25(57):7505-11.
[69] Varea O, Garrido JJ, Dopazo A, Mendez P, Garcia-Segura LM, Wandosell F. Estradiol activates beta-catenin dependent transcription in neurons. *PLoS One*. 2009;4(4):e5153.
[70] Varea O, Arevalo MA, Garrido JJ, Garcia-Segura LM, Wandosell F, Mendez P. Interaction of estrogen receptors with insulin-like growth factor-I and Wnt signaling in the nervous system. *Steroids*. 2010;75(8-9):565-9.
[71] Kouzmenko AP, Takeyama K, Ito S, Furutani T, Sawatsubashi S, Maki A, et al. Wnt/beta-catenin and estrogen signaling converge in vivo. *Journal of Biogical Chemistry*. 2004;279(39):40255-40258.
[72] Ray S, Xu F, Wang H, Das SK. Cooperative control via lymphoid enhancer factor 1/T cell factor 3 and estrogen receptor-alpha for uterine gene regulation by estrogen. *Molecular Endocrinology*. 2008;22(5):1125-40.
[73] Pap M, Cooper GM. Role of glycogen synthase kinase-3 in the phosphatidylinositol 3-Kinase/Akt cell survival pathway *Journal of Biogical Chemistry*. 1998;273(32):19929-32.
[74] Dubal DB, Shughrue PJ, Wilson ME, Merchenthaler I, Wise PM. Estradiol modulates bcl-2 in cerebral ischemia: a potential role for estrogen receptors. *Journal of. Neurosciences*. 1999;19(15):6385-6393.
[75] Culmsee C, Vedder H, Ravati A, Junker V, Otto D, Ahlemeyer B, et al. Neuroprotection by estrogens in a mouse model of focal cerebral ischemia and in cultured neurons: evidence for a receptor-independent antioxidative mechanism. *Journal of. Cerebral Blood Flow & Metabolism*. 1999;19(11):1263-1269.
[76] Wang CN, Chi CW, Lin YL, Chen CF, Shiao YJ. The neuroprotective effects of phytoestrogens on amyloid beta protein- induced toxicity are mediated by abrogating the activation of caspase cascade in rat cortical neurons. *Journal of Biogical Chemistry*. 2001;276(7):5287-95.
[77] Wise P. Estradiol exerts neuroprotective actions against ischemic brain injury: insights derived from animal models. *Endocrine*. 2003;21(1):11-5.
[78] Yu X, Rajala RV, McGinnis JF, Li F, Anderson RE, Yan X, et al. Involvement of insulin/phosphoinositide 3-kinase/Akt signal pathway in 17 beta-estradiol-mediated neuroprotection. *Journal of Biogical Chemistry*. 2004;279(13):13086-13094.
[79] Lucas JJ, Hernandez F, Gomez-Ramos P, Moran MA, Hen R, Avila J. Decreased nuclear beta-catenin, tau hyperphosphorylation and neurodegeneration in GSK-3beta conditional transgenic mice. *Embo Journal*. 2001;20(1-2):27-39.
[80] Xu H, Gouras GK, Greenfield JP, Vincent B, Naslund J, Mazzarelli L, et al. Estrogen reduces neuronal generation of Alzheimer beta-amyloid peptides. *Nature Medicine*. 1998;4(4):447-51.
[81] Jamora C, DasGupta R, Kocieniewski P, Fuchs E. Links between signal transduction, transcription and adhesion in epithelial bud development. *Nature*. 2003;422(6929):317-322.

[82] Tetsu O, McCormick F. Beta-catenin regulates expression of cyclin D1 in colon carcinoma cells. *Nature.* 1999;398(6726):422-6.

[83] Sansom OJ, Reed KR, van de Wetering M, Muncan V, Winton DJ, Clevers H, et al. Cyclin D1 is not an immediate target of beta-catenin following Apc loss in the intestine. *Journal of Biogical Chemistry.* 2005;280(31):28463-28467.

[84] Shtutman M, Zhurinsky J, Simcha I, Albanese C, D'Amico M, Pestell R, et al. The cyclin D1 gene is a target of the beta-catenin/LEF-1 pathway. *Proceedings of the National Academy of Sciences USA*. 1999;96(10):5522-7525.

[85] He MX, Wangler RD, Dillon PF, Romig GD, Sparks HV. Phosphorylation potential and adenosine release during norepinephrine infusion in guinea pig heart. *American Journal of Physiology*. 1987;253(5 Pt 2):H1184-91.

[86] Díaz H, Lorenzo A, Carrer HF, Cáceres A. Time lapse study of neurite growth in hypothalamic dissociated neurons in culture: Sex differences and estrogen effects. *Journal of Neuroscience Research.* 1992;33(2):266-81.

[87] Lenz KM, McCarthy MM. Organized for sex – steroid hormones and the developing hypothalamus. *European Journal of Neuroscience.* 2010;32(12):2096-104.

[88] Beyer C, Karolczak M. Estrogenic stimulation of neurite growth in midbrain dopaminergic neurons depends on cAMP/protein kinase A signalling. *Journal of Neuroscience Research.* 2000;59(1):107-16.

[89] Tsutsui K. Biosynthesis and organizing action of neurosteroids in the developing Purkinje cell. *The Cerebellum.* 2006;5(2):89-96.

[90] Tsutsui K. Neurosteroid Biosynthesis and Action During Cerebellar Development. *The Cerebellum.* 2012;11(2):414-5.

[91] Bender RA, Zhou L, Wilkars W, Fester L, Lanowski J-S, Paysen D, et al. Roles of 17β-Estradiol Involve Regulation of Reelin Expression and Synaptogenesis in the Dentate Gyrus. *Cerebral Cortex.*2010; 20:2985-2995.

[92] Hu R, Cai WQ, Wu XG, Yang Z. Astrocyte-derived estrogen enhances synapse formation and synaptic transmission between cultured neonatal rat cortical neurons. *Neuroscience.* 2007;144(4):1229-40.

[93] Arevalo MA, Ruiz-Palmero I, Scerbo MJ, Acaz-Fonseca E, Cambiasso MJ, Garcia-Segura LM. Molecular mechanisms involved in the regulation of neuritogenesis by estradiol: Recent advances. *The Journal of Steroid Biochemistry and Molecular Biology.* 2012;131:52-6.

[94] Fester L, Zhou L, Bütow A, Huber C, von Lossow R, Prange-Kiel J, et al. Cholesterol-promoted synaptogenesis requires the conversion of cholesterol to estradiol in the hippocampus. *Hippocampus.* 2009;19(8):692-705.

[95] Kretz O, Fester L, Wehrenberg U, Zhou L, Brauckmann S, Zhao S, et al. Hippocampal Synapses Depend on Hippocampal Estrogen Synthesis. T*he Journal of Neuroscience.* 2004; 24:5913-21.

[96] Von Schassen C, Fester L, Prange-Kiel J, Lohse C, Huber C, Böttner M, et al. Oestrogen Synthesis in the Hippocampus: Role in Axon Outgrowth. *Journal of Neuroendocrinology*. 2006;18(11):847-56.

[97] Maki PM, Rich JB, Shayna Rosenbaum R. Implicit memory varies across the menstrual cycle: estrogen effects in young women. *Neuropsychologia*. 2002;40(5):518-29.

[98] Savonenko AV, Markowska AL. The cognitive effects of ovariectomy and estrogen replacement are modulated by aging. *Neuroscience*. 2003;119(3):821-30.

[99] Yaffe K, Lui L-Y, Grady D, Cauley J, Kramer J, Cummings SR. Cognitive decline in women in relation to non-protein-bound oestradiol concentrations. *The Lancet*. 2000;356(9231):708-12.

[100] Sandstrom N, Williams C. Memory retention is modulated by acute estradiol and progesterone replacement. *Behavioral. Neuroscience*. 2001;115(2):384-93.

[101] Rissman EF, Wersinger SR, Taylor JA, Lubahn DB. Estrogen Receptor Function as Revealed by Knockout Studies: Neuroendocrine and Behavioral Aspects. *Hormones and Behavior*. 1997;31(3):232-43.

[102] Day M, Sung A, Logue S, Bowlby M, Arias R. Beta estrogen receptor knockout (BERKO) mice present attenuated hippocampal CA1 long-term potentiation and related memory deficits in contextual fear conditioning. *Behavioural Brain Research*. 2005;164(1):128-31.

[103] Rhodes ME, Frye CA. ERβ-selective SERMs produce mnemonic-enhancing effects in the inhibitory avoidance and water maze tasks. *Neurobiology of Learning and Memory*. 2006;85(2):183-91.

[104] Woolley CS, McEwen BS. Estradiol mediates fluctuation in hippocampal synapse density during the estrous cycle in the adult rat. *The Journal of Neuroscience*. 1992;12:2549-2554.

[105] Li C, Brake WG, Romeo RD, Dunlop JC, Gordon M, Buzescu R, et al. Estrogen alters hippocampal dendritic spine shape and enhances synaptic protein immunoreactivity and spatial memory in female mice. *Proceedings of the National Academy of Sciences*. 2004;101:2185-2190.

[106] Smith CC, McMahon LL. Estradiol-Induced Increase in the Magnitude of Long-Term Potentiation Is Prevented by Blocking NR2B-Containing Receptors. *The Journal of Neuroscience*. 2006;26:8517-8522.

[107] Kitay JI. Pituitary-Adrenal Function in the Rat After Gonadectomy and Gonadal Hormone Replacement. *Endocrinology* 1963;76:253-260.

[108] Handa RJ, Burgess LH, Kerr JE, O'Keefe JA. Gonadal Steroid Hormone Receptors and Sex Differences in the Hypothalamo-Pituitary-Adrenal Axis. *Hormones and Behavior*. 1994;28(4):464-76.

[109] Sencar-Cupović I, Milković S. The development of sex differences in the adrenal morphology and responsiveness in stress of rats from birth to the end of life. *Mechanisms of Ageing and Development* 1976;5(1):1-9.

[110] Figueiredo HF, Dolgas CM, Herman JP. Stress Activation of Cortex and Hippocampus Is Modulated by Sex and Stage of Estrus. *Endocrinology*. 2002;143:2534-2540.

[111] Ochedalski T, Subburaju S, Wynn PC, Aguilera G. Interaction Between Oestrogen and Oxytocin on Hypothalamic-Pituitary-Adrenal Axis Activity. *Journal of Neuroendocrinology*. 2007;19(3):189-97.

[112] Young EA, Altemus M, Parkison V, Shastry S. Effects of Estrogen Antagonists and Agonists on the ACTH Response to Restraint Stress in Female Rats. *Neuropsychopharmacology*. 2001;25(6):881-91.

[113] Lund TD, Rovis T, Chung WCJ, Handa RJ. Novel Actions of Estrogen Receptor-β on Anxiety-Related Behaviors. *Endocrinology* 2005;146:797-807.

[114] Kornstein S. Gender differences in depression: implications for treatment. *Journal of Clinical Psychiatry*. 1997;58(15):12-22.

[115] Fink G, Sumner B, McQueen J, Wilson H, Rosie R. Sex steroid control of mood, mental state and memory. *Clinical and Experimental Pharmacology and Physiology*. 1998;25(10):764-775

[116] Morgan MA, Pfaff DW. Effects of Estrogen on Activity and Fear-Related Behaviors in Mice. *Hormones and Behavior*. 2001;40(4):472-82.

[117] Toufexis DJ, Myers KM, Bowser ME, Davis M. Estrogen Disrupts the Inhibition of Fear in Female Rats, Possibly through the Antagonistic Effects of Estrogen Receptor α (ERα) and ERβ. *The Journal of Neuroscience* 2007; 27:9729-9735.

[118] Sugiyama N, Barros RPA, Warner M, Gustafsson JA. ERβ: recent understanding of estrogen signaling. *Trends in Endocrinology & Metabolism*. 2010;21(9):545-52.

[119] McQueen JK, Wilson H, Sumner BEH, Fink G. Serotonin transporter (SERT) mRNA and binding site densities in male rat brain affected by sex steroids. *Molecular Brain Research*. 1999;63(2):241-7.

[120] McQueen JK, Wilson H, Fink G. Estradiol-b increase serotonin transporter (SERT) mRNA levels and the density of SERT-binding sites in female rat brain. *Molecular Brain Research*. 1997;45(1):13-23.

[121] Nomura M, Durbak L, Chan J, Smithies O, Gustafsson J-A, Korach KS, et al. Genotype/Age Interactions on Aggressive Behavior in Gonadally Intact Estrogen Receptor β Knockout (βERKO) Male Mice. *Hormones and Behavior*. 2002;41(3):288-296.

[122] Lucas S-M, Rothwell NJ, Gibson RM. The role of inflammation in CNS injury and disease. *British Journal of Pharmacology*. 2006;147(S1):S232-S40.

[123] Ogawa S, Chan J, Chester AE, Gustafsson J-A, Korach KS, Pfaff DW. Survival of reproductive behaviors in estrogen receptor β gene-deficient (βERKO) male and female mice. Proceedings *of the National Academy of Sciences*1999;96:12887-12892.

[124] Spooner MF, Robichaud P, Carrier JC, Marchand S. Endogenous pain modulation during the formalin test in estrogen receptor beta knockout mice. *Neuroscience*. 2007;150(3):675-80.

[125] Gardell LR, Hyldtoft L, Del Tredici AL, Andersen CB, Fairbairn LC, Lund BW, et al. Differential modulation of inflammatory pain by a selective estrogen receptor beta agonist. *European Journal of Pharmacology*. 2008;592:158-9.

[126] Bourque M, Dluzen DE, Di Paolo T. Neuroprotective actions of sex steroids in Parkinson's disease. *Frontiers in Neuroendocrinol*. 2009;30(2):142-57.

[127] Schreihofer DA, Ma Y. Estrogen receptors and ischemic neuroprotection: Who, what, where and when? *Brain Research*. 2013.

[128] Simpkins JW, Wen Y, Perez E, Yang S, Wang X. Role of nonfeminizing estrogens in brain protection from cerebral ischemia: an animal model of Alzheimer's disease neuropathology. *Annals of the New York Academy of Science*. 2005;1052:233-242.

[129] Perez-Alvarez MJ, Maza Mdel C, Anton M, Ordonez L, Wandosell F. Post-ischemic estradiol treatment reduced glial response and triggers distinct cortical and hippocampal signaling in a rat model of cerebral ischemia. *Journal of Neuroinflammation*. 2012;9:157-170.

[130] Dye RV, Miller KJ, Singer EJ, Levine AJ. Hormone replacement therapy and risk for neurodegenerative diseases. *International Journal of Alzheimer's Disease*. 2012;2012:258454.

[131] Azcoitia I, Arevalo MA, De Nicola AF, Garcia-Segura LM. Neuroprotective actions of estradiol revisited. *Trends in Endocrinology and Metabolism.* 2011;22(12):467-474.

[132] Weintraub D, Comella CL, Horn S. Part 1: Pathophysiology, Symptoms, Burden, Diagnosis, and Assessment. *American Journal of Managed Care.* 2008;14:S40-S48.

[133] Shulman LM, Bhat V. Gender disparities in Parkinson's disease. *Expert Review of Neurotherapeutics.* 2006;6(3):407-16.

[134] Bower JH, Maraganore DM, McDonnell SK, WA. R. Incidence and distribution of parkinsonism in Olmsted County, Minnesota, 1976-1990. *Neurology.* 1999;52(6):1274.

[135] Baldereschi M, Di Carlo A, Rocca WA, Vanni P, Maggi S, Perissinotto E, et al. Parkinson's disease and parkinsonism in a longitudinal study: two-fold higher incidence in men. ILSA Working Group. Italian Longitudinal Study on Aging. *Neurology.* 2000;55(9):1358-1363.

[136] Scott B, Borgman A, Engler H, Johnels B, Aquilonius SM. Gender differences in Parkinson's disease symptom profile. *Acta. Neurologica Scandinavica.* 2000;102(1):37-43.

[137] Bourque M, Dluzen DE, Di Paolo T. Signaling pathways mediating the neuroprotective effects of sex steroids and SERMs in Parkinson's disease. *Frontiers in Neuroendocrinology.* 2012;33(2):169-78.

[138] Brann D, Raz L, Wang R, Vadlamudi R, Zhang Q. Oestrogen Signalling and Neuroprotection in Cerebral Ischaemia. *Journal of Neuroendocrinology.* 2012;24(1): 34-47.

[139] Gillies GE, McArthur S. Estrogen Actions in the Brain and the Basis for Differential Action in Men and Women: A Case for Sex-Specific Medicines. *Pharmacological Reviews* 2010;62:155-198.

[140] Perry V, Anthony D. Axon damage and repair in multiple sclerosis. Philosophical *Transactions of the Royal Society B: Biological Sciences.* 1999;354:1641–1647.

[141] Duquette P, Girard M. Hormonal factors in susceptibility to multiple sclerosis. *Current Opinion in Neurology and Neurosurg*ery. 1993;6(2):195-201.

[142] Runmarker B, Andersen O. Pregnancy is associated with a lower risk of onset and a better prognosis in multiple sclerosis. *Brain* 1995. p. 253-61.

[143] Dong Y, Benveniste EN. Immune function of astrocytes. *Glia.* 2001;36(2):180-90.

[144] Rebenko-Moll NM, Liu L, Cardona A, Ransohoff RM. Chemokines, mononuclear cells and the nervous system: heaven (or hell) is in the details. *Current Opinion in Immunology.* 2006;18(6):683-9.

[145] Vegeto E, Belcredito S, Ghisletti S, Meda C, Etteri S, Maggi A. The Endogenous Estrogen Status Regulates Microglia Reactivity in Animal Models of Neuroinflammation. *Endocrinology* 2006;147:2263-2272.

[146] Vegeto E, Benedusi V, Maggi A. Estrogen anti-inflammatory activity in brain: A therapeutic opportunity for menopause and neurodegenerative diseases. Frontiers in *Neuroendocrinology.* 2008;29(4):507-519.

[147] Baker AE, Brautigam VM, Watters JJ. Estrogen Modulates Microglial Inflammatory Mediator Production via Interactions with Estrogen Receptor β. *Endocrinology* 2004;145:5021-5032.

[148] Bruce-Keller AJ, Keeling JL, Keller JN, Huang FF, Camondola S, Mattson MP. Antiinflammatory Effects of Estrogen on Microglial Activation. *Endocrinology* 2000;141:3646-3656.

[149] Vegeto E, Bonincontro C, Pollio G, Sala A, Viappiani S, Nardi F, et al. Estrogen Prevents the Lipopolysaccharide-Induced Inflammatory Response in Microglia. *The Journal of Neuroscience* 2001;21:1809-1818.

[150] Go AS, Mozaffarian D, Roger VL, Benjamin EJ, Berry JD, Borden WB, et al. Heart Disease and Stroke Statistics- 2013 Update A Report From the American Heart Association. *Circulation* 2013;127:e6-e245.

[151] Scott E, Zhang Q-g, Wang R, Vadlamudi R, Brann D. Estrogen neuroprotection and the critical period hypothesis. *Frontiers in Neuroendocrinology.* 2012;33(1):85-104.

[152] Dirnagl U, Iadecola C, Moskowitz MA. Pathobiology of ischaemic stroke: an integrated view Trends in Neuroscience. 1999;22:391-398.

[153] Green RA, Odergren T, Ashwood T. Animal models of stroke: do they have value for discovering neuroprotective agents? *Trends in Pharmacological Sciences.* 2003;24(8):402-8.

[154] Alkayed N, Harukuni I, Kimes A, London E, Traystman R, Hurn P. Gender-linked brain injury in experimental stroke. *Stroke* 1998;29:159-165.

[155] Rusa R, Alkayed NJ, Crain BJ, Traystman RJ, Kimes AS, London ED, et al. 17beta-estradiol reduces stroke injury in estrogen-deficient female animals. *Stroke.* 1999;30(8):1665-70.

[156] Liao S, Chen W, Kuo J, Chen C. Association of serum estrogen level and ischemic neuroprotection in female rats. *Neuroscience Lettes.* 2001;297(3):159-62.

[157] Dubal DB, Kashon ML, Pettigrew LC, Ren JM, Finklestein SP, Rau SW, et al. Estradiol protects against ischemic injury. *Journal of Cerebral Blood Flow & Metabolism* 1998;18(11):1253-1258.

[158] Toung TJK, Traystman RJ, Hurn PD. Estrogen-Mediated Neuroprotection After Experimental Stroke in Male Rats. *Stroke* 1998;29:1666-1670.

[159] Inagaki T, Etgen AM. Neuroprotective action of acute estrogens: Animal models of brain ischemia and clinical implications. *Steroids.* 2013;78(6):597-606.

[160] Sawada M, Alkayed NJ, Goto S, Crain BJ, Traystman RJ, Shaivitz A, et al. Estrogen receptor antagonist ICI182,780 exacerbates ischemic injury in female mouse. *Journal of Cerebral Blood Flow & Metabolism* 2000;20(1):112-8.

[161] McCullough LD, Blizzard K, Simpson ER, Oz OK, Hurn PD. Aromatase cytochrome P450 and extragonadal estrogen play a role in ischemic neuroprotection. *Journal of Neuroscience.* 2003;23(25):8701-5.

[162] Weaver CE, Park-Chung M, Gibbs TT, Farb DH. 17beta-Estradiol protects against NMDA-induced excitotoxicity by direct inhibition of NMDA receptors. *Brain Research.* 1997;761(2):338-41.

[163] Singer CA, Rogers KL, Strickland TM, Dorsa DM. Estrogen protects primary cortical neurons from glutamate toxicity. *Neuroscience Letters.* 1996;212(1):13-6.

[164] Connell BJ, Crosby KM, Richard MJ, Mayne MB, Saleh TM. Estrogen-mediated neuroprotection in the cortex may require NMDA receptor activation. *Neuroscience.* 2007;146(1):160-9.

[165] Chen H, Yoshioka H, Kim GS, Jung JE, Okami N, Sakata H, et al. Oxidative stress in ischemic brain damage: mechanisms of cell death and potential molecular targets for neuroprotection. *Antioxidants & Redox Signaling.* 2011;14(8):1505-17.

[166] Suh SW, Shin BS, Ma H, Van Hoecke M, Brennan AM, Yenari MA, et al. Glucose and NADPH oxidase drive neuronal superoxide formation in stroke. *Annals of Neurology*. 2008;64(6):654-63.

[167] Behl C, Widmann M, Trapp T, Holsboer F. 17-beta estradiol protects neurons from oxidative stress-induced cell death in vitro. *Biochemical and Biophysical Research Communications* 1995;216(2):473-82.

[168] Vedder H, Anthes N, Stumm G, Wurz C, Behl C, Krieg JC. Estrogen hormones reduce lipid peroxidation in cells and tissues of the central nervous system. *Journal of Neurochemistry*. 1999;72(6):2531-8.

[169] Jover-Mengual T, Zukin RS, Etgen AM. MAPK signaling is critical to estradiol protection of CA1 neurons in global ischemia. *Endocrinology*. 2007;148(3):1131-43.

[170] Koh PO. Estradiol prevents the injury-induced decrease of 90 ribosomal S6 kinase (p90RSK) and Bad phosphorylation. *Neuroscience Letters*. 2007;412(1):68-72.

[171] De Butte-Smith M, Zukin RS, Etgen AM. Effects of global ischemia and estradiol pretreatment on phosphorylation of Akt, CREB and STAT3 in hippocampal CA1 of young and middle-aged female rats. *Brain Research*. 2012;1471:118-128.

[172] Dubal DB, Shughrue PJ, Wilson ME, Merchenthaler I, Wise PM. Estradiol Modulates bcl-2 in Cerebral Ischemia: A Potential Role for Estrogen Receptors. *The Journal of Neuroscience*1999;19:6385-6393.

[173] Rau SW, Dubal DB, Böttner M, Gerhold LM, Wise PM. Estradiol Attenuates Programmed Cell Death after Stroke-Like Injury. *The Journal of Neuroscience*. 2003;23(36):11420-6.

[174] Jia J, Guan D, Zhu W, Alkayed NJ, Wang MM, Hua Z, et al. Estrogen inhibits Fas-mediated apoptosis in experimental stroke. *Experimental Neurology*. 2009;215:48-53.

[175] Zhang QG, Wang R, Khan M, Mahesh V, Brann DW. Role of Dickkopf-1, an antagonist of the Wnt/beta-catenin signaling pathway, in estrogen-induced neuroprotection and attenuation of tau phosphorylation. *The Journal of Neuroscience*. 2008;28(34):8430-8441.

[176] Sawe N, Steinberg G, Zhao H. Dual roles of the MAPK/ERK1/2 cell signaling pathway after stroke. *Journal of Neuroscience Research*. 2008;86(8):1659-1669.

[177] Wen Y, Yang S, Liu R, Perez E, Yi KD, Koulen P, et al. Estrogen attenuates nuclear factor-kappa B activation induced by transient cerebral ischemia. *Brain Research*. 2004;1008(2):147-154.

[178] Koerner IP, Zhang W, Cheng J, Parker S, Hurn PD, Alkayed NJ. Soluble epoxide hydrolase: regulation by estrogen and role in the inflammatory response to cerebral ischemia. *Frontiers in Bioscience*. 2008;13:2833-2841.

[179] Arevalo MA, Santos-Galindo M, Acaz-Fonseca E, Azcoitia I, Garcia-Segura LM. Gonadal hormones and the control of reactive gliosis. *Hormones and Behavior*. 2013;63(2):216-221.

[180] Dhandapani KM, Wade FM, Mahesh VB, Brann DW. Astrocyte-derived transforming growth factor-{beta} mediates the neuroprotective effects of 17{beta}-estradiol: involvement of nonclassical genomic signaling pathways. *Endocrinology*. 2005;146(6):2749-2759.

[181] O'Donnell ME, Lam TI, Tran LQ, Foroutan S, Anderson SE. Estradiol reduces activity of the blood-brain barrier Na-K-Cl cotransporter and decreases edema formation in

permanent middle cerebral artery occlusion. *Journal of Cerebral Blood Flow & Metabolism* 2006;26(10):1234-1249.

[182] Dubal DB, Rau SW, Shughrue PJ, Zhu H, Yu J, Cashion AB, et al. Differential modulation of estrogen receptors (ERs) in ischemic brain injury: a role for ERalpha in estradiol-mediated protection against delayed cell death. *Endocrinology.* 2006;147(6):3076-3084.

[183] Dubal DB, Zhu H, Yu J, Rau SW, Shughrue PJ, Merchenthaler I, et al. Estrogen receptor alpha, not beta, is a critical link in estradiol-mediated protection against brain injury. *Proceedings of the National Academy of Sciences*. 2001;98(4):1952-1957.

[184] Farr TD, Carswell HV, Gsell W, Macrae IM. Estrogen receptor beta agonist diarylpropiolnitrile (DPN) does not mediate neuroprotection in a rat model of permanent focal ischemia. *Brain Research*. 2007;1185:275-282.

[185] Zhao L, Brinton RD. Estrogen receptor alpha and beta differentially regulate intracellular Ca(2+) dynamics leading to ERK phosphorylation and estrogen neuroprotection in hippocampal neurons. *Brain Research*. 2007;1172:48-59.

[186] Connell BJ, Saleh TM. Differential Neuroprotection of Selective Estrogen Receptor Agonists against Autonomic Dysfunction and Ischemic Cell Death in Permanent versus Reperfusion Injury. *Advances in Pharmacology Science*. 2011;2011:976951.

[187] Zhang B, Subramanian S, Dziennis S, Jia J, Uchida M, Akiyoshi K, et al. Estradiol and G1 Reduce Infarct Size and Improve Immunosuppression after Experimental Stroke. *The Journal of Immunology*. 2010;184(8):4087-4094.

[188] Kosaka Y, Quillinan N, Bond CT, Traystman RJ, Hurn PD, Herson PS. GPER1/GPR30 Activation Improves Neuronal Survival Following Global Cerebral Ischemia Induced by Cardiac Arrest in Mice. *Translational Stroke Research*. 2012;3(4):500-507.

[189] Ng KM, Catalano MG, Pinos T, Selva DM, Avvakumov GV, Munell F, et al. Evidence that fibulin family members contribute to the steroid-dependent extravascular sequestration of sex hormone-binding globulin. *Journal of Biological Chemistry.* 2006;281(23):15853-15861.

[190] Avvakumov GV, Cherkasov A, Muller YA, Hammond GL. Structural analyses of sex hormone-binding globulin reveal novel ligands and function. *Molecular and Celular Endocrinology*. 2010;316(1):13-23.

[191] Selkoe DJ. Biochemistry and molecular biology of amyloid beta-protein and the mechanism of Alzheimer's disease. *Handbook of Clinical Neurology*. 2008;89:245-260.

[192] Selkoe DJ. The molecular pathology of Alzheimer's disease. *Neuron.* 1991;6(4):487-98.

[193] Avila J, Wandosell F, Hernandez F. Role of glycogen synthase kinase-3 in Alzheimer's disease pathogenesis and glycogen synthase kinase-3 inhibitors. *Expert Review of Neurotheraphy*. 2010;10(5):703-710.

[194] Mucke L, Masliah E, Johnson WB, Ruppe MD, Alford M, Rockenstein EM, et al. Synaptotrophic effects of human amyloid beta protein precursors in the cortex of transgenic mice. *Brain Researc*. 1994;666(2):151-167.

[195] Wang J, Tanila H, Puolivali J, Kadish I, van Groen T. Gender differences in the amount and deposition of amyloidbeta in APPswe and PS1 double transgenic mice. *Neurobiology of Disease*. 2003;14(3):318-327.

[196] Trushina E, Nemutlu E, Zhang S, Christensen T, Camp J, Mesa J, et al. Defects in mitochondrial dynamics and metabolomic signatures of evolving energetic stress in mouse models of familial Alzheimer's disease. *PLoS One*. 2012;7(2):e32737.

[197] Sarsoza F, Saing T, Kayed R, Dahlin R, Dick M, Broadwater-Hollifield C, et al. A fibril-specific, conformation-dependent antibody recognizes a subset of Abeta plaques in Alzheimer disease, Down syndrome and Tg2576 transgenic mouse brain. *Acta Neuropathogica.* 2009;118(4):505-517.

[198] Morinaga A, Ono K, Takasaki J, Ikeda T, Hirohata M, Yamada M. Effects of sex hormones on Alzheimer's disease-associated beta-amyloid oligomer formation in vitro. *Experimental Neurology.* 2011;228(2):298-302.

[199] Greenfield JP, Leung LW, Cai D, Kaasik K, Gross RS, Rodriguez-Boulan E, et al. Estrogen lowers Alzheimer beta-amyloid generation by stimulating trans-Golgi network vesicle biogenesis. *Journal of Biological Chemistry.* 2002;277(14):12128-12136.

[200] Honjo H, Kikuchi N, Hosoda T, Kariya K, Kinoshita Y, Iwasa K, et al. Alzheimer's disease and estrogen. *The Journal of Steroid Biochemistry and Molecular Biology.* 2001;76(1-5):227-230.

[201] Li R, He P, Cui J, Staufenbiel M, Harada N, Shen Y. Brain Endogenous Estrogen Levels Determine Responses to Estrogen Replacement Therapy via Regulation of BACE1 and NEP in Female Alzheimer's Transgenic Mice. *Molecular Neurobiology.* 2013;47(3):857-867.

[202] Henderson VW, Paganini-Hill A, Miller BL, Elble RJ, Reyes PF, Shoupe D, et al. Estrogen for Alzheimer's disease in women: randomized, double-blind, placebo-controlled trial. *Neurology.* 2000;54(2):295-301.

[203] Zandi PP, Carlson MC, Plassman BL, Welsh-Bohmer KA, Mayer LS, Steffens DC, et al. Hormone replacement therapy and incidence of Alzheimer disease in older women: the Cache County Study. *JAMA*. 2002;288(17):2123-9.

[204] Resnick SM, Coker LH, Maki PM, Rapp SR, Espeland MA, Shumaker SA. The Women's Health Initiative Study of Cognitive Aging (WHISCA): a randomized clinical trial of the effects of hormone therapy on age-associated cognitive decline. *Clinical Trials*. 2004;1(5):440-50.

[205] Sherwin BB, Henry JF. Brain aging modulates the neuroprotective effects of estrogen on selective aspects of cognition in women: a critical review. *Frontiers in Neuroendocrinology*. 2008;29(1):88-113.

[206] Taylor HS, Manson JE. Update in hormone therapy use in menopause. *The Journal of Clinical Endocrinology & Metabolism.* 2011;96(2):255-264.

[207] Selvamani A, Sohrabji F. The Neurotoxic Effects of Estrogen on Ischemic Stroke in Older Female Rats Is Associated with Age-Dependent Loss of Insulin-Like Growth Factor-1. *The Journal of Neuroscience.*2010;30:6852-6861.

[208] De Butte-Smith M, Gulinello M, Zukin RS, Etgen AM. Chronic estradiol treatment increases CA1 cell survival but does not improve visual or spatial recognition memory after global ischemia in middle-aged female rats. *Hormones and Behavior.* 2009;55(3):442-453.

[209] Traub ML, De Butte-Smith M, Zukin RS, Etgen AM. Oestradiol and Insulin-Like Growth Factor-1 Reduce Cell Loss after Global Ischaemia in Middle-Aged Female Rats. *Journal of Neuroendocrinology*. 2009;21(12):1038-44.

[210] Suzuki S, Brown CM, Dela Cruz CD, Yang E, Bridwell DA, Wise PM. Timing of estrogen therapy after ovariectomy dictates the efficacy of its neuroprotective and antiinflammatory actions. *Proceedings of the National Academy of Sciences.* 2007;104(14):6013-6018.

[211] Zhang Q-G, Raz L, Wang R, Han D, De Sevilla L, Yang F, et al. Estrogen Attenuates Ischemic Oxidative Damage via an Estrogen Receptor α-Mediated Inhibition of NADPH Oxidase Activation. *The Journal of Neuroscience*. 2009;29(44):13823-13836.

In: Estradiol: Synthesis, Health Effects and Drug Interactions ISBN: 978-1-62808-962-2
Editors: Ricco Palmeri and Sal Grimaudo

Chapter 3

Effects of Estradiol on Male and Female Reproductive Tissues and the Influence of Endocrine Disruptors

Luiz Gustavo de Almeida Chuffa[1,*], Beatriz Aparecida Fioruci-Fontanelli[1], Elaine Manoela Porto-Amorim[2] and João Paulo de Arruda Amorim[2]

[1]Department of Anatomy - IBB/UNESP – Univ Estadual Paulista, Sao Paulo, Brazil
[2]Department of Anatomy - UNIOESTE – Univ Estadual do Oeste do Paraná, PR, Brazil

Abstract

Estradiol (E2) is the major steroid hormone which is involved in several organic functions, such as physiological sexual behavior, development and maintenance of male and female reproductive organs, control of visceral secretion, modulation of immune system, tumorigenesis, and others. This hormone is essential for the acquisition of secondary sexual characteristics and hypothalamic release of gonadotropin-releasing hormone (GnRH) in mammals. In women, E2 is primarily synthesized by the granulosa cells of the ovary during aromatization of androstenedione (produced in the theca cells) to estrone, and finally to E2. An additional but not significant E2 contribution is derived from liver, adrenal and mammary glands. In both sex, testosterone can be converted into estradiol by aromatization. In females, E2 has a key role on the functioning of reproductive organs, supporting the lining of the endometrium, cervix, uterine tubes, and vagina. Also, E2 is essential for the growth and maturation of oocytes and to orchestrate folliculogenesis. During menstrual cycle, E2 triggers the hypothalamic-pituitary events via feedback system to induce ovulation, besides participating with progesterone in the preparation of endometrium for blastocyst implantation. In males, the effect of E2 seems to be more complex. E2 is produced by the activity of aromatase mainly in leydig cells of

* Corresponding author: Luiz Gustavo de Almeida Chuffa, Email: guchuffa@yahoo.com.br, Department of Anatomy, Bioscience Institute, Univ. Estadual Paulista, Address: Distrito de Rubião Júnior s/n, Botucatu - São Paulo/SP.

the testis. Current researches have provided evidences that E2 is not only responsible for differentiation and function of the testes, but it may also exert actions in the epididymis, efferent ductules, prostate, seminal vesicles, and even the penis. Furthermore, excessive estrogen exposure has been postulated to be the main cause of low sperm counts which can lead to subfertility or infertility-related disorders.

E2 binds to estrogen receptors (namely ERα and ERβ subunits) at nuclear level and stimulates selective genes transcription in a tissue and cell-specific manner. The effective activation of the ERs by E2 is strongly associated with an estrogen responsive element (ERE) in the promoter region of the target genes to control its activation and/or repression. There is a variety of medications that preferentially act on one of these ER to exert such effects. Notably, endocrine-disrupting chemicals (EDCs) are synthetic or natural compounds found in the environment which interfere with hormone production and physiological functions of the reproductive organs. The most EDCs affecting reproductive function include synthetic agents used as polychlorinated biphenyls, polybrominated-biphenyls, methoxychlor-(MXC), phthalates, dichloro-diphenyl-trichloroethane (DDT), diethylstilbestrol (DES), and other related compounds. The naturally occurring agents with estrogenic activity are originated from phytoestrogens (e.g., genistein and coumestrol). This chapter will give attention to the main actions of E2 on both male and female reproductive organs and discuss on the specific toxicity of EDCs to the reproductive function.

Keywords: Estradiol (E2), ERα, ERβ, reproductive tissues, endocrine disruptors

Introduction

E2: A Brief Overview

E2 is the major steroid hormone which regulates several physiological events including sexual behaviour, reproductive organ development, cardiovascular function, bone formation and remodeling, immune and inflammation functions (Kousteni et al. 2003). Also, it is thought to be of fundamental importance for the acquisition of secondary sexual characteristics and for the hypothalamic regulation of expression and release of GnRH in mammals (Maffucci and Gori, 2009). In women, the production of E2 occurs within the ovarian follicle (mainly by the theca and granulosa cells) and is under the fine control of FSH and LH hormones (Gordon et al. 2008). In addition, E2 is produced by the corpus luteum, adrenal glands, liver and mammary glands, however the quantity is not significant (Simpson, 2003, Lee et al. 2012). In men, E2 has an important role on the differentiation and function of Leydig cells and during the development of testes (Murono et al. 2000). E2 modulates cell function and the activation of estrogen-dependent metabolism. The basic mechanism of ER activation by E2 binding is dependent on EREs in the promoter site to control either activation and/or repression of target genes (Simoncini et al. 2004, Wang et al. 2006). After the formation of E2-ER complex, the ER undergoes a conformational change allowing interactions with cofactors, coactivators and corepressors related to gene expression (Ambrosino et al. 2010). While nuclear ER-meadiated transactivation is referred to as genomic pathway and require several hours for activation, membrane ERs can activate ligand-independent pathways (non-genomic pathways) within few minutes after a given ligand exposure (Jepsen et al. 2000, Suzuki et al. 2008). In addition, membrane ERs need activation of secondary messengers by tyrosine kinases receptors, such as the epidermal growth factor receptor (EGFR) (Filardo et al. 2002, Levin, 2005). Differently, the transcriptional activation of ERα and ERβ is dependent on the promoter, ligand affinity and specific cell type (Samudio et al. 2001). Figure 1 indicates the main functions of E2 on female and male reproductive tissues.

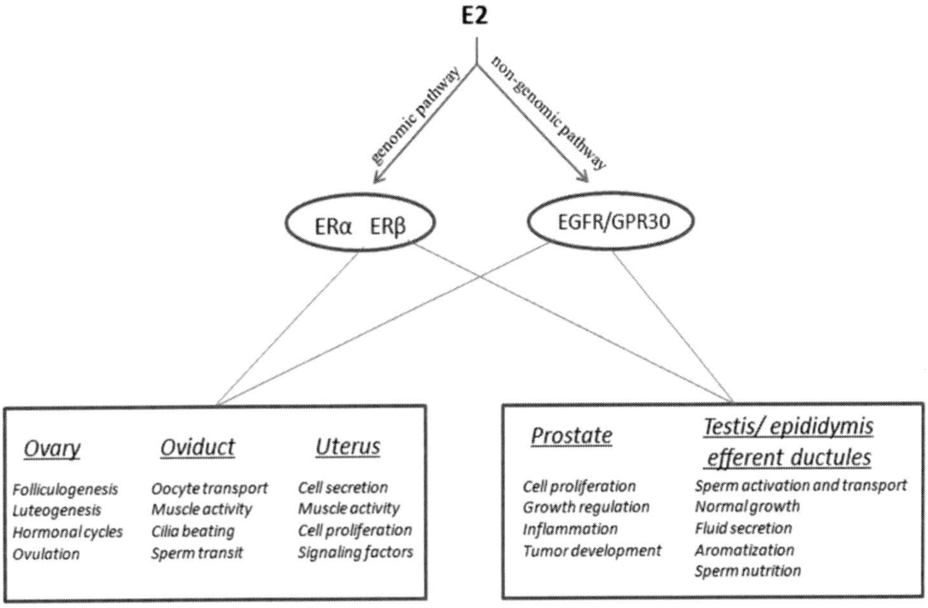

Figure 1. Normal activity of E2 via genomic and non-genomic pathways on female (ovary, oviduct and uterus) and male (prostate, testis, epididymis and efferent ductules) reproductive organs. E2: estradiol; ERα: estrogen receptor subunit α; ERβ: estrogen receptor subunit β; EGFR: epidermal growth factor receptor; GPR30: G protein-coupled receptor.

The Role of E2 and ERs on Female Reproductive Tissues

Ovary

The effects of E2 on folliculogenesis are mediated by both ERα and β and the membrane-bound G protein-coupled receptor, GPR30, can mediate rapid non-genomic E2 signaling (Prossnitz et al. 2008) involved in the maintenance of meiotic arrest and oocyte maturation (Pang et al. 2008). In ovaries from GPR30-deficient mice, the fertility is undisturbed and folliculogenesis arises normal with the presence of follicles in all stages and corpus luteum (Otto et al. 2009). In contrast, mice lacking ERα and β exhibits several ovarian disorders consistent with their patterns of expression (Lubahn et al. 1993, Krege et al. 1998, Couse et al. 1999, Dupont et al. 2000).

ERβ is expressed in granulosa cells of growing follicles and is regulated by gonadotropins, while ERα is predominantly expressed in thecal and interstitial cells (Britt and Findlay, 2003). Absence of ERα causes infertility and mutant ovaries contain an increase of cystic and hemorrhagic follicles with no corpus luteum (similar to polycystic ovary syndrome

"PCOS"). The increased levels of androgen, E2 and luteinizing hormone (LH) in the serum of ER-α null mice indicate that loss of ER-alpha affects the negative feedback of estradiol on the HPG axis. In addition, intraovarian feedback of estradiol on thecal cell androgen production also appears to be disrupted in ERα null follicles, which occurs through loss of repression of CYP17A1 by ERα, with subsequent increase of androstenedione synthesis (Taniguchi et al. 2007).

Mice lacking ERβ are subfertile, where the main detrimental effect is attributed to a reduced ovulation. This may be accompanied by a reduced expression of LH/choriogonadotrophin receptor (LHCGR) in granulosa cells (Couse et al. 2005) because the induction of LHCGR in these cells is highest in preovulatory follicles and depends on the synergistic interactions between follicle stimulating hormone (FSH) and E2 (Richards et al. 1976). Ovaries from adult ERβ-knockout mice have follicles at all stages of development and fewer corpora lutea. Based on ER knockouts, mice lacking both ERα and ERβ (α- and β-ERKO) develops anovulatory cycles, and they also exhibit a distinct phenotype depending on each single ER knockout. Ovaries from pre-pubertal α- and β-ERKO mice present early signs of maturation. Importantly, ovaries displaying α- and β-ERKO have most follicles only reaching the antral stage while the corpus luteum are absent (Fisher et al. 1998). Briefly, the ERs and CYP19A1 knockout models suggest that unlike FSH, estradiol is not essential for antral follicle formation, but is critical for granulosa cell growth and differentiation in order to maintain follicular activity and perform ovulation (Edson et al. 2009).

Oviduct

The oviduct comprises four distinct regions (infundibulum, ampulla, isthmus and intramural) with different roles in the processes of oocyte pickup, transport of gametes, fertilization and transport of embryos (Jansen, 1984; Abe, 1996). The function of the oviduct during the oocyte transport has been classically attributed to the cilia beating and muscular wall activity, both the events controlled by E2 and progesterone (Chang, 1966). It is not clear if differences exist in the expression of the ERα and β among the oviductal regions that would relate to their functions (Cárdenas and Pope, 2012); however, it seems true that the oviduct ERα is more expressed in some cell types than ERβ (Wang et al. 2000, Okada et al. 2003, Ulbrich et al. 2003). More recently, ERα was localized in the nuclei of various cell types, including the mucosal epithelium, stromal cells of the subepithelial layer, smooth muscle cells of the tunica muscularis and endothelial cells. Conversely, the ERβ was not detected in the oviduct through immunohistochemical assay (Cárdenas and Pope, 2012).

In the oviduct, both ER-α protein and mRNA were found in almost all epithelial cells throughout the oestrous cycle, with a similar pattern of expression. Also, ERα immunostaining is absent in ciliated epithelial cells or the intensity of positive immunoreactions is less than that of non-ciliated cells (Press et al. 1986, Cooke et al. 1998). In another study, ERα was increased during mid-cycle in the ampulla, whereas it was unrelated in other segments of the oviduct (Amso et al. 1994). The lack of ERα in oviduct may support the concept that ERα has cyclical fluctuations and is associated with dramatic morphological changes in the reproductive tract during the oestrous and menstrual cycles (Brenner et al. 1979). In contrast, only a few cells containing ERβ mRNA were found in the oviduct, especially in the smooth muscle cells.

The ERβ protein was either absent or very low to be detected by immunohistochemistry in oviduct epithelium (Wang et al. 2000). E2 effectively regulates peristalsis and muscular contractions which promotes formation of sperm reservoirs, transit of sperm to the ampulla, and retention of oocytes in the ampulla–isthmus junction (Puri and Roy, 1981, Hawk, 1987, Suarez and Pacey, 2006). Interestingly, the relationship between E2 and nitric oxide synthase (NOS) has been implicated in oviductal motility and oocyte transport. Lapointe et al. (2006) showed that expression of NOS is upregulated by E2 during oocyte transport in the bovine oviduct. The regulation of NOS by E2 suggests a equilibrium of the oviductal motility, and this process seems to be mediated by the non-genomic pathway of E2 which leads to cAMP activation (Perez Martinez et al. 2000, Orihuela et al. 2003).

Uterus

In the uterus, ERα has been highly expressed in various cell types, whereas the ERβ has been undetectable or significantly less abundant (Taylor and Al-Azzawi, 2000, Cárdenas and Pope, 2004). It has been shown that ERα mRNA expression is markedly changed in glandular epithelium (GE) and stromal cells of human and monkey endometrium during the menstrual cycle (Matsuzaki et al. 1999, Koji and Brenner, 1993). In luminal epithelium (LE) of the rat uterus, ERα was higher in proestrus, diestrus and estrus phases. More than 90% of the epithelium nuclei were positive for ERα. In GE, the number of ERα positive cells was lowest in metestrus and significantly higher in diestrus. Also, the presence of ERα was observed in both circular and longitudinal muscle layers of myometrium in all stages of the cycle (Wang et al. 2000).

In contrast, the intensity of nuclear ERβ immunostaining was lower than that of ERα in the stroma, GE, LE and myometrium during estrus phase (Wang et al. 2000). A recent study reported that relative amounts of ERα expressed in LE, stroma, GE and myometrium did not change during the estrous cycle while ERβ were not evident in the uterus (Cárdenas and Pope, 2012). These regulatory activities may be attributed to the E2-ER complex.

The Role of E2 and ERs on Male Reproductive Tissues

Prostate

The E2 exert important roles in several male reproductive tissues. Importantly, a lack of circulating E2 and consequent elevation of testosterone and gonadotrophins can lead to various pathologies including infertility (Grumbach and Auchus, 1999, Rochira et al. 2002). In aged men, the level of E2 remains unchanged (Vermeulen et al. 1972, 2002), however, the testosterone levels decrease within the testis and blood serum (Baulieu, 2002). In this context, there is an imbalance between testosterone and E2 ratio (E/T) that is temporally related to the onset of prostate diseases, such as prostate cancer (PCa) (Ellem and Risbridger, 2009).

In the prostate, E2 is responsible for the growth regulation throughout the life. E2 may acts on the prostate through indirect mechanisms, such as altering the androgen production by suppression of the hypothalamic–pituitary–gonadal axis, via prolactin and even directly in the Leydig cells of the testis or through direct mechanism including local aromatization of testosterone into E2 (Härkönen and Mäkelä, 2004).

The aromatase enzyme is encoded by the *CYP19* gene and expressed within the prostatic stroma. E2 binds to their receptors (ERα and ERβ) for controlling cellular events, such as proliferation, inflammation and cancer (Ellem and Risbridger, 2009). In the late 1950s, Elwood Jensen discovered and started the characterization of an E2 binding protein (ER-α).

Only in 1996s, the second ER (ERβ) was isolated from rat and human tissues (Kuiper et al. 1996, Mosselman et al. 1996). It is well-known that the cellular response to E2 is mediated through nuclear estrogen receptor (ER) in the prostate (Katzenellenbogen et al. 2000). In normal prostate tissue, ERα is expressed in stroma but, during administration of E2, the ERα can also be readily detected in the epithelia (Ellem and Risbridger, 2009). Also, ERα has been characterized as a positive regulator of secondary branching of stromal growth (Omoto et al. 2005).

Several studies have shown that high levels of E2 stimulates the DNA synthesis and induces metaplastic epithelial morphology both in human and rat prostate (Nevalainen et al. 1991, 1993). Furthermore, elevation in E2 cause proliferation of the prostatic epithelium which is characterized by the so called squamous metaplasia (SQM). Additionally, increased levels of E2 have other responses to prostatic epithelium, such as local inflammation and cancer (Ellem and Risbridger, 2009), and the ERα subtype is involved in all of these molecular events (Ellem and Risbridger, 2009). A study with ERα knockout mice (αERKO) demonstrated that E2-induced squamous metaplasia is strongly associated with ERα (Risbridger et al. 2001). To date, ERα is reported to be an inductor of proliferation, inflammation and tumor (Ellem and Risbridger, 2009). Conversely, ERβ is expressed at high levels in the rat prostate and testis (Prins and Korach, 2008). It is primarily located in different epithelial cells, which may preclude formation of ERα:ERβ heterodimers in this organ (Prins et al. 1998, 2001; Makela et al. 2000). Unlike the ERα, the expression of ERβ in the rodent prostate gland are up-regulated by androgens while E2 do not regulate the expression ERβ (Prins et al. 1998, Chang et al. 1999, Asano et al. 2003). Although ERβ is the predominant receptor expressed in the adult prostate gland, its role has not yet been clearly established. Indirect evidence exists for a role of ERβ in the differentiated state of the prostate epithelium. It has also been suggested that ERß has an antiproliferative role in the prostate besides reducing the androgenic stimulation of prostate growth (Weihua et al. 2001). Finally, ERβ has also been proposed to regulate immunomodulatory (Prins and Korach, 2008) and antioxidant functions (Montano et al. 1998).

Testis, Epididymis and Efferent Ductules

In several species, E2 is present at high concentrations in the testis, seminal fluids and in semen (Hess et al. 2001). In the testis, both Leydig cells and germ cells can synthesize E2 (Nitta et al. 1993, Carreau et al. 1999, Hess, 2000). This fact is supported by the presence of cytochrome P450 aromatase (CYP19A1) in both germ cells and spermatozoa of several species. However, the major source of E2 in male reproductive tract is located in the upper epididymis (Nitta et al. 1993, Carreau et al. 1999, Hess, 2000).

Danzo et al. (1975) first described the presence of an ER protein in epididymal tissues. Both ERα and ERβ are present in the epididymis (Hess et al. 1997), but the highest concentration of ER is evidenced in cauda epididymis (Danzo et al. 1981, 1983). Early studies have confirmed the presence of a protease in the adult epididymis, which is responsible for removing the DNA-binding portion from ER, thus making E2 less active in this organ (Hendry and Danzo, 1986).

However, later E2-binding activity was largely shown in epididymis of other species such as human (Murphy et al. 1980). Moreover, Schleicher et al. (1989) have described that aromatase activity is absent in the epididymis.

The efferent ductules, a series of small tubules that transport sperm from the testis to the epididymis, are known to express high amounts of ERα and low amounts of ERβ (Hess et al. 1997, Fisher et al. 1997. Ilio and Hess, 1994). The ERα is important for normal growth and for the function of the efferent ductules. Conversely, studies with mice have revealed that ERα is required for both male fertility and sexual behavior (Kooy et al. 1996). Other data suggest that E2 deficiency might also result in accumulation of fluid into the efferent ductules and subsequent atrophy of the testis (Hess et al. 1997).

The Endocrine Disruptors: General Aspects

Over the past decades, special attention has been given to EDCs effects which have been closely related to the human environment. There are various EDCs present in the environment as they are widely used by industries throughout the world, and found in some pesticides. These compounds may interfere with either regulation of hormone synthesis or receptor binding by changing the homeostasis of endocrine system (Fowler et al. 2012). Its effects are associated with exacerbated reproductive development and sexual behaviour dysfunction in both humans and animals. Because natural or synthetic EDCs share similar structures to those of steroid hormones, such as E2 or androgen, they can affect the ligation of steroid hormones via binding to the specific hormone receptors. Constant exposure to EDCs may cause severe injuries to reproductive function, including the formation of different hormone-dependent cancers (Fernandez and Russo, 2010, Hwang et al. 2011). Furthermore, EDCs may alter other estrogen-dependent tissues leading to impaired bone integrity, adipogenesis and behaviour (Byrnes et al. 2011, Ijichi et al. 2007).

Most of the synthetic and natural compounds are designated as xeno-estrogen capable of binding to the ER with 1000-fold lower affinity than estrogen. Notably, these EDCs can exhibit estrogenic responses as an ER agonist or antagonist. Interestingly, many estrogenic EDCs have been used as drugs to treat hormone disorders. For example, diethylstilbestrol (DES), a non-steroid estrogen acting via ER-signaling, was used in combination with other medications to block spontaneous abortion between the 1940s and 1970s (Couse and Korach, 2004). However, it is known to induce tumorigenesis in estrogen-dependent-tissues (e.g., breast cancer; Fischer et al. 2008). Other related chemicals and pesticides- like compounds used for plastic manufacturing, such as dichlorodiphenyltrichloroethane (DDT), bisphenol A (BPA), octyl-phenol (OP), methoxychlor (MXC) and nonylphenol (NP) can pass through the placenta reaching high levels in the fetus (Maffini et al. 2006). The main activating receptors by which they bind include ER, progesterone receptors (PRs) and androgen receptors (AR). Recent studies reported that OP, BPA and NP may alternatively act through nongenomic pathways in some cells. These EDCs are strongly related with G-proteins, ERK1/2 and AKT1/2/3, and other ER-mediated signaling pathway via cascade regulated by phosphorylation (Bouskine et al. 2009, Watson et al. 2012). Non-genomic action of EDCs include a rapid pathway to activate membrane ERs coupled tyrosine kinase receptor, which is given a signal through GPR30, a novel seven-transmembrane estrogen receptor displaying both 17-beta estradiol and EDCs-binding sites (Figure 2).

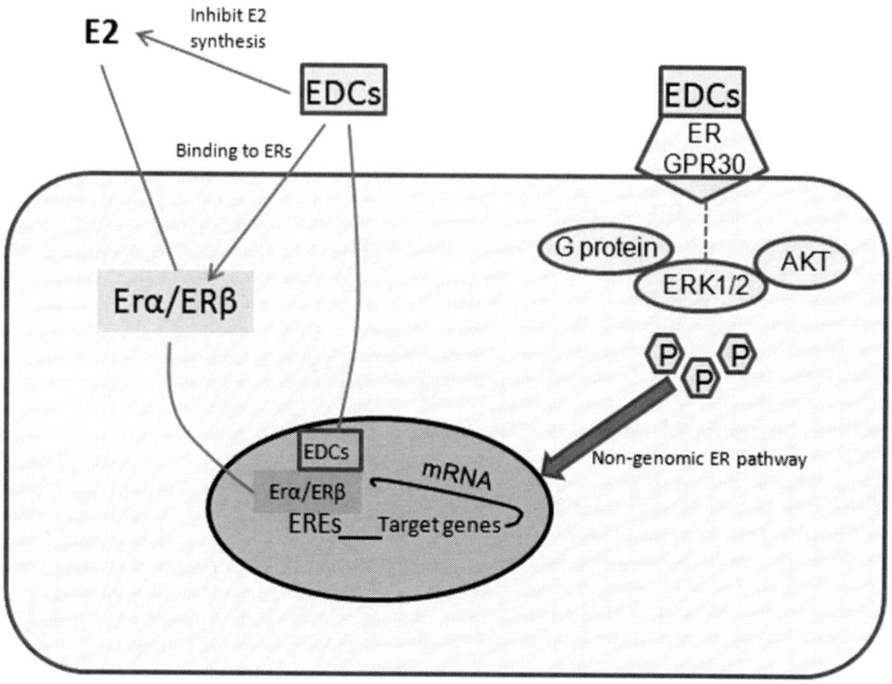

Figure 2. Potential mechanisms involving EDCs action. EDCs interfere with E2 synthesis and also can bind directly to estrogen receptors (ERα and ERβ) through the genomic pathway. After EDCs bind to ERs instead of E2, they can alter the transcription of target genes by binding to the EREs into the nucleus. The non-genomic pathway of EDCs action include the association with GPR30 located in the cell membrane. This activation leads to rapid downstream cellular signaling through protein kinases activation and phosphorylation, which in turn affect the transcription of target genes. Interaction between ERs and GPR30 may produce adverse effects of EDCs in several E2-dependent organs due to changes in gene expression. E2: estradiol; ERα: estrogen receptor subunit α; ERβ: estrogen receptor subunit β; ERE: estrogen response elements; EDCs: endocrine-disrupting chemicals; GPR30: G protein-coupled receptor, ERK: extracellular signal-regulated kinases; AKT: serine/threonine-specific protein kinase.

EDCs are responsible for innumerous endocrine and reproductive dysfunctions in both males and females; however, the exact effects on human are still obscure. It seems true that function and maturation of the sexual glands are dramatically affected by EDCs during the development. Although EDCs are potential dangerous agents with global concern, only a few in vitro and in vivo studies have been conducted to clarify the capacity of a chemical in disrupting endocrine system. Because EDCs are chemicals mimicking estrogen effects and affecting target cells in a dose-dependent manner, it will be discussed about some reproductive abnormalities in males and females, animals and humans exposed to EDCs considering a subset of chemical agents.

Polychlorinated Biphenyls (PCBs)

PCBs are synthetic organic compounds whose exposure levels are associated with various health hazards. They are persistent and bioaccumulative environmental pollutants that elicit a number of adverse health effects including neurotoxicity, carcinogenesis, teratogenesis, reproductive toxicity, and endocrine disruption (Diamanti-Kandarakis et al. 2008). Despite being banned in the US since the 1970s, these compounds are still detected in the environment (Kodavanti and Curras-Collazo et al. 2010). Because of their lipophilic structures, PCBs are easily absorbed from the environment into the food chain (Steinberg et al. 2008). The specific mechanisms underlying the observed reproductive effects are not well understood, but PCBs are thought to act through steroid hormone receptors, particularly ERs (Dickerson et al. 2011). It has been identified about 40 mono-hydroxylated polychlorinated biphenyls (OH-PCBs) which can contribute with estrogenic activity of the PCBs (Ruiz et al. 2013). These metabolites may act as agonists and/or antagonists of the ERα and ERβ to induce ER-mediated responses (Takeuchi et al. 2011). Human exposure to PCBs is associated with increased risk of breast cancer (Holford et al. 2000), pregnancy disorders (Pollack et al. 2011), increased menstrual cycle length (Cooper et al. 2005), increased risk of testicular germ cell tumors (McGlynn et al. 2008), delayed puberty (Grandjean et al. 2012) and poor semen quality (Hauser, 2006).

Adverse effects of the PBCs has also been demonstrated in animal models. Walker et al. (2013) reported that administration of Aroclor (1 mg/kg) during gestation of Sprague Dawley rats cause sexual dimorphic effects to their offspring. While PBCs induced longer estrous cycles, no reproductive effect was observed in male rat. Other effects of exposure to PCBs in female rat include: increased uterine wet weights (Hany et al. 1999) and increased ovarian weights (Ceccatelli et al. 2006). Dickerson et al. (2011) showed that prenatal exposure to PCBs leads to precocious puberty, irregularity in estrous cycle and impairs sexual differentiation of the hypothalamus in Sprague-Dawley rats. In addition, high doses of PCBs severely affect the development of spermatogonia and spermatids in adult rat (Akagi et al. 2005).

Polybrominated Diphenyl Ethers (PBDEs)

PBDEs are members of a large super family of environmental pollutants known as polyhalogenated aromatic hydrocarbons (Miller et al. 2012). They are synthetic compounds used as additive to retard fire and flames in a variety of commercial and household products, such as in foam furniture padding, paints, plastics, curtains, textiles, televisions, automobiles and airplanes (Siddiqi et al. 2003). PBDEs are persistent lipophilic contaminants widely distributed around the world and have a high potential for bioaccumulation (Kuo et al. 2010). The main routes of human exposure include dietary intake, inhalation of indoor air ingestion and dermal absorption (Frederiksen et al. 2009, Polder et al. 2010). They can cross through the placenta resulting in fetal exposure (Doucet et al. 2009) or even being passed during lactation (Gascon et al. 2012).

Epidemiological and experimental studies showed associations between PBDEs exposure and the adverse effects in neuropsychological development (Boucher et al. 2009, Fitzgerald et al. 2012, Forns et al. 2012) and thyroid function (Ren et al. 2013, Blanco et al. 2013). *In vitro* study has shown that PBEDs exposure can increase the proliferation of cancer cells (Ukpebor et al. 2011). Studies regarding the reproductive effects of exposure to PBDEs in humans and animals are limited.

Previous studies have proposed that a direct effect of PBDE congeners (BDE-47, BDE-99 and BDE -100) on the ovarian follicles is able to increase testosterone secretion, but not affect the E2 secretion (Karpeta et al. 2011). Recently, Karpeta et al. (2013) demonstrated that two hydroxylated PBDE metabolites, 5-OH-BDE-47 and 6-OH-BDE-47, have a stimulatory effect on E2 secretion, and this increase occurs by the high expression and activity of aromatase. Both 5-OH-BDE-47 and 6-OH-BDE-47 did not affected testosterone secretion.

Ceccatelli et al. (2006) showed that female rats exposed to 1 or 10 mg/kg/day PBDE 99 had increased ovarian weight and alteration of E2 gene regulation in uterus. In adult male rats, exposure to low-dose of PBDE-99 (60 and 300 μg/kg b.w) led to impaired spermatogenesis, reduced spermatid in testis and epididymis, and decreased daily sperm production. Lilienthal at al. (2006) showed that PBDE exposure reduces the anogenital distance, the number of primordial/primary ovarian follicles and decreases circulating sex steroids in male offspring.

Methoxychlor (MXC)

MXC is a pesticide structurally similar to DDT and considered to be an alternative insecticide to replace DDT due to its low toxicity and reduced persistence in the environment. MXC is primarily used to prevent against various species of insects that attack crops, vegetables, fruits and home garden (Gupta et al. 2006), as it is present in air, soil and contaminated water. MXC has weak estrogenic activity and binds to both ER-α and ER-β. In addition to E2, MXC is able to increase uterine weight in ovariectomized rats, and it was also reported to adversely affect the development and reproduction of laboratory animals (Kwack et al. 2002). In contrast to E2, the MXC does not increase FSH or LH concentrations, and furthermore, MXC seems to act as an ER-agonist in the uterus and an ER-antagonist in the ovary. Because that, excessive exposure to MXC alter normal ovarian function via mechanisms of DNA methylation (Zama and Uzumcu, 2009). Also, MXC specifically targets antral follicles and its exposure leads to persistent estrus, ovarian atrophy and follicular atresia (Eroschenko et al. 1997). In vivo and in vitro studies demonstrated the toxicity of MXC in reducing the percentage of antral follicles while increasing atresia. In these follicles, MXC may induce atresia by altering Bcl-2 factors and subsequent activation of downstream caspases (Basavarajappa et al. 2012). MXC is predominantly metabolized into mono-and bis-demethylated metabolites, including HPTE, which has a 100-fold higher affinity for the ER-α than that observed for MXC (Kapoor et al. 1970). More recently, HPTE has been associated with greater reproductive toxicity in both sexes than MXC compound (Gupta et al. 2007). In female rats, HPTE inhibited FSH and cAMP-stimulated steroid production by regulating mRNA expression of some steroidogenic enzymes in granulosa cells (Harvey et al. 2009). In male rats, both MXC and HPTE were shown to inhibit testosterone synthesis in Leydig cells (Akingbemi et al. 2000). This was attributed to a direct inhibition of the biosynthetic enzymes, mainly the 3β-hydroxysteroid dehydrogenase (3β-HSD). Moreover, Guo et al. (2013) have proposed that MXC and HPTE inhibited both isoforms of 11β-HSD in a species- and chemical structure-dependent manner. Because HPTE has showed a weak AR antagonist activity, its daily exposure may lead to reproductive organ abnormalities and hormone disturbances (Harvey et al. 2009).

Phthalates

Di-(2-ethylhexyl)-phthalate (DEHP), one of the EDCs, affects humans greatly in industry due to its extensive use in manufacture of plastic and non-polymer materials like paints, adhesives, fillers and printing inks and cosmetics (Heudorf et al. 2007). DEHP poses severe public health hazard as it can pass through inhalation, ingestion and dermal absorption.

The competitive binding of phthalates to the ER was first reported for hepatic receptors. DEHP did not affect E2 binding at a concentration of 2 μM, however there was a decrease in E2 binding at higher concentrations. Di-n-butyl phthalate (DBP) showed no effect at concentration of 80 nM, but induced a decrease in E2 binding at higher concentrations. Benzyl n-butyl phthalate (BBP) inhibited E2 binding at all concentrations (estimated between 80 nM and 50 μM; Moore, 2000). Interestingly, a study involving eight competitive phthalate diesters (DBP, DEHP, BBP, di-n-hexyl (DHP), di-iso-heptyl (DiHpP), di-n-octyl (DnOP), di-iso-nonyl (DiNP), and di-iso-decyl (DiDP)) showed that only DBP, BBP and DHP was effective to displace E2 (Zacharewski et al. 1998).

The continuous use of DEHP has drawn attention due to its adverse effects on reproductive system. DEHP has been extensively correlated with a decrease in concentration- and duration-dependent sperm viability (Pant et al. 2011). Epidemiological studies have focused on exposure to phthalates and their ability to compromise semen quality in men (Pant et al. 2008, Swan, 2008). Studies on experimental animals have shown that exposure to 500-750 mg di-n-butyl phthalate (DBP)/kg during critical periods of development, results in altered phenotype of normal development (Mylchreest et al. 2000).

These phenotypes may include cryptorchidism, epididymal agenesis, testicular atrophy, hypospadias, and absence of seminal vesicle and prostate. In contrast, when mice are exposed to 500 mg DBP/kg during gestation, some signs of testicular dysgenesis were common such as increased number of multinucleated germ cells and increased seminiferous cord diameter, with no decrease in testosterone levels (Gaido et al. 2007). Surprisingly, plasma E2 levels were increased approximately two-fold in males exposed to DEHP compared to controls. Further assays are needed to determine the exact source of E2, i.e. high aromatase activity by the Sertoli cells, the Leydig cells, or both types (Klinefelter et al. 2012).

In laboratory animals, phthalates disrupt oocyte maturation, impair intraovarian steroidogenesis, and alter the normal development of female reproductive organs (Anas et al. 2003, Lovekamp and Davis, 2001, Stoker et al. 2008).

In women, phthalates have been detected in blood, urine and breast milk (Hogberg et al. 2008). Also, the levels of phthalates in human follicular fluid are several orders of magnitude below the minimum levels known to cause toxicity to the oocytes of laboratory animals. Lenie et al. (2008) demonstrated that 50 μM mono-(2-ethylhexyl) phthalate (MEHP) was sufficient to induce abnormal increase in the testosterone/E2 ratio, and in the overall levels of progesterone.

Exposure to DEHP was associated with decreased number of primordial follicles at pubertal and adult age by possibly enhancing the follicle recruitment dynamics. Furthermore, there was a reduction in the weights of pups and litter size of mothers compared to controls (Zhang et al. 2013).

Dichlorodiphenyltrichloroethane (DDT)

Pesticides are widely used as environmental chemicals which have a role in many adverse human health outcomes such as tumorigenesis, reproductive and developmental conditions (Turusov et al. 2002). DDT is a well-known organochlorine pesticide used for the control of mosquitoes and it has been banned in North America since 1972. Previous studies have indicated DDT as having estrogenic activity (Sonnenschein and Soto, 1998, De Jager et al. 2006), and its main metabolite p,p-DDE, may interact synergistically with other disrupting agents to alter the homeostasis of sexual steroid hormone, such as increasing the expression of hepatic aromatase in adult male rats, and also impairing sexual development in young male rats after in-utero exposure (You et al. 2002). This metabolite persists in the environment and is consequently found in reproductive fluids of women (e.g., breast milk, cervical mucus and amniotic fluid, Dewailly et al. 1996, Wagner et al. 1990, Foster et al. 2000). A study reporting the different doses of 50 and 100 mg DDT/kg body weight (b.w)/day for 10 consecutive days showed a dose-dependent reductions in both testicular and seminal vesicles weights and in sperm numbers and motility, as well as decreased testosterone levels, and increased serum levels of LH and FSH (Rhouma et al. 2001). Furthermore, Kelce et al. (1997) demonstrated that p,p-DDE at doses of 200 mg/kg b.w/day is able to induce anti-androgenic effects by downregulating the expression of a testosterone-induced prostatic message C3 mRNA23. In female mice, a direct exposure to 200 and 300 ppm of DDT during gestational period resulted in death of male and female offspring (Cannon and Holcomb, 1968). This may be due to the lethal dose during the developmental period in treated mice. Younglai et al. (2004) have demonstrated that DDE levels can enhance FSH stimulation of aromatase activity in human granulosa cells. While its effects might be beneficial to the oocyte since estradiol plays an important role in its maturation, it could also be detrimental in producing high amount of estradiol early in folliculogenesis and accelerate oocyte maturation which can results in failed fertilization. DDT is known to interfere with endocrine system homeostasis because of its binding to the ER-α in several reproductive tissue. It has been described that DDT binds to ER-α and induces transcriptional activity in ER-α-positive breast cancer MCF-7 cells (Lemaire et al. 2006). Satisfactorily, the effects of DDT on ER-α signalling pathways can be blocked by the anti-estrogens (Villa et al. 2004). Both DDT and DDE severely impair estrogen biosynthesis and DDE also enhances aromatase activity. Some studies involving metabolized extracts of organochlorines mixtures, including DDT, showed that concentrations of 5,000 to 10,000-fold lower than that environmentally relevant is capable of inducing marked effects on male reproductive function in vivo (Anas et al. 2005). However, in vitro studies found that exposure to organochlorine mixture at higher levels than those of human fluids alters normal sperm fertility parameters.

Diethylstilbestrol (DES)

DES was the first synthetic E2 produced for the treatment of pregnant women in their first trimester during the 1940s–1970s in order to facilitating placental steroidogenesis and to prevent miscarriage or spontaneous abortion (Marselos and Tomatis, 1992). The exposure caused injuries both to the pregnant mother that was treated as well as to their offspring, besides having detrimental effects on fertility and increased risks for several types of cancer in humans.

In laboratory animals, exposure to ≥8 μg DES day^{-1} animal^{-1} for 12 days significantly reduced the weights of all reproductive organs, including the testis, caput, corpus and cauda of the epididymis, and seminal vesicle. Functionally, DES has produced estrogenic effects in many reproductive processes, such as reducing the epididymal sperm numbers and sperm transit time but did not affect daily sperm production or sperm morphology (Goyal et al. 2001). Furthermore, no influence of DES on the sperm counts and reproductive organs weights at 26 and 52 weeks of age were detected. In the rodent, a neonatal DES exposure induced a permanent decrease in the prostate AR levels, which led to an inability of the tissue to fully respond to endogenous androgens during adulthood (Prins et al. 1993)

Ohta et al. (2012) showed that doses of 5 μg DES/kg/day for 5 days after birth promote estrous cycle irregularities while doses of 0.5 μg DES/kg significantly decrease the weight of the ovaries. Conversely, low doses of DES did not accelerated sex maturation but stimulated the aging process in estrous cycle, conception rate and ovulation in female rats. In neonate mice exposed to DES, the vaginal lining epithelium exhibited persistent proliferation and stratification even after ovariectomy. Also, studies with tissue recombination suggest that neonatally-estrogenized vaginal stroma may induce vaginal epithelial hyperplasia (Katoh et al. 2013). Additionally, perinatal DES exposure in rodents leads to an attenuated uterine response to E2 during adulthood, characterized by a decrease in both uterine growth and secretory activity as well as abnormal E2-induced cellular differentiation (Medlock et al. 1988, Medlock et al. 1992). This resistance to E2 treatment may be attributed to a continuous decrease in ER levels.

Bisphenol A (BPA)

BPA, a compound used as a plasticizer for the production of polycarbonate and epoxy resins, is a well-characterized chemical proposed to have estrogenic activity. BPA exposure in the perinatal period causes physiological and morphological underdevelopment of male and female genitalia, tracts and glands that may result in reduced fertility, immature reproductive tissues and even growth of several cancers such as ovary, breast and prostate cancer (Singh and Li, 2011). Normally, the binding affinity of BPA for ER is approximately 1000-fold lower than that of E2, and it can stimulates both ER-α and ER-β signalling with estrogen activity (Gaido et al. 2000). In female mice, prenatal exposure to BPA induced reproductive abnormalities such as polyovular follicles and vaginal epithelial cornification (An et al. 2003, Nadzialek et al. 2011). Furthermore, exposure to low dose BPA (2.4 μg/kg b.w) accelerated body weight gain and puberty in female CF-1 mice. BPA has been reported to promote the proliferation of MCF-7 breast cancer cells, and also the increase of progesterone receptors (PRs) expression in human ovarian, endometrial and breast cancer (Park et al. 2009). Studies have proposed that BPA directly activates ERE promoter and cotreatment with ER antagonists seems to block the complex (Wetherill et al. 2007). In female rodents, BPA caused a significant increase of uterine weight and induce vaginal phenotypic alteration (Nah et al. 2012).

In male rats, prenatal exposure to BPA leads to a decrease in the weights of the seminal vesicle and epididymis, and a decrease in sperm density (Vom Saal et al. 1998). Additionally, oral administration of 200-950 mg BPA/kg/b.w/day for 44 days caused a decrease in the seminal vesicle, prostate, and preputial gland, seminiferous tubule disarrangement, and spermospore deletion in adult male F344 rats (Takahashi and Oishi, 2001). Recently, while the concentration of 50 mg BPA/kg/b.w has not been caused reproductive toxicity in rats (Doerge et al. 2011), doses of BPA ranging from 10 to 40 mg/kg/b.w produced a significant dose-dependent reduction in sperm density and quality in mice (Dobrzynska and Radzikowska, 2012). Sun et al. (2006) have showed that the dose of 3 mg BPA/kg/b.w per day, via s.c., for 2 weeks is able to cause a reduction of testosterone levels, and a increase of LH levels in adult rat serum and testes. Ultimately, Qiu et al. (2013) have reported that low BPA concentration can induce spermatogenesis disorders mainly through a decrease of the androgen receptor expression.

Phytoestrogens

Phytoestrogens are diphenolic compounds derived from the metabolism of plants, which can modulate or disrupt the actions of endogenous E2 (Woclawek-Potocka et al. 2013) or even affect the activity of steroidogenesis (Whitehead and Rice, 2006). They can be divided into isoflavones (e.g., genistein and daidzein), flavones (e.g., luteolin), coumestans (e.g., coumestrol), stilbenes (e.g., resveratrol) and lignans (e.g., matairesinol and lariciresinol) (Moutsatsou, 2007). Phytoestrogens are abundant in legumes, vegetables, fruit, whole grains and especially soy products. There is an increasing number of recent reports that suggest phytoestrogens as an endocrine-disrupting molecule (Waring et al. 2008, Jefferson et al. 2012). Diets rich in phytoestrogens represent a significant source of additional estrogens to human and animals (Yum et al. 2013).

Genistein is one of the most active isoflavones found in soy-bean with weak estrogenic activity due to its ability to act as an ER ligand (especially the ERβ), thus producing estrogenic or anti-estrogenic effect on the reproductive organs (Setchell, 2001, Schmidt et al. 2006). Experimental studies have shown that neonatal exposure to genistein cause adverse effects on the female reproductive system, including alterations in the ovarian function, estrous cycle, early reproductive senescence and subfertility/infertility (Jefferson et al. 2005). Padilla-Banks et al. (2012) demonstrated that female CD-1 mice treated with genistein at doses of 50 mg/kg/day developed hypospadias, suggesting that prenatal exposure to environmental estrogens can promote alterations or gynecological pathologies that become apparent later. In addition, genistein exposure in post-pubertal rats has increased the uterine weight, fluid secretion and hyperplasia of the uterine glands (Salleh et al. 2013). Other important soy-derived isoflavone is daidzein. *In vitro* studies have demonstrated that daidzein inhibits the progesterone secretion by luteinized granulosa cells and increases the expression of ERβ protein (Nynca et al. 2013). Equol, a biologically active metabolite of daidzein, is thought to increase the uterine weight, endometrial thickness and uterine epithelial proliferation (Wood et al. 2006, Rachoń et al. 2007), besides stimulating EREs mRNA levels in the uteri and pituitaries of adult ovariectomized rats (Rachoń et al. 2007). Importantly, a continuous exposure of male rats to low-dose phytoestrogens is related to decreased sperm counts and low sperm motion (Eustache et al. 2009). During developmental period, exposure to genistein may lead to a decreased prostate weight and ductal hyperplasia in contrast to a hypertrophy of the mammary glands (Delcos et al. 2001).

Conclusion

E2 is a steroid hormone extremely important for maintaining the homeostasis of male and female reproductive tissues. It may orchestrate essential reproductive function after binding to its ERα and ERβ, such as secretion, cell proliferation, tissue development, production of signaling factors and others. Any internal or external disturbance on the E2-ER regulation is associated with severe disorders including male and female reproductive cancers. Unlike E2, EDCs can lead to adverse biological effects in both humans and animals. The mechanism underlying such effects may rely on the alteration of E2 synthesis or after changing the E2 binding sites. Exposure to these chemical agents has detrimental effects on metabolism along with endocrine and reproductive systems that can persist for several generations due to its accumulative properties. Furthermore, EDCs may stimulate carcinogenesis and potentially alter the immune systems. There is an incessant necessity for describing the exact mechanism(s) by which these compounds can affect the reproduction and development. Particularly, the impact of combinations of EDCs generally released into environment as mixtures is more deleterious than individual reagents. Therefore, it is needed to disclose the synergistic effects of exposure to multiple EDCs action and their repercussions on reproductive tissues.

References

Abe, H., (1996). The mammalian oviductal epithelium: regional variations in cytological and functional aspects of the oviductal secretory cells. *Histology and Histopathology,* 11, 743-768.

Akagi, Y., Yokoo, K., Takahashi, H., Muto, T., Suzuki, Y., Hano, H., Furusato, M., Endou, H., Wakui, S. (2005). Evaluation of testicular toxicology in puberty to adult rats with prenatal exposure to 3′,4,4′,5-pentachlorobiphenyl. *The Journal of Toxicological Sciences,* 30, 75.

Akingbemi, B.T., Ge, R.S., Klinefelter, G.R., Gunsalus, G.L., Hardy, M.P. (2000). A metabolite of methoxychlor, 2,2-bis(p-hydroxyphenyl)-1,1, 1-trichloroethane, reduces testosterone biosynthesis in rat leydig cells through suppression of steady-state messenger ribonucleic acid levels of the cholesterol side-chain cleavage enzyme. *Biology of Reproduction,* 62, 571-578.

Ambrosino, C., Tarallo, R., Bamundo, A., Cuomo, D., Franci, G., Nassa, G., Paris, O., Ravo, M., Giovane, A., Zambrano, N., Lepikhova, T., Janne, O.A., Baumann, M., Nyman, T.A., Cicatiello, L., Weisz, A. (2010). Identification of a hormone-regulated dynamic nuclear actin network associated with estrogen receptor alpha in human breast cancer cell nuclei. *Molecular & Cellular Proteomics,* 9, 1352-1367.

Amso, N.N., Crow, J., Shaw, W.R. (1994). Comparative immunohistochemical study of oestrogen and progesterone receptors in fallopian tube and uterus at different stages of the menstrual cycle and the menopause. *Human Reproduction,* 9, 1027-1037.

An, B.S., Choi, K.C., Kang, S.K., Hwang, W.S., Jeung, E.B. (2003). Novel Calbindin-D(9k) protein as a useful biomarker for environmental estrogenic compounds in the uterus of immature rats. *Reproductive Toxicology,* 17, 311-319.

Anas, M.K., Guillemette, C., Ayotte, P., Pereg, D., Giguere, F., Bailey, J.L. (2005). In utero and lactational exposure to an environmentally relevant organochlorine mixture disrupts reproductive development and function in male rats. *Biology of Reproduction* 73, 414-426.

Anas, M.K., Suzuki, C., Yoshioka, K., Iwamura, S. (2003). Effect of mono-(2- ethylhexyl) phthalate on bovine oocyte maturation in vitro. Reproductive Toxicology, 17, 305-310.

Asano, K., Maruyama, S., Usui, T., Fujimoto, N. (2003). Regulation of estrogen receptor alpha and beta expression by testosterone in the rat prostate gland. *Endocrinology Journal,* 50(3), 281-287.

Basavarajappa, M.S., Karman, B.N., Wang, W., Gupta, R.K., Flaws, J.A. (2012). Methoxychlor induces atresia by altering Bcl2 factors and inducing caspase activity in mouse ovarian antral follicles in vitro. *Reproductive Toxicology,* 34, 545-551.

Baulieu, E.E. (2002). Androgens and aging men. *Molecular and Cellular Endocrinology,* 198, 41-49.

Blanco, J., Mulero, M., Heredia, L., Pujol, A., Domingo, J.L., Sánchez, D.J. (2013). Perinatal exposure to BDE-99 causes learning disorders and decreases serum thyroid hormone levels and BDNF gene expression in hippocampus in rat offspring. *Toxicology,* 308, 122-128.

Bouskine, A., Nebout, M., Brucker-Davis, F., Benahmed, M., Fenichel, P. (2009). Low doses of bisphenol A promote human seminoma cell proliferation by activating PKA and PKG via a membrane Gprotein-coupled estrogen receptor. *Environmental Health Perspectives,* 117, 1053-1058.

Brenner, R.M., West, N.B., Norman, R.L., Sandow, B.A., Verhage, H.G. (1979). Progesterone suppression of the estradiol receptor in the reproductive tract of macaques, cats and hamsters. *Advances in Experimental Medicine and Biology,* 117, 173-196.

Britt, K.L., Findlay, J.K. (2003). Regulation of the phenotype of ovarian somatic cells by estrogen. *Molecular and Cellular Endocrinology,* 202, 11-17.

Byrnes, E.M., Casey, K., Bridges, R.S. (2011). Reproductive experience modifies the effects of estrogen receptor alpha activity on anxietylike behavior and corticotropin releasing hormone mRNA expression. *Hormone and Behavior,* 61, 44-49.

Cannon, M.S., Holcomb, L.C. (1968). The Effect of DDT on Reproduction in Mice. *The Ohio Journal of Science,* 68, 19.

Cárdenas, H., Pope, W.F. (2004). Attenuation of estrogenic effects by dihydrotestosterone in the pig uterus is associated with down regulation of the estrogen receptors. *Biology of Reproduction,* 70, 297-302.

Cárdenas, H., Pope, W.F. (2012). Amounts of an estrogen receptor β isoform increased in the theca of preovulatory follicles of sheep. *Animal Reproduction Science,* 131, 143-152.

Carreau, S., Genissel, C., Bilinska, B., and Levallet, J. (1999). Sources of oestrogen in the testis and reproductive tract of the male. *International Journal of Andrology,* 22, 211–23.

Ceccatelli, R., Faass, O., Schlumpf, M., Lichtensteiger, W. (2006). Gene expression and estrogen sensitivity in rat uterus after developmental exposure to the polybrominated diphenylether PBDE 99 and PCB. *Toxicology,* 220, 104-116.

Chang, M.C. (1966). Transport of eggs from the fallopian tube to the uterus as a function of oestrogen. *Nature,* 212, 1048-1049.

Chang, W., Prins, G. (1999). Estrogen receptor-β: Implications for the prostate gland. *Prostate,* 40, 115-124.

Cooke, P.S., Buchannan, D.L., Lubahn, D.B., Cunha, G.R. (1998). Mechanism of estrogen action: lessons from the estrogen receptor-knockout mouse. *Biology of Reproduction,* 59, 470-475.

Cooper, G.S., Klebanoff, M.A., Promislow, J., Brock, J.W., Longnecker, M.P. (2005). Polychlorinated biphenyls and menstrual cycle characteristics. *Epidemiology,* 16, 191-200.

Couse, J.F., Hewitt, S.C., Bunch, D.O., Sar, M., Walker, V.R., Davis, B.J., Korach, K.S. (1999). Postnatal sex reversal of the ovaries in mice lacking estrogen receptors alpha and beta. *Science,* 286, 2328-2331.

Couse, J.F., Korach, K.S. (2004). Estrogen receptor alpha mediates the detrimental effects of neonatal diethylstilbestrol (DES) exposure in the murine reproductive tract. *Toxicology,* 205, 55–63.

Couse, J.F., Yates, M.M., Deroo, B.J., Korach, K.S. (2005) Estrogen receptor-beta is critical to granulosa cell differentiation and the ovulatory response to gonadotropins. *Endocrinology,* 146, 3247-3262.

Danzo, B. J., Eller, B. C., Hendry, W. J. D. (1983). Identification of cytoplasmic estrogen receptors in the accessory sex organs of the rabbit and their comparison to the cytoplasmic estrogen receptor in the epididymis. *Molecular and Cellular Endocrinology,* 33, 197-209.

Danzo, B. J., Eller, B. C., Judy, L. A., Trautman, J. R., Orgebin-Crist, M. C. (1975). Estradiol binding in cytosol from epididymides of immature rabbits. *Molecular and Cellular Endocrinology,* 2, 91-105.

Danzo, B. J., St. Raymond, P. A., Davies, J. (1981). Hormonally responsive areas of the reproductive system of the male guinea pig. III. Presence of cytoplasmic estrogen receptors. *Biology of Reproduction,* 25, 1159–68.

De Jager, C., Farias, P., Barraza-Villarreal, A., Avila, M.H., Ayotte, P., Dewailly, E., Dombrowski, C., Rousseau, F., Sanchez, V.D., Bailey, J.L. (2006). Reduced Seminal Parameters Associated With Environmental DDT Exposure and p,p-DDE Concentrations in Men in Chiapas, Mexico: A Cross-Sectional Study. *Journal of Andrology,* 27, 16-27.

Delclos, K.B., Bucci, T.J., Lomax, L.G., Latendresse, J.R., Warbritton, A., Weis, C.C., Newbold, R.R. (2001). Effects of dietary genistein exposure during development on male and female CD (Sprague-Dawley) rats. *Reproductive Toxicology,* 15, 647-663.

Dewailly, E., Ayotte, P., Laliberte, C., Weber, J-P, Gingras, S. Nantel, A.J. (1996). Polychlorinated biphenyl (PCB) and dichlorodiphenyldichloroethylene (DDE) concentrations in breast milk of women in Quebec. American Journal of Public Health, 86, 1241-*1246.*

Diamanti-Kandarakis, E., Bourguignon, J.P., Giudice, L.C., Hauser, R., Prins, G.S., Soto, A.M., Zoeller, R.T., Gore, A.C. (2009). Endocrine-disrupting chemicals: an Endocrine Society scientific statement. *Endocrine Reviews,* 30, 293-342.

Dickerson, S.M., Cunningham, S.L., Patisaul, H.B., Woller, M.J., Gore, A.C. (2011). Endocrine disruption of brain sexual differentiation by developmental PCB exposure. *Endocrinology,* 152, 581-594.

Dobrzynska, M.M., Radzikowska, J. (2012). Genotoxicity and reproductive toxicity of bisphenol A and X-ray/bisphenol A combination in male mice. *Drug and Chemical Toxicology,* 36, 19-26.

Doerge, D.R., Twaddle, N.C., Vanlandingham, M., Brown, R.P., Fisher, J.W. (2011). Distribution of bisphenol A into tissues of adult, neonatal, and fetal Sprague-Dawley rats. *Toxicology and Applied Pharmacology,* 255, 261-270.

Doucet, J., Tague, B., Arnold, D.L., Cooke, G.M., Hayward, S., Goodyer, C.G. (2009). Persistent organic pollutant residues in human fetal liver and placenta from Greater Montreal, Quebec: a longitudinal study from 1998 through 2006. *Environmental Health Perspectives,* 117, 605-611.

Dupont, S., Krust, A., Gansmuller, A., Dierich, A., Chambon, P., Mark, M. (2000) Effect of single and compound knockouts of estrogen receptors alpha (ERalpha) and beta (ERbeta) on mouse reproductive phenotypes. *Development,* 127, 4277-4291.

Edson, M.A., Nagaraja, A.K., Matzuk, M.M. (2009). The mammalian ovary from genesis to revelation. *Endocrine Reviews,* 30, 624-712.

Ellem, S. J., Risbridger, G. P. (2009). The Dual, Opposing Roles of Estrogen in the Prostate. Steroid Enzymes and Cancer: *Ann. N.Y. Acad. Sci.,* 1155, 174-186.

Eroschenko, V.P., Swartz, W.J., Ford, L.C. (1997). Decreased superovulation in adult mice following neonatal exposures to technical methoxychlor. *Reproductive Toxicology,* 11, 807-814.

Eustache, F., Mondon, F., Canivenc-Lavier, M.C., Lesaffre, C., Fulla, Y., Berges, R., Cravedi, J.P., Vaiman, D., Auger, J. (2009). Chronic dietary exposure to a low-dose mixture of genistein and vinclozolin modifies the reproductive axis, testis transcriptome, and fertility. *Environmental Health Perspectives,* 117, 1272-1279.

Fernandez, S.V., Russo, J. (2010). Estrogen and xenoestrogens in breast cancer. *Toxicology and Pathology,* 38, 110-122.

Filardo, E.J. (2002). Epidermal growth factor receptor (EGFR) transactivation by estrogen via the G-protein-coupled receptor, GPR30: a novel signaling pathway with potential significance for breast cancer. *The Journal of Steroid Biochemistry and Molecular Biology*, 80, 231–238.

Fischer, T., Schomacker, K., Schicha, H. (2008). Diethylstilbestrol (DES) labeled with Auger emitters: potential radiopharmaceutical for therapy of estrogen receptor-positive tumors and their metastases? *International Journal of Radiation Biology,* 84, 1112–1122.

Fisher, C.R., Graves, K.H., Parlow, A.F., Simpson, E.R. (1998). Characterization of mice deficient in aromatase (ArKO) because of targeted disruption of the cyp19 gene. *Proceedings of the National Academy of Sciences of the United States of America,* 95, 6965-6970.

Fisher, J. S., Millar, M. R., Majdic, G., Saunders, P. T., Fraser, H. M., Sharpe, R. M. (1997). Immunolocalisation of oestrogen receptor-a within the testis and excurrent ducts of the rat and marmoset monkey from perinatal life to adulthood. *The Journal of Endocrinology,* 153, 485-495.

Fitzgerald, E.F., Shrestha, S., Gomez, M.I., McCaffrey, R.J., Zimmerman, E.A., Kannan, K., Hwang, S.A. (2012). Polybrominated diphenyl ethers (PBDEs), polychlorinated biphenyls (PCBs) and neuropsychological status among older adults in New York. *Neurotoxicology,* 33, 8-15.

Forns, J., Torrent, M., Garcia-Esteban, R., Grellier, J., Gascon, M., Julvez, J., Guxens, M., Grimalt, J.O., Sunyer, J. (2012). Prenatal exposure to polychlorinated biphenyls and child neuropsychological development in 4-year-olds: an analysis per congener and specific cognitive domain. *The Science of the Total Environment,* 432, 338-343.

Foster, W., Chan, S., Platt, L., Hughes, C. (2000). Detection of endocrine disrupting chemicals in samples of second trimester human amniotic fluid. The journal of Clinical *Endocrinology and Metabolism,* 85, 2954-2957.

Fowler, P.A., Bellingham, M., Sinclair, K.D., Evans, N.P., Pocar, P., Fischer, B., Schaedlich, K., Schmidt, J.S., Amezaga, M.R., Bhattacharya, S., Rhind, S.M., O'Shaughnessy, P.J. (2012). Impact of endocrine-disrupting compounds (EDCs) on female reproductive health. *Molecular and Cellular Endocrinology,* 355, 213-219.

Frederiksen, M., Vorkamp, K., Thomsen, M., Knudsen, L.E. (2009). Human internal and external exposure to PBDEs–a review of levels and sources. *International Journal of Hygiene and Environmental Health,* 212, 109–134.

Gaido, K.W., Henslely, J.B., Liu, D., Wallace, D.G., Borghoff, S., Johnson, K.J., Hall, S.J., Boekelheide, K. (2007). Fetal mouse phthalate exposure shows that gonocyte multinucleation is not associated with decreased testicular testosterone. *Toxicological Sciences,* 97, 491-503.

Gaido, K.W., Maness, S.C., McDonnell, D.P., Dehal, S.S., Kupfer, D., Safe, S. (2000). Interaction of methoxychlor and related compounds with estrogen receptor alpha and beta, and androgen receptor: structure-activity studies. *Molecular Pharmacology,* 58, 852-858.

Gascon, M., Fort, M., Martínez, D., Carsin, A.E., Forns, J., Grimalt, J.O., Santa-Marina, L., Lertxundi, N., Sunyer, J., Vrijheid, M. (2012). Polybrominated diphenyl ethers (PBDEs) in breast milk and neuropsychological development in infants. *Environmental Health Perspectives,* 120, 1760-1765.

Gordon A, Garrido-Gracia JC, Aguilar R, Bellido, C., Velasco, J.A., Millan, Y., Tena-Sempere, M., Martín de Las Mulas, J., Sánchez-Criado, J.E. (2008). The ovary-mediated FSH attenuation of the LH surge in the rat involves a decreased gonadotroph progesterone receptor (PR) action but not PR expression. *Journal of Endocrinology,* 196, 583–592.

Goyal, H.O., Braden, T.D., Mansour, M., Williams, C.S., Kamaleldin, A., Srivastava, K.K. (2001). Diethylstilbestrol-Treated Adult Rats with Altered Epididymal Sperm Numbers and Sperm Motility Parameters, but Without Alterations in Sperm Production and Sperm Morphology. *Biology of Reproduction,* 64, 927-934.

Grandjean, P., Grønlund, C., Kjær, I.M., Jensen, T.K., Sørensen, N., Andersson, A.M., Juul, A., Skakkebæk, N.E., Budtz-Jørgensen, E., Weihe, P. (2012). Reproductive hormone profile and pubertal development in 14-year-old boys prenatally exposed to polychlorinated biphenyls. *Reproductive Toxicology,* 34, 498-503.

Grumbach, M. M., Auchus, R.J. (1999). Estrogen: Consequences and implications of human mutations in synthesis and action. *The* Journal *of Clinical Endocrinology &* Metabolism, 84, 4677-4694.

Guo, J., Deng, H., Li, H., Zhu, Q., Zhao, B., Chen, B., Chu, Y., Ge, R.S. (2013). Effects of methoxychlor and its metabolite 2,2-bis (p-hydroxyphenyl)-1,1,1-trichloroethane on 11β-hydroxysteroid dehydrogenase activities in vitro. *Toxicology Letters,* 27, 18-23.

Gupta, R.K., Aberdeen, G., Babus, J.K. Albrecht, E.D., Flaws, J.A. (2007). Methoxychlor and its metabolites inhibit growth and induce atresia of baboon antral follicles. *Toxicologic Pathology,* 35, 649-656.

Hany, J., Lilienthal, H., Sarasin, A., Roth-Härer, A., Fastabend, A., Dunemann, L., Lichtensteiger, W., Winneke, G. (1999). Developmental exposure of rats to a reconstituted PCB mixture or aroclor 1254: effects on organ weights, aromatase activity, sex hormone levels, and sweet preference behavior. *Toxicology and Applied Pharmacology,* 158, 231-243.

Härkönen, P. L., Mäkelä, S. I. (2004). Role of estrogens in development of prostate cancer. *Journal of Steroid Biochemistry & Molecular Biology,* 92, 297-305.

Harvey, C.N., Esmail, M., Wang, Q., Brooks, A.I., Zachow, R., Uzumcu, M. (2009). Effect of the methoxychlor metabolite HPTE on the rat ovarian granulosa cell transcriptome in vitro. *Toxicological Sciences,* 110, 95-106.

Hauser, R. (2006). The environment and male fertility: recent research on emerging chemicals and semen quality. *Seminars in Reproductive Medicine,* 24, 156-167.

Hawk, H.W. (1987). Transport and fate of spermatozoa after insemination of cattle. *Journal of Dairy Science,* 70, 1487-1503.

Hendry, W. J. D., and Danzo, B. J. (1986). Further characterization of a steroid receptor-active protease from the mature rabbit epididymis. *Journal of Steroid Biochemistry,* 25, 433-43.

Hess, R. A. (2000). Oestrogen in fluid transport and reabsorption in efferent ducts of the male reproductive tract. *Review of Reproduction,* 5, 84-92.

Hess, R. A., Bunick, D., Lee, KH., Bahr, J., Taylor, J. A., Korach, K. S., Lubahn, D. B. (1997). A role for oestrogens in the male reproductive system. *Nature,* 390, 509-512.

Hess, R.A., Gist, D. H., Bunick, D., Lubahn, D. B., Farrell, A., Bahr, J., Cooke, P. S., Greene, G. L. (1997). Estrogen receptor (a & b) expression in the excurrent ducts of the adult male rat reproductive tract. *Journal of Andrology,* 18, 602-611.

Heudorf, U., Mersch-Sundermann, V., Angerer, J. (2007). Phthalates: toxicology and exposure. *International Journal of Hygiene and Environmental Health,* 210, 623-634.

Högberg, J., Hanberg, A., Berglund, M., Skerfving, S., Remberger, M., Calafat, A.M., Filipsson, A.F., Jansson, B., Johansson, N., Appelgren, M., Håkansson, H. (2008). Phthalate diesters and their metabolites in human breast milk, blood or serum, and urine as biomarkers of exposure in vulnerable populations. *Environmental Health Perspectives,* 116, 334-339.

Holford, T.R., Zheng, T., Mayne, S.T., Zahm, S.H., Tessari, J.D., Boyle, P. (2000). Joint effects of nine polychlorinated biphenyl (PCB) congeners on breast cancer risk. *International Journal of Epidemiology,* 29, 975-982.

Hwang, K.A., Park, S.H., Yi, B.R., Choi, K.C. (2011). Gene alterations of ovarian cancer cells expressing estrogen receptors by estrogen and bisphenol a using microarray analysis. *Laboratory Animals Research,* 27, 99–107.

Ijichi, N., Ikeda, K., Horie-Inoue, K., Yagi, K., Okazaki, Y., Inoue, S. (2007). Estrogen-related receptor alpha modulates the expression of adipogenesis-related genes during adipocyte differentiation. *Biochemical and Biophysical Research Communications,* 358, 813–818.

Ilio, K., Hess, R. (1994). Structure and function of the ductuli efferentes: A review. *Microscopy Research and Technique,* 29, 432–467.

Jansen, R.P. (1984). Endocrine response in the fallopian tube. *Endocrine Reviews,* 5, 525-551.

Jefferson, W.N., Padilla-Banks, E., Newbold, R.R. (2005). Adverse effects on female development and reproduction in CD-1 mice following neonatal exposure to the phytoestrogen genistein at environmentally relevant doses. *Biology of Reproduction,* 73, 798-806.

Jefferson, W.N., Patisaul, H.B., Williams, C,J. (2012). Reproductive consequences of developmental phytoestrogen exposure. *Reproduction,* 143, 247-60.

Jensen, E. V. (1962). On the mechanism of estrogen action. *Perspectives in Biology and Medicine,* 6, 47-54.

Jepsen, K., Hermanson, O., Onami, T.M., Gleiberman, A.S., Lunyak, V., McEvilly, R.J., Kurokawa, R., Kumar, V., Liu, F., Seto, E., Hedrick, S.M., Mandel, G., Glass, C.K., Rose, D.W., Rosenfeld, M.G. (2000). Combinatorial roles of the nuclear receptor corepressor in transcription and development. *Cell,* 102, 753-763.

Kapoor, I.P., Metcalf, R.L., Nystrom, R.F., Sangha, G.K. (1970). Comparative metabolism of methoxychlor, methiochlor, and DDT in mouse, insects, and in a model ecosystem. *Journal of Agricultural and Food Chemistry,* 18, 1145-1152.

Karpeta, A., Rak-Mardyła, A., Jerzak, J., Gregoraszczuk, E.L. (2011). Congener-specific action of PBDEs on steroid secretion, CYP17, 17β-HSD and CYP19 activity and protein expression in porcine ovarian follicles. *Toxicology Letters.* 206, 258-263.

Karpeta, A., Barc, J., Ptak, A., Gregoraszczuk, E.L. (2013). The 2,2',4,4'-tetrabromodiphenyl ether hydroxylated metabolites 5-OH-BDE-47 and 6-OH-BDE-47 stimulate estradiol secretion in the ovary by activating aromatase expression. *Toxicology,* 305, 65-70.

Katoh, T., Hayashi, S., Iguchi, T., Sato, T. (2013). Epithelial-stromal Interactions in the mouse vagina exposed neonatally to diethylstilbestrol. *In Vivo,* 27, 333-337.

Katzenellenbogen, B. S., Montano, M. M., Ediger, T. R., Sun, J., Ekena, K., Lazennec, G., Martini, P. G., Mclnerney, E. M., Delage-Mourroux, R., Weis, K., Katzenellenbogen, J. A. (2000). Estrogen receptors: selective ligands, partners, and distinctive pharmacology. *Recent Progress in Hormone Research,* 55, 163-65.

Kelce, W.R., Lambright, C.R., Gray, L.E., Roberts, K.P. (1997). Vinclozolin and p, p'-DDE alter androgen dependent gene expression: in vivo confirmation of an androgen receptor-mediated mechanism. *Toxicology and Applied Pharmacology,* 142, 192-200.

Klinefelter, G.R., Laskey, J.W., Winnik, W.M., Suarez, J.D., Roberts, N.L., Strader, L.F., Riffle, B.W., Rao Veeramachaneni, D.N. (2012). Novel molecular targets associated with testicular dysgenesis induced by gestational exposure to diethylhexyl phthalate in the rat: a role for estradiol. *Reproduction,* 144, 747-761.

Kodavanti, P.R., Curras-Collazo, M.C. (2010). Neuroendocrine actions of organohalogens: thyroid hormones, arginine vasopressin, and neuroplasticity. *Frontiers in neuroendocrinology,* 31, 479-496.

Koji, T., Brenner, R.M. (1993). Localization of estrogen receptor messenger ribonucleic acid in rhesus monkey uterus by nonradioactive in situ hybridization with digoxigenin-labeled oligodeoxynucleotides. *Endocrinology,* 132, 382-392.

Kooy, R. F., D'Hooge, R., Reyniers, E., Bakker, C. E., Nagels, G., Boulle, K. D., Storm, K., Clincke, G., Deyn, P. P. D., Oostra, B. A., Willems, P. J. (1996). Transgenic mouse model for the fragile X syndrome. *American Journal of Medical Genetics,* 64, 241-245.

Kousteni, S., Han, L., Chen, J.R, Almeida, M., Plotkin, L.I., Bellido, T., Manolagas, S.C. (2003). Kinasemediated regulation of common transcription factors accounts for the bone-protective effects of sex steroids. *Journal of Clinical Investigation,* 111, 1651–1664.

Krege, J.H., Hodgin, J.B., Couse, J.F., Enmark, E., Warner, M., Mahler, J.F., Sar, M., Korach, K.S., Gustafsson, J.A., Smithies, O. (1998). Generation and reproductive phenotypes of mice lacking estrogen receptor beta. *Proceedings of the National Academy of Sciences of the United States of America,* 95, 15677-15682.

Kuiper, G. G. J. M., Enmak, E., Pelto-Huikko, M., Nilsson, S., Gustaffson, J. A. (1996). Cloning of a novel estrogen receptor expressed in rat prostate and ovary. *Proceedings of the National Academy of Science of the United States of America,* 93, 5925-5930.

Kuo, Y.M., Sepúlveda, M.S., Hua, I., Ochoa-Acuña, H.G., Sutton, T.M. (2010). Bioaccumulation and biomagnification of polybrominated diphenyl ethers in a food web of Lake Michigan. *Ecotoxicology*, 19, 623-634.

Kwack, S.J., Kwon, O., Kim, H.S., Kim, S.S., Kim, S.H., Sohn, K.H., Lee, R.D., Park, C.H., Jeung, E.B., An, B.S., Park, K.L. (2002). Comparative evaluation of alkylphenolic compounds on estrogenic activity in vitro and in vivo. *Journal of Toxicology and Environmental Health A,* 65, 419-431.

Lapointe, J., Roy, M., St-Pierre, I., Kimmins, S., Gauvreau, D., MacLaren, L.A., Bilodeau, J.F. (2006). Hormonal and spatial regulation of nitric oxide synthases (NOS) (neuronal NOS, inducible NOS, and endothelial NOS) in the oviducts. *Endocrinology,* 147, 5600-5610.

Lee, H.R., Kim, T.H., Choi, K.C. (2012). Functions and physiological roles of two types of estrogen receptors, ERalpha and ERbeta, identified by estrogen receptor knockout mouse. *Laboratory Animal Research*, 28, 71–76.

Lemaire, G., Mnif, W., Mauvais, P., Balaguer, P., Rahmani, R. (2006). Activation of alpha- and beta estrogen receptors by persistent pesticides in reporter cell lines. *Life Sciences,* 79, 1160-1169.

Lenie, S., Cortvrindt, R., Eichenlaub-Ritter, U., Smitz, J. (2008). Continuous exposure to bisphenol A during in vitro follicular development induces meiotic abnormalities. *Mutation Research,* 651, 71-81.

Levin, E.R. (2005). Integration of the extranuclear and nuclear actions of estrogen. *Molecular Endocrinology,* 19, 1951-1959.

Lilienthal, A., Hack, A., Roth-Härer, A., Grande, W., Talsness, C.E. (2006). Effects of developmental exposure to 2,2́,4,4́,5-pentabromodiphenyl ether (PBDE-99) on sex steroids, sexual development, and sexually dimorphic behavior in rats. *Environmental Health Perspectives,* 114, 194–201.

Lovekamp, T.N., Davis, B.J. (2001). Mono-(2-ethylhexyl) phthalate suppresses aromatase transcript levels and estradiol production in cultured rat granulosa cells. *Toxicology and Applied Pharmacology,* 172, 217-224.

Lubahn, D.B., Moyer, J.S., Golding, T.S., Couse, J.F., Korach, K.S., Smithies, O. (1993). Alteration of reproductive function but not prenatal sexual development after insertional disruption of the mouse estrogen receptor gene. *Proceedings of the National Academy of Sciences of the United States of America,* 90, 11162-11166.

McGlynn, K.A., Quraishi, S.M., Graubard, B.I., Weber, J.P., Rubertone, M.V., Erickson, R.L. (2008). Persistent organochlorine pesticides and risk of testicular germ cell tumors. *Journal of the National Cancer Institute,* 100, 663-671.

Maffini, M.V., Rubin, B.S., Sonnenschein, C., Soto, A.M. (2006). Endocrine disruptors and reproductive health: the case of bisphenol-A. *Molecular and Cellular Endocrinology,* 254, 179–186.

Maffucci, J.A., Gore, A.C. (2009). Chapter 2: hypothalamic neural systems controlling the female reproductive life cycle gonadotropin-releasing hormone, glutamate, and GABA. *International Review of Cell & Molecular Biology,* 274, 69–127.

Makela, S., Strauss, L., Kuiper, G., Valve, E. M., Salmi, S., Santti, R., Gustasson, J. A. (2000). Differential expression of estrogen receptors alpha and beta in adult rat accessory sex glands and lower urinary tract. *Molecular and Cellular Endocrinology,* 164, 109-116.

Marselos, M., Tomatis, L. (1992). Diethylstilboestrol: I, pharmacology, toxicology and carcinogenicity in humans. European. *Journal of Cancer*, 28A, 1182–1189.

Martikainen, P., Härkönen, P., Vanhala, T., Mäkelä, S., Viljanen, M., Suominen, J. (1987). Multihormonal control of synthesis and secretion of prostatein in cultured rat ventral prostate, *Endocrinology,* 121, 604-611.

Matsuzaki, S., Fukaya, T., Suzuki, T., Murakami, T., Sasano, H., Yajima, A. (1999). Oestrogen receptor α and β mRNA expression in human endometrium throughout the menstrual cycle. *Molecular Human Reproduction,* 5, 559-564.

Medlock, K.L., Branham, W.S., Sheehan, D.M. (1992). Long-term effects of postnatal exposure to diethylstilbestrol on uterine estrogen receptor and growth. *The Journal of Steroid Biochemistry and Molecular Biology,* 42, 23-28.

Medlock, K.L., Sheehan, D.M., Nelson, C.J., Branham, W.S. (1988). Effects of postnatal DES treatment on uterine growth, development, and estrogen receptor levels. *Journal of Steroid Biochemistry,* 29, 527-532.

Miller, V.M., Sanchez-Morrissey, S., Brosch, K.O., Seegal, R.F. (2012). Developmental coexposure to polychlorinated biphenyls and polybrominated diphenyl ethers has additive effects on circulating thyroxine levels in rats. *Toxicological Science,* 127, 76-83.

Montano, M., Jaiswal, A., Katzenellenbogen, B. (1998). Transcriptional regulation of the human quinine reductase gene by antiestrogen-liganded estrogen receptor-α and estrogen receptor-α. *Fertility and Sterility,* 273, 25443-25449.

Moore, N.P. (2000). The oestrogenic potential of the phthalate esters. *Reproductive Toxicology*, 14, 183-192.

Mosselman, S., Polman, J., Dijkema, R. (1996). ER-beta: identification and characterization of a novel human estrogen receptor. *FEBS letter,* 392, 49-53.

Moutsatsou, P. (2007). The spectrum of phytoestrogens in nature: our knowledge is expanding. *Hormones,* 6, 173-193.

Murono, E.P., Derk, R.C., de Leon, J.H. (2000). Octylphenol inhibits testosterone biosynthesis by cultured precursor and immature Leydig cells from rat testes. *Reproductive Toxicology,* 14, 275-288.

Murphy, J. B., Emmott, R. C., Hicks, L. L., and Walsh, P. C. (1980). Estrogen receptors in the human prostate, seminal vesicle, epididymis, testis, and genital skin a marker for estrogen-responsive tissues? *The Journal of Clinical Endocrinology & Metabolism,* 50, 938-48.

Mylchreest, E., Wallace, D.G., Cattley, R.C., Foster, P.M.D. (2000). Dose-dependent alterations in androgen-regulated male reproductive development in rats exposed to di(n-butyl) phthalate during late gestation. *Toxicological Sciences,* 55, 143-151.

Nadzialek, S., Depiereux, S., Mandiki, S.N., Kestemont, P. (2011). In vivo biomarkers of estrogenicity: limitation of interpretation in wild environment. *Archives of Environmental Contamination and Toxicology,* 60, 471-478.

Nah, W.H., Park, M.J., Gye, M.C. (2012). Effects of early prepubertal exposure to bisphenol A on the onset of puberty, ovarian weights, and estrous cycle in female mice. *Clinical and Experimental Reproductive Medicine,* 38, 75-81.

Nevalainen, M.T., Härkönen, P. L., Valve, E.M., Wu, P., Nurmi, M., Martikainen, P.M. (1993). Hormone regulation of human prostate in organ culture, *Cancer Research,* 53, 5199-5207.

Nevalainen, M.T., Valve, E.M., Mäkelä, S. I., Bläuer, M., Tuohimaa, P.J., Härkönen, P. L. (1991). Estrogen and prolactin regulation of rat dorsal and lateral prostate in organ culture, *Endocrinology,* 129, 612-622.

Nitta, H., Bunick, D., Hess, R. A., Janulis, L., Newton, S. C., Millette, C. F., Osawa, Y., Shizuta, Y., Toda, K., and Bahr, J. M. (1993). Germ cells of the mouse testis express P450 aromatase. *Endocrinology,* 132, 1396-401.

Nynca, A., Słonina, D., Jablońska, O., Kamińska, B., Ciereszko, R.E. (2013). Daidzein affects steroidogenesis and oestrogen receptor expression in medium ovarian follicles of pigs. *Acta veterinaria Hungarica,* 61, 85-98.

Ohta, R., Ohmukai, H., Marumo, H., Shindo, T., Nagata, T., Ono, H. (2012). Delayed reproductive dysfunction in female rats induced by early life exposure to low-dose diethylstilbestrol. *Reproductive Toxicology,* 34, 323-330.

Okada, A., Ohta, Y., Inoue, S., Hiroi, H., Muramatsu, M., Iguchi, T. (2003). Expression of estrogen, progesterone and androgen receptors in the oviduct of developing, cycling and pre-implantation rats. *Journal of Molecular Endocrinology,* 30, 301-315.

Omoto, Y., Imamov, O., Warner, M., Gustafsson, J. A. (2005). Estrogen receptor alpha and imprinting of the neonatal mouse ventral prostate by estrogen. *Proceedings of the National Academy of Science of the United States of America,* 102, 1484-1489.

Orihuela, P.A., Parada-Bustamante, A., Corte´s, P.P., Gatica, C., Croxatto, H.B. (2003). Estrogen receptor, cyclic adenosine monophosphate, and protein kinase A are involved in the nongenomic pathway by which estradiol accelerates oviductal oocyte transport in cyclic rats. *Biology of Reproduction,* 68, 1225-1231.

Otto, C., Fuchs, I., Kauselmann, G., Kern, H., Zevnik, B., Andreasen, P., Schwarz, G., Altmann, H., Klewer, M., Schoor, M.,Vonk, R., Fritzemeier,K.H. (2009). GPR30does not mediate estrogenic responses in reproductive organs in mice. *Biology of Reproduction,* 80, 34-41.

Padilla-Banks, E., Jefferson, W.N., Myers, P.H., Goulding, D.R., Williams, C.J. (2012). Neonatal phytoestrogen exposure causes hypospadias in female mice. *Molecular Reproduction and Development,* 79, 3.

Pang, Y., Dong, J., Thomas, P. (2008). Estrogen signaling characteristics of Atlantic croaker G protein-coupled receptor 30 (GPR30) and evidence it is involved in maintenance of oocyte meiotic arrest. *Endocrinology,* 149, 3410-3426.

Pant, N., Pant, A., Shukla, M., Mathur, N., Gupta, Y., Saxena, D. (2011). Environmental and experimental exposure of phthalate esters: the toxicological consequence on human sperm. *Human & Experimental Toxicology,* 30, 507-514.

Pant, N., Shukla, M., Patel, D.K., Shukla, Y., Mathur, N., Gupta, Y.K., Saxena, D.K. (2008). Correlation of phthalate exposures with semen quality. *Toxicology and Applied Pharmacology,* 23, 1112-1116.

Park, S.H., Kim, K.Y., An, B.S., Choi, J.H., Jeung, E.B., Leung, P.C., Choi, K.C. (2009). Cell growth of ovarian cancer cells is stimulated by xenoestrogens through an estrogen-dependent pathway, but their stimulation of cell growth appears not to be involved in the activation of the mitogen-activated protein kinases ERK-1 and p38. *Journal of Reproductive Development*, 55, 23-29.

Perez-Martinez, S., Viggiano, M., Franchi, A., Herrero, M., Ortiz, M., Gimeno, M., Villalo´n, M. (2000). Effect of nitric oxide synthase inhibitors on ovumtransport and oviductal smooth muscle activity in the rat oviduct. *Journal of Reproduction and Fertility,* 118, 111-117.

Polder, A., Avinova, T.N., Tkachev, A., Løken, K.B., Odland, J.O., Skaare, J.U. (2010). Levels and patterns of Persistent Organic Pollutants (POPS) in selected food items from Northwest Russia (1998-2002) and implications for dietary exposure. *The Science of the Total Environment,* 408, 5352-5361.

Pollack, A.Z., Buck Louis, G.M., Lynch, C.D., Kostyniak, P.J. (2011). Persistent Organochlorine Exposure and Pregnancy Loss: A Prospective Cohort Study. *Journal of Environmental Protection,* 2, 683-691.

Press, M.F., Nousek-Goebl, N.A., Bur, M., Green, G.L. (1986). Estrogen localization in the female genital tract. *The American Journal of Pathology,* 123, 280-292.

Prins, G.S., Birch, L., Couse, J. F., Choi, I., Katzenellenbogen, B., Korach, K. S. (2001). Estrogen imprinting of the developing prostate gland in mediated through stromal estrogen receptor α: studies with αERKO and βERKO mice. *Cancer Research,* 61, 6089-6097.

Prins, G. S., Korach, K. S. (2008). The Role of Estrogens and Estrogen Receptors in Normal Prostate Growth and Disease. *Steroids,* 73(3), 233-244.

Prins, G.S., Marmer, M., Woodham, C., Chang, W. Y., Kuiper, G., Gustafsson, J. A., Birch, L. (1998). Estrogen receptor-β messenger ribonucleic acid ontogeny in the prostate of normal and neonatally estrogenized rats. *Endocrinology,* 139(3), 874-883.

Prins, G.S., Woodham, C., Lepinske, M., Birch, L. (1993). Effects of neonatal estrogen exposure on prostatic secretory genes and their correlation with androgen receptor expression in the separate prostate lobes of the adult rat. *Endocrinology,* 132, 2387-2398.

Prossnitz, E.R., Arterburn, J.B., Smith, H.O., Oprea, T.I., Sklar, L.A., Hathaway, H.J. (2008). Estrogen signaling through the transmembrane G protein-coupled receptor GPR30. *Annual Review of Physiology,* 70, 165-190.

Puri, R.K., Roy, S.K. (1981). Estradiol binding in different parts of the rabbit oviduct during egg transport. *Endokrinologie,* 78, 12-20.

Qiu, L-L., Wang, X., Zhang, X-H., Zhang, Z., Gu, J., Liu, L., Wang, Y., Wang, X., Wang, S-L. (2013). Decreased androgen receptor expression may contribute to spermatogenesis failure in rats exposed to low concentration of bisphenol A. *Toxicological Letters,* 23, 116-124.

Rachoń, D., Vortherms, T., Seidlová-Wuttke, D., Menche, A., Wuttke, W. (2007). Uterotropic effects of dietary equol administration in ovariectomized Sprague-Dawley rats. *Climacteric,* 10, 416-426.

Ren, X.M., Guo, L.H., Gao, Y., Zhang, B.T., Wan, B. (2013). Hydroxylated polybrominated diphenyl ethers exhibit different activities on thyroid hormone receptors depending on their degree of bromination. *Toxicology and Applied Pharmacology,* 268, 256-263.

Richards, J.S., Ireland, J.J., Rao, M.C., Bernath, G.A., Midgley Jr, A.R., Reichert Jr, L.E. (1976). Ovarian follicular development in the rat: hormone receptor regulation by estradiol, follicle stimulating hormone and luteinizing hormone. *Endocrinology,* 99, 1562-1570.

Risbridger, G. P., Wang, H., Young, P., Takeshi, K., Wong, Y. Z., Lubahn, D., Gustafsson, J. A., Cunha, G. (2001). Evidence that epithelial and mesenchymal estrogen receptor-α mediates effects of estrogen on prostatic epithelium. *Developmental Biology,* 229, 432-444.

Rhouma, B.K., Tebourbi, O., Krichah, R., Sakly, M. (2001). Reproductive toxicity of DDT in adult male rats. *Human Exposure and Toxicology,* 20, 393-397.

Rochira, V., Balestrieri, A., Madeo, B., Spaggiari, A., Carani, C. (2002). Congenital estrogen deficiency in men: A new syndrome with different phenotypes; clinical and therapeutic implications in men. *Molecular and Cellular Endocrinology,* 193, 19-28.

Ruiz, P., Myshkin, E., Quigley, P., Faroon, O., Wheeler, J.S., Mumtaz, M.M., Brennan, R.J. (2013). Assessment of hydroxylated metabolites of polychlorinated biphenyls as potential xenoestrogens: a QSAR comparative analysis*. SAR and QSAR in Environmental Research. [Epub ahead of print].

Salleh, N., Helmy, M.M., Fadila, K.N., Yeong, S.O. (2013). Isoflavone genistein induces fluid secretion and morphological changes in the uteri of post-pubertal rats. *International Journal Medical Sciences,* 10, 665-675.

Samudio, I., Vyhlidal, C., Wang, F., Stoner, M., Chen, I., Kladde, M., Barhoumi, R., Burghardt, R., Safe, S. (2001). Transcriptional activation of deoxyribonucleic acid polymerase alpha gene expression in MCF-7 cells by 17 beta-estradiol. *Endocrinology,* 142, 1000-1008.

Schleicher, G., Drews, U., and Stumpf, W. E. (1989). No evidence for aromatization of [3H] testosterone in oestrogen receptor containing cells of the epididymis. *Journal Steroid Biochemistry,* 32, 299-302.

Schmidt, S., Degen, G.H., Seibel, J., Hertrampf, T., Vollmer, G., Diel, P. (2006). Hormonal activity of combinations of genistein, bisphenol A and 17beta-estradiol in the female Wistar rat. *Archives of Toxicology,* 80, 839-845.

Selvaraj,V., Zakroczymski, M.A., Naaz, A., Mukai, M., Ju, Y.H., Doerge, D.R., Katzenellenbogen, J.A., Helferich, W.G., Cooke, P.S. (2004). Estrogenicity of the isoflavone metabolite equol on reproductive and non-reproductive organs in mice. *Biology of Reproduction,* 71, 966-972.

Setchell, K.D. (2001). Soy isoflavones-benefits and risks from nature's selective estrogen receptor modulators (SERMs). *Journal of the American College of Nutrition,* 20, 354S-362S.

Siddiqi, M.A., Laessig, R.H., Reed, K,D. (2003). Polybrominated diphenyl ethers (PBDEs): new pollutants-old diseases. *Clinical Medicine & Research,* 1, 281-290.

Simoncini, T., Mannella, P., Fornari, L., Caruso, A., Varone, G., Genazzani, A.R. (2004). Genomic and non-genomic effects of estrogens on endothelial cells. *Steroids,* 69, 537–542.

Simpson, E.R. (2003). Sources of estrogen and their importance. *The Journal of Steroid Biochemistry and Molecular Biology,* 86, 225–230.

Singh, S., Li, S.S. (2011). Bisphenol A and phthalates exhibit similar toxicogenomics and health effects. *Gene,* 494, 85-91.

Sonnenschein, C., Soto, A.M. (1998). An updated review of environmental estrogen and androgen mimics and antagonists. *Journal of Steroids Biochemicals and Molecular Biology,* 65, 143-150.

Steinberg, R.M., Walker, D.M., Juenger, T.E., Woller, M.J., Gore, A,C. (2010). Effects of perinatal polychlorinated biphenyls on adult female rat reproduction: development, reproductive physiology, and second generational effects. *Biology of Reproduction,* 78, 1091-1101.

Stoker, C., Beldoménico, P.M., Bosquiazzo, V.L., Zayas, M.A., Rey, F., Rodríguez, H., Muñoz-de-Toro, M., Lugue, E.H. (2008). Developmental exposure to endocrine disruptor chemicals alters follicular dynam-ics and steroid levels in Caiman latirostris. *General and Comparative Endocrinology,* 156, 603-612.

Suarez, S.S., Pacey, A.A. (2006). Sperm transport in the female reproductive tract. *Human Reproduction Update,* 12, 363-372.

Suzuki, T., Yu, H.P., Hsieh, Y.C., Choudhry, M.A., Bland, K.I., Chaudry, I.H. (2008). Estrogen-mediated activation of non-genomic pathway improves macrophages cytokine production following trauma-hemorrhage. *Journal of Cellular Physiology,* 214, 662-672.

Sun, H., Xu, L.C., Chen, J.F., Song, L., Wang, X.R. (2006). Effect of bisphenol A, tetrachlorobisphenol A and pentachlorophenol on the transcriptional activities of androgen receptor-mediated reporter gene. *Food and Chemical Toxicology,* 44, 1916-1921.

Swan, S. (2008). Environmental phthalate exposure in relation to reproductive outcomes and other health endpoints in humans. *Environmental Research,* 108, 177-184.

Takahashi, O., Oishi, S. (2001). Testicular toxicity of dietary 2,2-bis(4 hydroxyphenyl)propane (bisphenol A) in F344 rats. *Archives of Toxicology,* 75, 42-51.

Takeuchi, S., Shiraishi, F., Kitamura, S., Kuroki, H., Jin, K., Kojima, H. (2011). Characterization of steroid hormone receptor activities in 100 hydroxylated polychlorinated biphenyls, including congeners identified in humans. *Toxicology,* 289, 112-121.

Taniguchi, F., Couse, J.F., Rodriguez, K.F., Emmen, J.M., Poirier, D., Korach, K.S. (2007). Estrogen receptor-alpha mediates an intraovarian negative feedback loop on thecal cell steroidogenesis via modulation of Cyp17a1 (cytochrome P450, steroid 17 alpha-hydroxylase/17,20 lyase) expression. *FASEB Journal,* 21, 586-595.

Taylor, A.H., Al-Azzawi, F. (2000). Immunolocalisation of oestrogen receptor beta in human tissues. *Journal of Molecular Endocrinology,* 24, 145-155.

Tsubota, T., Nitta, H., Osawa, Y., Mason, I., Kita, I., Tiba, T., and Bahr, J. (1993). Immunolocalization of steroidogenic enzymes, P450scc, 3β-HSD, P450c17, and P450arom in the Hokkaido brown bear. *General and Comparative Endocrinology,* 92, 439-44.

Turusov, V., Rakitsky, V., Tomatis, L. (2002). Dichlorodiphenyltrichloro ethane (DDT): ubiquity, persistence and risks. *Environmental Health Perspectives,* 110, 125-128.

Ukpebor, J., Llabjani, V., Martin, F.L., Halsall, C.J. (2011). Sublethal genotoxicity and cell alterations by organophosphorus pesticides in MCF-7 cells: implications for environmentally relevant concentrations. *Environmental Toxicology and Chemistry,* 30, 632–639.

Ulbrich, S.E., Kettler, A., Einspanier, R. (2003). Expression and localization of estrogen receptor α, estrogen receptor β, and progesterone receptor in the bovine oviduct in vivo and in vitro. *The Journal of Steroid Biochemistry and Molecular Biology,* 84, 279-289.

Vermeulen, A., Kaufman, J. M., Goemaere, S., van Pottelberg, I. (2002). Estradiol in elderly men. *Aging Male,* 5(2), 98-102.

Vermeulen, A., Rubens, R., Verdonck, L. (1972). Testosterone secretion and metabolism in male senescence. *The Journal of Clinical Endocrinology & Metabolism,* 34, 730-735.

Villa, R., Bonetti, E., Penza, M.L., Iacobello, C., Bugari, G., Bailo, M., Parolini, O., Apostoli, P., Caimi, L., Ciana, P., Maggi, A., Di Lorenzo, D. (2004). Target specific action of organochlorine compounds in reproductive and nonreproductive tissues of estrogen-reporter male mice. *Toxicology Applied Pharmacology,* 201, 137-148.

Vom Saal, F.S., Cooke, P.S., Buchanan, D.L., Palanza, P., Thayer, K.A., Nagel, S.C., Parmigiani, S., Welshons, W.V. (1998). A physiologically based approach to the study of bisphenol A and other estrogenic chemicals on the size of reproductive organs, daily sperm production, and behavior. *Toxicology and Industrial Health,* 14, 239-260.

Wagner, U., Schlebusch, H., van der Ven, H., van der Ven, K., Diedrich, K., Krebs, D. (1990). Accumulation of pollutants in the genital tract of sterility patients. *Journal of Clinical Chemistry & Clinical Biochemistry*, 28, 683–688.

Walker, D.M., Kermath, B.A., Woller, M.J., Gore, A.C. (2013). Disruption of reproductive aging in female and male rats by gestational exposure to estrogenic endocrine disruptors. *Endocrinology,* 154, 2129-2143.

Wang. H., Eriksson, H., Sahlin, L. Estrogen receptors alpha and beta in the female reproductive tract of the rat during the estrous cycle. (2000). *Biology of reproduction,* 63, 1331-1340.

Wang, Z., Zhang, X., Shen, P., Loggie, B.W., Chang, Y., Deuel, T.F. (2006). A variant of estrogen receptor-{alpha}, hER {alpha} 36: transduction of estrogen- and antiestrogen-dependent membrane-initiated mitogenic signaling. *Proceedings of the National Academy of Sciences USA,* 103, 9063–9068.

Waring, R.H., Ayers, S., Gescher, A.J., Glatt, H.R., Meinl, W., Jarratt, P., Kirk, C.J., Pettitt, T., Rea, D., Harris, R.M. (2008). Phytoestrogens and xenoestrogens: the contribution of diet and environment to endocrine disruption. *The Journal of Steroid Biochemistry and Molecular Biology,* 108, 213-220.

Watson, C.S., Jeng, Y.J., Hu, G., Wozniak, A., Bulayeva, N., Guptarak, J. (2012). Estrogen- and xenoestrogen-induced ERK signaling in pituitary tumor cells involves estrogen receptor-alpha interactions with G protein-alphai and caveolin I. *Steroids,* 77, 424-432.

Weihua, Z., Makela, S., Andersson, L. C., Salmi, S., Saji, S., Webster, J. I., Jensen, E. V., Nilsson, S., Warner, M., Gustafsson, J. A. (2001). A role for estrogen receptor beta in the regulation of growth of the ventral prostate. *Proceedings of the National Academy of Science,* 98(11), 6330-6335.

Wetherill, Y.B., Akingbemi, B.T., Kanno, J., McLachlan, J.A., Nadal, A., Sonnenschein, C., Watson, C.S., Zoeller, R.T., Belcher, S.M. (2007). In vitro molecular mechanisms of bisphenol A action. *Reproductive Toxicology,* 24, 178-198.

Whitehead, S.A., Rice, S. (2006). Endocrine-disrupting chemicals as modulators of sex steroid synthesis. Best Practice and Research. *Clinical Endocrinology and Metabolism,* 20, 45-61.

Wocławek-Potocka, I., Mannelli, C., Boruszewska, D., Kowalczyk-Zieba, I., Waśniewski, T., Skarżyński, D.J. (2013). Diverse effects of phytoestrogens on the reproductive performance: cow as a model. *International Journal of Endocrinology,* 2013, 650984.

Wood, C.E., Appt, S.E., Clarkson, T.B., Franke, A.A., Lees, C.J., Doerge, D.R., Cline, J.M. (2006). Effects of high-dose soy isoflavones and equol on reproductive tissues in female cynomolgus monkeys. *Biology of Reproduction,* 75, 477-486.

You, L., Sar, M., Bartolucci, E., Ploch, S., Whitt, M. (2002). Induction of hepatic aromatise by p,p - DDE in adult male rats. *Molecular Cellular Endocrinology,* 178, 207-214.

Younglai, E.V., Holloway, A.C., Lim, G.E., Foster, W.G. (2004). Synergistic effects between FSH and 1,1-dichloro-2,2-bis (P-chlorophenyl)ethylene (P,P'-DDE) on human granulosa cell aromatase activity. Human Reproduction, 19, 1089-1093.

Yum, T., Lee, S., Kim, Y. (2013). Association between precocious puberty and some endocrine disruptors in human plasma. Journal of Environmental Science and Health. Part A, Toxic/*Hazardous Substances and Environmental Engineering,* 48, 912-917.

Zacharewski, T.R., Meek, M.D., Clemons, J.H., Wu, Z.F., Fielden, M.R., Matthews, J.B. (1998). Examination of the in vitro and in vivo estrogenic activities of eight commercial phthalate esters. *Toxicological Sciences,* 46, 282-293.

Zama, A.M., Uzumcu, M. (2009). Fetal and neonatal exposure to the endocrine disruptor methoxychlor causes epigenetic alterations in adult ovarian genes. *Endocrinology,* 150, 4681-4691.

Zhang, X.F., Zhang, L.J., Li, L., Feng, Y.N., Chen, B., Ma, J.M., Huynh, E., Shi, Q.H., De Felici, M., Shen, W. (2013). Diethylhexyl phthalate exposures impairs follicular development and affects oocyte maturation in the mouse. *Environmental and Molecular Mutagenesis,* 54, 354-361.

In: Estradiol: Synthesis, Health Effects and Drug Interactions ISBN: 978-1-62808-962-2
Editors: Ricco Palmeri and Sal Grimaudo

Chapter 4

Estrogens and Prostate Cancer: From Biosynthesis to Physiological Effects

Inês M. Gomes, Cátia V. Vaz, Daniel B. Rodrigues, Sandra M. Rocha, Sílvia Socorro, Cecília R. Santos and Cláudio J. Maia*

CICS-UBI - Health Sciences Research Centre, University of Beira Interior, Portugal

Abstract

Although the most impressive characteristic of prostate cancer is its androgen dependence, several studies support that 17β-estradiol (E_2) also plays an important role in onset and progression of prostate cancer. Regarding the effects of E_2 in prostate carcinogenesis, we can highlight the carcinogenic properties of several products derived from E_2 metabolism, which play an important role on cell malignant transformation. Several polymorphisms in estrogen-related genes such as estrogen receptors (ERs) and enzymes involved in E_2 biosynthesis and metabolism have been described to favour carcinogenesis. Also, both isoforms of ERs (ERα and ERβ), which act on cells in order to maintain the normal physiology of prostate gland, are differentially expressed between neoplastic and non-neoplastic prostate cells. Therefore, this deregulation may conduct to alterations on normal gene expression in prostate cells, which may favour the progression and migration of cancer cells. On the other hand, other studies have been pointing the anti-carcinogenic activity of E_2 in prostate. These contradictory effects are based on the role of ERβ, which has been shown to exhibit anti-proliferative and anti-oxidant functions. Taking into account the scientific evidences that relate E_2 with prostate cancer, several therapeutic approaches based on ERs are being explored. This chapter summarizes the main knowledge on how E_2 may contribute to the pathophysiology of prostate gland.

* Corresponding author: Cláudio J Maia, Faculdade de Ciências da Saúde, Av. Infante D. Henrique, 6200-506 Covilhã, Portugal, Phone: +351 275 329 068, FAX: +351-275 329 099, E-mail: cmaia@fcsaude.ubi. ptIntroduction.

In developed countries, prostate cancer (PCa) is the most frequently diagnosed malignancy in men [1]. The aetiology of this disease is complex and remains unclear. Risk factors for a high morbidity of PCa can be classified as endogenous (family history, hormones, race, aging and oxidative stress) or exogenous (dietary factors, physical inactivity, obesity, environmental factors, occupation, smoking, sexual activity, vasectomy). However, a positive family history is the strongest epidemiological risk factor for PCa [1-3].

The relationship between hormones and the pathogenesis of PCa has been extensively studied. PCa is generally considered a paradigm of androgen-dependent tumour. However, estrogens role appears to be equally important in both normal and malignant prostate. Recent epidemiologic and experimental data have clearly pinpointed the key roles of estrogens in PCa development and progression [4, 5]. PCa risk in adulthood could be determined by exposure to estrogens during embryonic, perinatal/neonatal, or peripubertal development, a phenomenon referred to as ''estrogen imprinting'' [6]. Estrogens action should be considered both at a systemic endocrine level, because these steroid hormones are able to act through the pituitary gland to indirectly lower androgens, and locally within the prostate tissue [4, 7]. Salonia and collaborators demonstrated for the first time that the circulating 17β-estradiol (E_2, the most potent subtype of estrogens) levels are associated with a greater incidence of high grade PCa. Patients with high E_2 levels have an increased risk to develop PCa [8]. Another study also demonstrated that E_2 exposure could neoplastically transform the rat prostatic epithelial cells *in vitro* [9]. These results support the idea that estrogens have long been implicated in the prostate carcinogenesis. In addition, high estrogens levels and low testosterone levels induce the development of inflammation upon aging and the onset of premalignant lesions [10].

Understanding how estrogens are synthesized and act on prostate cells, will indubitably contribute to better understand the molecular mechanisms underlying PCa onset and progression, as well as to delineate novel strategies in diagnosis and treatment of PCa.

Biosynthesis and Metabolism of 17β-Estradiol in Prostate Cells

Estrogens are stereogenic-derived hormones which encompass natural and synthetic compounds. Natural estrogens are composed of 18-carbons steroids with an aromatic ring containing the CH_3 group in the 13th carbon. These natural estrogens can be divided into three basic and biologically active subtypes: estrone (E_1), E_2 and estriol (E_3) [11].

Using cholesterol as precursor, steroidogenic enzymes are responsible for the biosynthesis of various steroid hormones (Figure 1). Some of these steroids include glucocorticoids, mineralocorticoids, progestins and androgens which will lead to the biosynthesis of estrogens. These enzymes belong to the family of cytochrome P450 (CYPs), hydroxysteroid dehydrogenases (HSDs), and steroid reductases [12].

Androgen precursors for the biosynthesis of estrogens can be derived from various pathways. 17α-hydroxylase/17,20-lyase (P450c17, CYP17) is considered a crucial enzyme in the steroidogenic pathway, possessing dual enzymatic activity, namely 17α-hydroxylase and 17,20-lyase, that converts C21-steroids (pregnenolone and progesterone) into 17α-hydroxypregnenolone and 17α-hydroxyprogesterone, which are the precursors of cortisol biosynthesis in the human, as well as into C19-steroids (dehydroepiandrosterone (DHEA) and 4-androstenedione) that are precursors of potent sex steroid hormones [13, 14]. Biosynthesis of estrogens precursors is achieved through the high level of circulating adrenal pro-hormones DHEA and DHEA sulphate (DHEAS) in humans. This pathway is well recognized as an additional source of active sex steroids in peripheral tissues [13-16]. Many of these steroidogenic enzymes, involved in estrogen biosynthesis and metabolism, are expressed in the human prostate [17], suggesting that E_1 and E_2 may be produced locally within the prostate via aromatization of androstenedione and testosterone, respectively, catalyzed within the prostate stroma by aromatase [18-20]. This conversion occurs due to the chemical structure of testosterone and androstenedione which allows these two precursors to act as substrates for aromatization to estrogens [20], and this process is irreversible under biological conditions [21].

Aromatase is a CYP-dependent enzyme which requires NADPH as a coenzyme. Aromatase action involves oxidation, removal of the methyl group at the carbon 19 position of testosterone or androstenedione, and removal of the hydrogen at the carbon 1β-position. For aromatase activity, three molecules of oxygen are required per molecule of steroid. Aromatase is encoded by the CYP19 gene, which encodes a protein that in many species consists of approximately 500 amino acids. The coding region of the gene spans nine exons beginning with exon II, and expression of the gene is determined by tissue-specific promoters, which lead to transcripts that are always the same regardless of the site of expression [21].

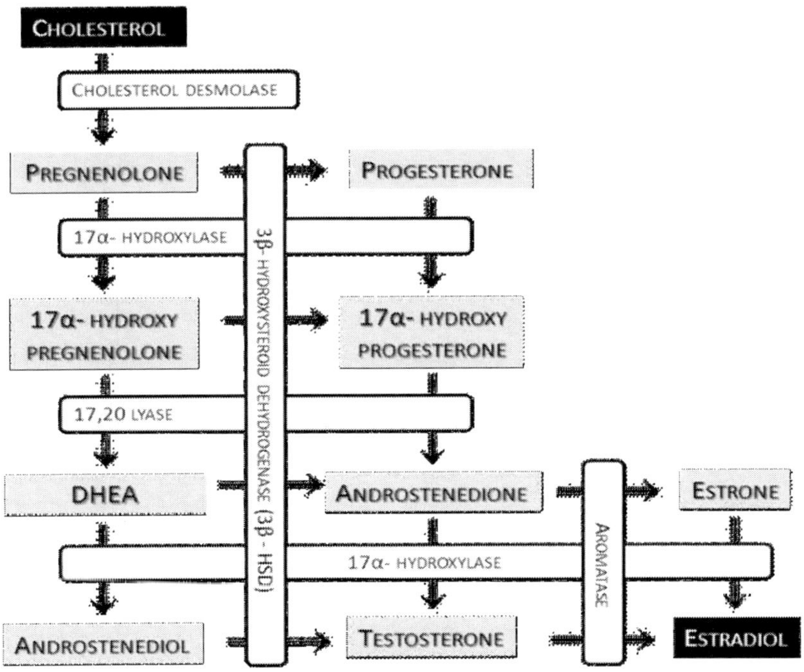

Figure 1. Biosynthesis of steroids hormones, starting with the oxidation of the side chain of cholesterol, which is catalyzed by the enzyme cholesterol desmolase. The next steps in the 17β-estradiol synthesis can proceed via different routes that are outlined in the figure. Abbreviation: DHEA – dehydroepiandrosterone.

The testis are the main source of testosterone that is delivered into all tissues of the body through the blood circulation, and it is believed that circulating testosterone is the main precursor for the biosynthesis of estrogens, namely E_2, via aromatase [22]. However, alternative pathways for the biosynthesis of E_2 have been suggested. Although aromatase uses testosterone as a substrate, it has been shown that 4-dione acts as a better substrate for this enzyme [23, 24] leading to the conversion of androstenedione to E_1, whereas reductive 17β-HSDs, namely the types 1, 7, and 12, convert E_1 to E_2 [25-27]. On the other hand, the oxidative 17β-HSDs types 2 and 4 convert E_2 into a weak estrogen, E_1. These two estrogens are biochemically interconvertable by the enzyme E_2 dehydrogenase. Although controversial, several reports [17, 28, 29] show that enzymes involved in the metabolism of estrogens are expressed in both epithelial (including basal cells) and stromal cells.

After the biosynthesis of estrogens, these can be eliminated from the body by metabolic conversion to hormonally inactive (or less active) water soluble metabolites. This metabolic deposition of estrogens includes oxidative metabolism and conjugative metabolism by glucuronidation, sulfonation and/or *O*-methylation [30]. The phase I enzymes, CYP1A1 and CYP1B1, catalyze the conversion of E_2 to 2-hydroxyestradiol and 4-hydroyestradiol, respectively. These two metabolites are also called catechol estrogens. An evidence has arisen that local E_2 metabolism may contribute to PCa and play an important role in tumour progression because some metabolites have been linked to free radical generation and direct genomic damage [31]. Studies have shown that the 2- and 4-hydroxyestradiol can be rapidly oxidized to 2,3- and 3,4-semiquinones and quinines [20, 32] , respectively, which are capable of forming DNA adducts, leading to DNA damage including single- and double stranded DNA breaks. In general, 2-hydroxyestradiol is considered less damaging, while 4-hydroxyestradiol and its respective quinine have greater toxicity. The catechol estrogens resultant from the CYP1A1 and CYP1B1 catalytic conversion are activated by conjugating reactions, such as glucuronidation and sulfonation [20]. To maintain intracellular homeostasis, the phase II enzyme, catechol-O-methyl transferase (COMT) converts these metabolites to 2- and 4-methoxyestrone, respectively, which are rapidly excreted. Importantly, while the human prostate expresses these enzymes [32], estrogens are capable of markedly increasing CYP1B1 expression in a variety of tissues, including prostate [33].

It is well characterized the association between androgens and the development of PCa, but recently, several studies have shown that aromatase expression is altered in PCa tissues [34], giving further support to a role of estrogens in this disease. Abnormal levels of E_2 and/or estrone and, especially, some of their hydroxylated derivates have also been implicated in tumour onset and progression [35]. In non-malignant prostate tissues, aromatase expression is confined to the stroma cells, while it is expressed throughout microdissected epithelial tumour cells and PCa cell lines [18].

In addition, it is important to have in consideration that polymorphisms of genes encoding the enzymes involved in estrogens biosynthesis, along with their epigenetic silencing or structural alterations may result in a profound disturbance of enzyme expression and activity. To date, at least three different polymorphisms in the CYP1A1 gene, encoding the 2-hydroxylase enzyme, have been associated with an increased risk of PCa [36]. Comparable findings were obtained for the CYP1B1 gene that encodes the 4-hydroxylase enzyme [37]. These polymorphisms usually induce a prolonged half-life and activity of both enzymes, and, hence, a sustained carcinogenic potential of their products, respectively 2- and 4-hydroxyestradiol. Moreover, a single nucleotide polymorphism (SNP) linked to the

CYP19A1 aromatase gene, is mildly through significantly associated with PCa risk, suggesting that this SNP may encode for a variant enzyme having higher activity and, hence, resulting in lower androgen levels [38].

Estrogens Receptors and Estrogens-Regulated Genes in Prostate Cells

Expression of ERs and Their Regulation in Prostate Cancer

The miscellaneous effects of estrogens in prostate may be explained by different expression patterns of estrogens receptors (ERs) in different cellular compartments of the prostate tissue. The classical ER, ERα, has been detected almost exclusively on the stroma and in subsets of basal cells [39-44]. Both in normal, high-grade prostatic intraepithelial neoplasia (HGPIN) and prostatic adenocarcinoma tissues, ERα maintains this restricted cellular expression. Interestingly, some studies show a positive correlation between ERα expression and high grade tumours (Gleason 4 and 5) as well as recurrent and metastatic tumours, leading to the assumption that the increase of receptor expression accompanies the development of PCa [45]. However, this is slightly controversial because although ERα is expressed in benign prostatic hyperplasia (BPH) and PCa cells, no clear or significant differences were found between the two pathologies, or even between hormone-responsive and refractory prostate carcinomas [46]. Epigenetic modifications have been pointed as one of the mechanisms involved in the regulation of ERα expression. It has been showed that the transcriptional activity of ERα gene is under control of methylation patterns, which is responsible to decrease ERα expression in higher grades of PCa [47].

ERβ expression, on the other hand, seems to be restricted to the luminal and basal epithelial cells, with lower or none expression in stromal cells [44, 48-51]. However, *in vitro* studies using normal and malignant prostate epithelial cell lines, show that this receptor is highly expressed [52]. In human prostate tissue specimens, ERβ expression pattern alters significantly across PCa progression, suggesting that it may have an important role on prostate carcinogenesis and metastasis. Diminished levels of ERβ have been associated with the appearance of HGPIN, and this receptor expression is progressively lost on primary PCa stages. Nonetheless, ERβ expression appears to be retained on tumours with higher rates of recurrence and regained in metastasis [44, 50, 53, 54]. The regulation of ERβ expression appears to be through epigenetic mechanisms, specifically by hypermethylation CpG islands in the ERβ promoter leading to gene silencing [52, 55]. This event seems to be in accordance with the proposed role of ERβ as a putative tumour suppressor gene [56].

Characterization and Expression of ER Splice Variants, and Their Association with Prostate Cancer Risk

There are at least five distinct mRNA isoforms of ERα, ERα-A-E, indicating that more than one promoter may control the ER transcriptional activity [57-59]. All these variants show deletions at the C-terminal ligand-binding domain (LBD), a domain essential for receptor dimerization, and partial or complete deletion leads to absence of transcriptional activity [59]. ERα-A and ERα-B mRNA transcripts originating from the proximal promoter A and distal promoter B, respectively, have distinct 5' untranslated regions and their transcriptional activity is tissue-specific [57, 60-63]. Common to these two promoters is the absence of TATA- and CAAT-boxes consensus sequences. The ERα-C isoform, has an even different 5' untranslated exon, with specific localization to the liver [58]. All these isoforms were found to have their expression controlled by epigenetic mechanisms in the prostate, namely through methylation of the gene promoter region. Of the three isoforms, ERα-A and ERα-B expression could only be noticed upon treatment with a demethylation agent. This methylation pattern associated to each isoform suggests that each one plays a specific role in prostate carcinogenesis [64]. Likewise, all other isoforms present low expression levels in PCa cell lines. Nonetheless, this fact does not exclude the possibility that these isoforms could be key regulatory elements or interact with other protein factors, regulating gene expression patterns and hormone sensitivity in normal and malignant prostate tissues [59].

In what concerns ERβ, five different human mRNA isoforms have been identified (ERβ1-5), which either have truncation or insertion in the LBD [44, 65]. Some studies have been performed to determine the expression and role of these splice variants in prostate tissue. Initially, it was thought that all isoforms acted individually, but recent data show that they depend of each other to enhance their transactivation activities and exert their physiologic functions, although only ERβ1 displays a fully functional activity as an ER [66]. The ERβ2 isoform (ERβcx), a C-terminal truncated splice variant, has been evaluated. This isoform is inversely associated with the expression pattern of the wild type ERβ, i.e., ERβ2 has no significant immunoreactivity in benign prostate epithelial cells, but it is greatly expressed in malignant lesions. Furthermore, its expression correlates with increasing Gleason score and poor survival, indicating that ERβ2 may potentiate PCa progression [44].

Genetic Polymorphisms of ER and Prostate Cancer Risk

The presence of polymorphisms in a gene sequence may reflect the risk of disease development. Several polymorphisms in ERα and ERβ have been identified, but not all have been implicated in PCa development. One of these polymorphisms in the ERα gene, which differs significantly from healthy and tumour bearing individuals, is located in intron 1 (GGGA sequence) and it is apparently associated with increased PCa risk. The length of this repeated sequence in the ERα gene could possibly alter the ability to bind transcription factors, and therefore the receptor transcriptional activity [67]. The genotypes of ERα *PvuII* (C/C, C/T or T/T) and *XbaI* (A/A, A/G or G/G) polymorphisms in intron 2 were analyzed on a Japanese population. Of these, the T/T genotype of ERα *PvuII* increased the risk of PCa development [68]. Previously, the G/G genotype of *XbaI* polymorphism and C/C genotype of *PvuII* polymorphism were also associated with increased risk of PCa [69]. Finally, the detected genotypic alterations (C/C, T/T or T/C) in codon 10 of the first exon of ERα gene were also associated with higher susceptibility to develop PCa [70]. Regarding ERβ, several SNPs were evaluated using the population-based case-control study CAPS (Cancer Prostate in Sweden). The selected SNPs were genotyped and one SNP located in the promoter region (-13950 C/T) was found to be associated with increased PCa risk, suggesting a role of ERβ promoter in PCa aetiology [71].

Animal Models to Study Gene Expression

Several animal models have been used to conduct studies in order to understand the role of estrogens and ERs in PCa. Present data lead us to believe that estrogens have a major role in prostate development and pathophysiology. Nowadays, there are distinct animal models with altered estrogenic response, ERα knockout (αERKO), ERβ knockout (βERKO), and the double ERα and ERβ knockout (DERKO), and estrogens-deficiency, the aromatase knockout (ArKO). Each animal model displays a unique phenotype and its usage to understand the role of estrogens in prostate is of great value [72]. To what it is known, only the βERKO mice display an abnormal prostate phenotype. These mice tend to develop severe epithelial hyperplasia with increasing age and display higher expression of androgen receptor [73-75]. The characteristics of the ArKO model include augmented androgen serum levels and total absence of E_2, and have also the particularity of being enabled to develop PCa [76]. Using this model, researchers are able to determine the rate of *de novo* E_2 synthesis from testosterone, through aromatase pathway [77].

Effects of Estrogens in Cell Cycle and Invasion of Prostate Cancer

It has been established the importance of estrogens in the normal growth, differentiation and development of prostate as well as in the uncontrolled growth and transformation observed in PCa [78, 79]. Experimental animal models support the view that estrogens, alone or in combination with androgens are potent inducers of cell growth and differentiation in PCa [80, 81]. The administration of estrogens at pharmacological doses, alone or with androgens, results in the development of benign lesions, known as squamous metaplasia in the prostates of various mammalian species, including humans [82, 83]. The treatment of Noble rats with estrogens plus androgens promoted the appearance of a pre-cancerous lesion similar to PIN and a high incidence of prostatic adenocarcinomas [84, 85]. In addition, estrogens lead to progression of human PCa and metastasis at distant organs in nude mice treated with E_2 and testosterone and transplanted with a recombinant tissue composed of mouse mesenchyme and human prostatic epithelial cell line [86]. *In vitro* studies also referred that both androgen and estrogens affect proliferation of cultured PCa cells. More specifically, physiological concentrations of estrogens stimulate LNCaP cell proliferation, and may decrease in a dose-dependent manner the growth of PC3 cells [87, 88]. The mechanisms underlying the action of estrogens in PCa development involve several growth factors-dependent signalling pathways that promote aberrant cell growth, e.g., TGFα/EGF receptor [89]; TGFβ [90]; IGF-1 and VEGF [91], ER [92], prolactin-receptor [93] and mitogen-activated protein kinase (MAPK) activation [94]. Furthermore, estrogens appear to have a stimulatory effect in the Src/Raf-1/Erks signal transducing pathway in LNCaP cells, allowing PCa cell survival [95].

Evasion of apoptosis is another mechanism of estrogens action, in which estrogens promote the overexpression of anti-apoptotic mediators, such as metallothionein and TRPM-2/clusterin [96, 97]. In addition, changes in gene-expression profiles related to cell proliferation, DNA damage, activation of proto-oncogenes and transforming factors are well established in *in vivo* studies [98].

The effect of estrogens in controlling cell growth appears to be mainly receptor-mediated [88]. ERα and ERβ seem to exert opposite effects in prostate cell proliferation (Figure 2). ERα stimulation has been described to result in hyperplasia, inflammation and dysplasia of prostate, and ERα inhibition prevents PCa progression [99-101]. On the other hand, ERβ exerts an anti-proliferative effect in the prostate, directly or through ERα inhibition, and a loss of ERβ expression has been related with PCa progression [102]. *In vivo* studies using the βERKO mice showed that these animals develop prostatic hyperplasia with aging, which is not observed in wild-type or αERKO mice [103]. In addition, treatment of neonatal rats with diethylstilbesterol (DES) leads to prostatic hyperplasia and dysplasia, which probably results from ERα upregulation and ERβ downregulation [104]. *In vitro* studies are well correlated with these data, as in prostate cells, ERβ caused a marked reduction of proliferation [56]. This mechanism involves, besides the ER activation, the recruitment of specific co-regulators, the interaction of the complex with estrogen-responsive elements (EREs) on the DNA and subsequently the activation of target gene transcription [105]. Furthermore, ERα and ERβ can interact with other DNA binding sites, such as AP-1 and Sp-1, which may regulate gene transcription in opposite directions [105].

The estrogen-ER complex regulates a set of genes involved in cell proliferation and cell cycle progression. It has been described that estrogens may exert their mitogenic effects regulating cyclin D1 expression, which increased expression causes aberrant G1 to S transition and lead to cell cycle progression [106]. In LNCaP cells, which are androgen-dependent, it was observed that ERβ expression increases from the G1 to the S phase and decreases previously to entry in the G2/M phase, and ERβ can activate transcription via ERE during the S phase in a ligand-dependent manner. In addition, ERβ overexpression caused an arrest in early G1 with a decrease in c-Jun phosphorylation and cyclin D1 expression [107]. Others refer that estrogens induce the expression of Cyclin D1 via ERβ by increasing c-fos and c-jun expression in PC3 cells. In PCa tissues, cyclin D1 is overexpressed and it is positively correlated with ERβ expression, while ERα was almost undetectable [108]. Pravettoni et al. showed that E_2 or a ERβ selective agonist, diarylpropionitrile, decrease DU145 cell proliferation, which is accompanied by an increase of p21, a nuclear protein and a key point in control of cell cycle progression due to its effect inhibiting cyclin-dependent kinases [109]. Also, another study using a flavonoid, shows that genistein arrests the cell cycle at the G2/M phases and also suppresses cyclin B and p21, and p21 is induced via both p53-dependent and p53-independent pathways [110].

ERα and ERβ can also regulate cell proliferation through the activation of specific kinase activity, regulating EGFR and the activation of PI3K and MAPK signalling pathway, or induction of calcium influx [111-113]. Previously, we identified regucalcin (RGN), a calcium-binding protein that maintains intracellular calcium levels, as an ER regulated gene in human prostate cell line [114]. Moreover, it was observed that RGN levels are diminished in human cases of PCa [115]. These findings suggest that ER may have a role controlling PCa progression by regulating proteins, such as RGN, which are involved in maintenance of calcium homeostasis.

ERβ inhibits cell growth and invasiveness of PCa cells, and strongly stimulates apoptosis regulating the expression of Bax, Poly(ADP-ribose) polymerase and caspase-3 [56]. In addition, ERβ induces apoptosis via caspase-8 in prostatic stromal, luminal and castrate-resistant basal epithelial cells of ArKO mice, in Gleason score 7 xenografted tissues and in PC3 and DU145 PCa cell lines [116].

The upregulation of AIB1 expression, an ER co-regulator associated with cell proliferation stimuli and cell motility and invasion, was significantly correlated with lymph node metastasis of PCa [117]. AIB1 directly regulates the transcription of matrix metalloproteinase (MMP)-2 and MMP-13 [117]. Interestingly, E_2 treatment leads to MMP2 production through stimulation of TGFβ1 expression in prostatic stromal cells which in turn promotes PCa cell invasion [118].

Although the effects of estrogens are known to be mainly mediated by ERα and ERβ, other alternative mediators may play important actions in PCa progression. ERβ2 and ERβ5 isoforms are reported to promote metastasis and their expression was associated with shorter metastasis in patients with PCa [119]. Recently, G-protein-coupled receptor-30 (GPR30) was referred to have estrogens-binding affinity, regulating cell growth [120]. Activation of GPR30 by its specific ligand G-1, inhibits PCa cell growth by activating Erk1/2 and also c-jun and c-fos, which in turn upregulates p21 that mediates G2-M arrest, suggesting GPR30 as a novel mediator of estrogenic actions in the prostate [120].

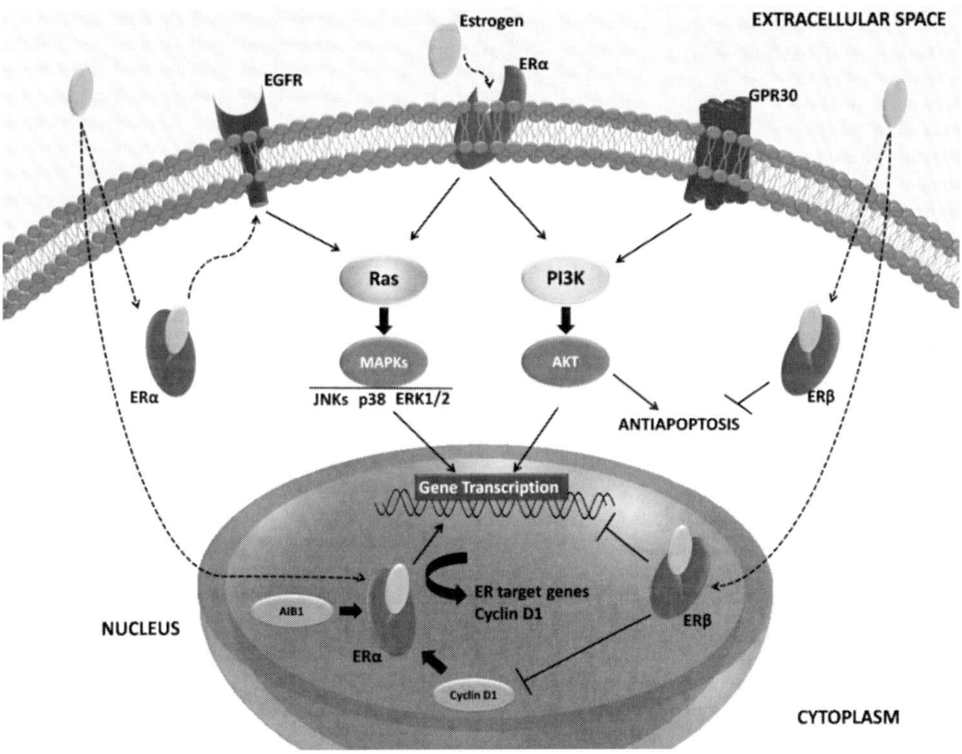

Figure 2. Schematic diagram of estrogen signalling in prostate cancer. Binding of Estrogen to the Estrogen Receptor α (ERα) promotes the translocation of this complex to the nucleus and the transcription of ER target genes along with a set of independent genes, including Cyclin D1. Estrogen-ERα complex also activates Ras-MAPK and PI3K signalling pathways, which in turn triggers cell proliferation and anti-apoptotic routes. Estrogen may stimulate the transcription of anti-apoptotic genes, via PI3K-AKT pathway, upon activation of G protein-coupled receptor 30 (GPR30). In addition, Cyclin D1 and AIB1 potentiate the transcription of ER-target genes. Contrarily, the binding of estrogen to ERβ seems to inhibit cell growth and anti-apoptotic events.

Estrogen Signalling as a Hallmark of Hormonal Therapy

The action of estrogenic therapeutic compounds has long been observed on several PCa cell lines, *in vivo* models and in clinical trials. From the two most expressed ER subtypes in prostate tissue, it is believed that only ERβ could mediate the anti-tumoural action in response to these compounds [52, 121]. Nonetheless, their action is not confined to restrain PCa development, when the tumour is only confined to the prostatic tissue, but also have anti-metastatic properties. The ultimate aim would be to prevent PCa by selectively induce apoptosis or restrain malignant cell proliferation, preferably by activation of ERβ signalling pathways avoiding undesirable side-effects. Nowadays, several new estrogenic/anti-estrogenic compounds are being studied.

Estrogens and Derivates

Estrogens-based hormonal therapy for PCa have been effectively used for over seventy years, since in 1941 Huggins et al. launched the first clinical trial to ascertain the effects of endocrine manipulation with the xenoestrogen, DES, in patients with advanced and metastatic prostate adenocarcinoma [122-124]. Since then, estrogens therapy became the standard treatment for PCa, minimally evolving for half a decade. The most commonly used was in fact 1-3mg of DES, but other compounds such as conjugated estrogens, poly-E_2 phosphate, ethinyl E_2, the synthetic estrogen chlorotrianisene or estramustine, a nor-nitrogen mustard carbamate derivate of E_2 phosphate were also considered. Although the majority of them presented mild to high toxicity, and the development of serious cardiovascular and thromboembolic complications, they showed relatively high efficacy on the treatment outcome, rivalling with those from surgical interventions [125]. Nonetheless, upon testing DES on a randomized controlled trial setting, its usage as a first-line medical treatment was discontinued on behalf of less toxic and equally effective agents [126]. Regardless, the European Organization for the Research and Treatment of Cancer (EORTC) established that 1mg of DES was effective and safe enough for clinical practices [127]. Several studies using cohorts of patients with advanced PCa recognized DES as an active drug and could still be seen as a useful treatment option, particularly when palliative chemotherapy is inappropriate or the life expectancy is poor [128-130]. The first proposed mechanism of action was based on a direct action of estrogens on the prostatic epithelium through the hypothalamic-pituitary axis by a negative feedback exerted on the pituitary, diminishing the secretion of gonadotropins leading to limited testicular testosterone production [123, 131]. Briefly, the hypothalamus production of the luteinizing hormone-releasing hormone (LHRH) induces the release of luteinizing hormone (LH) from the pituitary and consequently, the production of testosterone by the Leydig cells in testis [132]. Increasing estrogens levels exert a negative feedback on this pathway, impairing the release of LH and thus decreasing serum testosterone [123]. In the case of DES, a prolonged therapeutic approach will turn into a decline of serum LH levels and serum testosterone to a castrate level, due to irreversible damage of Leydig cells [133-135]. In fact, DES anti-tumoural effects do not involve just the direct regulation of androgen levels through negative feedback on the hypothalamic-pituitary axis, but also by induction of cytotoxicity [136]. More recently, DES was found to inhibit the activity of telomerase, synergistically with androgens in the case of the androgen-responsive LNCaP cells, disclosing a new possible therapeutic approach and showing that abolition of androgens is not always clinically beneficial [137]. Other estrogenic compounds are found to induce apoptosis through c-jun recruitment, increase the number of cells on the sub-G1 phase or by induction of death receptors, bind to tubulin causing microtubules depolymerization and impair cell cycle progression at G2/M phase [138-142].

Selective Estrogen Receptor Modulators (SERMs)

Selective ER modulators (SERMs) are synthetic compounds with weak estrogenic activity. According to the target tissue or cell, SERMs act either as agonists or antagonists, depending on the expression pattern of ERs and interaction with co-regulators that ultimately alter gene transcription [143, 144]. Different generations of SERMs have been used to suppress PCa progression, both on androgen- dependent and castration resistance stage. Pre-clinical studies using animal models revealed that SERMs such as toremifene and raloxifene tend to repress the androgen-dependent development of ventral prostate and seminal vesicles, reduce the appearance of HGPIN lesions and PCa incidence, as well as improve survival rates [99, 145]. Apparently, these effects are a reflection of ERα signalling activation and do not dependent on androgen action [99]. Usually, estrogens-based therapies are thought to be mediated by direct action on the hypothalamic-pituitary axis, inhibiting proliferation due to testosterone decline and preventing epigenetic silencing of anti-tumour genes. Nonetheless, several SERMs compounds act through pathways independent of this axis [5]. Their ability to suppress PCa development engages several events that ultimately culminate on anti-proliferative and pro-apoptotic activity [5, 146]. Accordingly, some of the described mechanisms of action include induction of apoptosis through increased nuclear fragmentation levels and induction of death receptors, proliferation arrest by inhibiting protein kinase C and induction of p21 (waf1/cip1) [121, 147, 148]. The differential expression of ERs is also central for SERMs action, as multiple signalling pathways leading to cell death and proliferation arrest are activated according to the expression levels of ERα and ERβ [149]. Recently, two novel SERMs were found to selectively activate ERβ, recruitment of TGFβ1 and members of the TNF family (Fas/Fas-L), increase of bax/bcl-2 ratio, decrease of ERα, AR and EGF receptor and impairment of IGF-I signalling and PARP cleaving [150]. The Food and Drug Administration (FDA) has approved the use of several SERMs in clinics. Unfortunately, these present some limitations and further studies are needed to undoubtedly prove that SERMs are the future for PCa prevention and as substitutes to DES in terms of efficiency [77, 151-156].

Phytoestrogens

Complementary and alternative medicine (CAM) strategies have been used for quite a while as potential adjuvant or alternative therapeutics on hormonal-dependent cancers, in order to improve the tolerance and efficacy of more conventional treatments [156]. Phytoestrogens are weak natural estrogens that display a similar structure to mammalian estrogens and can be found in a broad range of plants. These compounds are divided into three classes: isoflavones, flavones and lignans; being the isoflavones the most described and which major source is soybean, mainly in the form of genistein [155, 157]. Human diet has been pointed as an aetiological factor for PCa and the increased and widespread consumption of phytoestrogens provenient from soy appears to reduce the PCa risk [155, 158-160]. Studies suggest that genistein can activate ERβ, eliciting apoptosis or inhibiting cell proliferation and modulating genetic and epigenetic mechanisms [161-164]. Its ability to prevent PCa is believed to be achieved through downregulation of 5α-reductase, tyrosine-specific protein kinase, aromatase, and topoisomerase II activity and NF-κB activation, but also by increasing the levels of sex hormone-binding globulin, which decrease the free testosterone levels and induce G1 cell cycle arrest [155, 165-168]. Genistein induces the transcription of anti-angiogenic and anti-metastatic genes, as well as increases cell adhesion by stimulating the focal adhesion kinase pathway in PCa cells [169, 170]. Genistein is available in the market and it has been tested in clinical trials, although the results were not the most favourable [171]. Other phytoestrogens have been listed as PCa protectors, mostly by eliciting apoptosis and inhibiting proliferation [77, 172-174]. However, recent *in vivo* data produced contradictory effects of genistein compared to *in vitro*, requiring therefore a careful use [175-178]. Regardless of what is known, the use of CAMs for PCa prevention will require a more thorough control as they are usually unregulated commercially available formulations, with uncertain mechanisms of action, unconvincing safety, efficacy and effectiveness.

Conclusion

Estrogens are well known mitogenic agents whereas cancer is characterized by an uncontrolled cell proliferation and increased resistance to apoptosis. Thus, it is not surprising that several studies have pointed estrogens as players in prostate carcinogenesis. Several experimental studies showed that early exposure to estrogens predisposes individuals to later development of PCa and demonstrated the extremely genotoxic activity of several estrogens-derived metabolites. Moreover, the proliferative and anti-apoptotic role of ERα in prostate cells was defined. On the other hand, it was noticed that ERβ may act on prostate cells as an anti-proliferative agent and/or to favouring the apoptosis of PCa cells. Presently, experimentally and clinical evidences support the potential therapeutic application of estrogens-related targets which have a relevant role in prostate pathophysiology. Targeting the ERα and ERβ selectively, or in combination, with other anti-cancer molecules may represent a successful strategy as chemoprevention or treatment of PCa.

Funding

This work was partially supported by the COMPETE program (Pest-C/SAU/UI0709/2011) of Portuguese Foundation for Science and Technology (FCT). Inês Gomes and Cátia Vaz were funded by Banco Santander Totta and FCT fellowship (SFRH/BD/70316/2010), respectively.

References

[1] Hsing, AW; Chokkalingam, AP. Prostate cancer epidemiology. *Front Biosci*, 2006, 11, 1388-413.

[2] Bostwick, DG. et al. Human prostate cancer risk factors. *Cancer*, 2004, 101(10 Suppl), 2371-490.

[3] Simard, J. et al., Prostate cancer susceptibility genes, lessons learned and challenges posed. *Endocr Relat Cancer*, 2003, 10(2), 225-59.

[4] Carruba, G. Estrogen and prostate cancer, an eclipsed truth in an androgen-dominated scenario. *J Cell Biochem*, 2007, 102(4), 899-911.

[5] Ho, SM. et al., Estrogens and prostate cancer, etiology, mediators, prevention, and management. *Endocrinol Metab Clin North Am*, 2011, 40(3), 591-614, ix.

[6] Rajfer, J; Coffey, DS. Sex steroid imprinting of the immature prostate. Long-term effects. *Invest Urol*, 1978, 16(3), 186-90.

[7] Bonkhoff, H; Berges, R. The evolving role of oestrogens and their receptors in the development and progression of prostate cancer. *Eur Urol*, 2009, 55(3), 533-42.

[8] Salonia, A. et al. Circulating estradiol, but not testosterone, is a significant predictor of high-grade prostate cancer in patients undergoing radical prostatectomy. *Cancer*. 117(22), 5029-38.

[9] Yu, S. et al. 17-Beta-estradiol induces neoplastic transformation in prostatic epithelial cells. *Cancer Lett*. 304(1), 8-20.

[10] Ellem, SJ; Risbridger, GP. Aromatase and regulating the estrogen, androgen ratio in the prostate gland. *J Steroid Biochem Mol Biol*. 118(4-5), 246-51.

[11] Królik, M; Milnerowicz, H. The effect of using estrogens in the light of scientific research. Advances in Clinical and Experimental Medicine, *Official Organ Wroclaw Medical University*, 2012, 21(4), 535-543.

[12] Miller, WL. Molecular biology of steroid hormone synthesis. *Endocr Rev*, 1988. 9(3), 295-318.

[13] Labrie, F. Intracrinology. *Mol Cell Endocrinol*, 1991. 78(3), C113-8.

[14] Labrie, F. et al. History of LHRH agonist and combination therapy in prostate cancer. *Endocrine Related Cancer*, 1996. 3, p. 243-278.

[15] Labrie, F; Dupont, A; Belanger, A. Complete androgen blockade for the treatment of prostate cancer. *Important Adv Oncol*, 1985, 193-217.

[16] Labrie, F. et al. Is dehydroepiandrosterone a hormone? *J Endocrinol*, 2005, 187(2), 169-96.

[17] Takase, Y. et al., Expression of enzymes involved in estrogen metabolism in human prostate. *J Histochem Cytochem*, 2006. 54(8), 911-21.

[18] Ellem, SJ; Risbridger, GP. Aromatase and prostate cancer. *Minerva Endocrinol*, 2006. 31(1), 1-12.

[19] Matzkin, H; Soloway, MS. Immunohistochemical evidence of the existence and localization of aromatase in human prostatic tissues. *Prostate*, 1992, 21(4), 309-14.

[20] Rogan, EG; Cavalieri, EL. Estrogen metabolites, conjugates, and DNA adducts, possible biomarkers for risk of breast, prostate, and other human cancers. *Adv Clin Chem*, 2004. 38, 135-49.

[21] Schweikert, H-U. Estrogen in the Male, Nature, Sources, and Biological Effects Encyclopedia of Hormones, 2003, 584–591.
[22] Wilson, JD. Sexual differentiation. *Annu Rev Physiol*, 1978. 40, 279-306.
[23] Andersson, S; Russell, DW. Structural and biochemical properties of cloned and expressed human and rat steroid 5 alpha-reductases. *Proc Natl Acad Sci USA*, 1990. 87(10), 3640-4.
[24] Zhou, DJ; Pompon, D; Chen, SA. Structure-function studies of human aromatase by site-directed mutagenesis, kinetic properties of mutants Pro-308----Phe, Tyr-361----Phe, Tyr-361----Leu, and Phe-406----Arg. *Proc Natl Acad Sci USA*, 1991. 88(2), 410-4.
[25] Luu-The, V. Analysis and characteristics of multiple types of human 17beta-hydroxysteroid dehydrogenase. *J Steroid Biochem Mol Biol*, 2001. 76(1-5), 143-51.
[26] Simpson, ER; Davis, SR. Minireview, aromatase and the regulation of estrogen biosynthesis--some new perspectives. *Endocrinology*, 2001. 142(11), 4589-94.
[27] Mindnich, R; Moller, G; Adamski, J. The role of 17 beta-hydroxysteroid dehydrogenases. *Mol Cell Endocrinol*, 2004, 218(1-2), 7-20.
[28] El-Alfy, M. et al. Localization of type 5 17beta-hydroxysteroid dehydrogenase, 3beta-hydroxysteroid dehydrogenase, and androgen receptor in the human prostate by in situ hybridization and immunocytochemistry. *Endocrinology*, 1999. 140(3), 1481-91.
[29] Pelletier, G. et al. Immunocytochemical localization of type 5 17beta-hydroxysteroid dehydrogenase in human reproductive tissues. *J Histochem Cytochem*, 1999. 47(6), 731-8.
[30] Zhu, BT; Conney, AH. Functional role of estrogen metabolism in target cells, review and perspectives. *Carcinogenesis*, 1998. 19(1), 1-27.
[31] Cavalieri, E; et al. Estrogens as endogenous genotoxic agents--DNA adducts and mutations. *J Natl Cancer Inst Monogr*, 2000(27), 75-93.
[32] Martin, FL. et al. Constitutive expression of bioactivating enzymes in normal human prostate suggests a capability to activate pro-carcinogens to DNA-damaging metabolites. *Prostate*, 2010. 70(14), 1586-99.
[33] Tokizane, T. et al. Cytochrome P450 1B1 is overexpressed and regulated by hypomethylation in prostate cancer. *Clin Cancer Res*, 2005. 11(16), 5793-801.
[34] Ellem, SJ. et al., Local aromatase expression in human prostate is altered in malignancy. *J Clin Endocrinol Metab*, 2004. 89(5), 2434-41.
[35] Yager, JD; Davidson, NE. Estrogen carcinogenesis in breast cancer. *N Engl J Med*, 2006. 354(3), 270-82.
[36] Chang, BL. et al., Polymorphisms in the CYP1A1 gene are associated with prostate cancer risk. *Int J Cancer*, 2003. 106(3), 375-8.
[37] Nock, NL. et al., Polymorphisms in estrogen bioactivation, detoxification and oxidative DNA base excision repair genes and prostate cancer risk. *Carcinogenesis*, 2006. 27(9), 1842-8.
[38] Mononen, N. et al., Profiling genetic variation along the androgen biosynthesis and metabolism pathways implicates several single nucleotide polymorphisms and their combinations as prostate cancer risk factors. *Cancer Res*, 2006. 66(2), 743-7.
[39] Berney, D; Cheng, L. Prostate cancer, towards the standardization and synthesis of morphology, genetics, and prognosis. *Histopathology*. 60(1), 1-3.
[40] Joshua, AM. et al. Prostatic preneoplasia and beyond. *Biochim Biophys Acta*, 2008. 1785(2), 156-81.

[41] Kelloff, GJ; Sigman, CC. Cancer biomarkers, selecting the right drug for the right patient. *Nat Rev Drug Discov*. 11(3), 201-14.

[42] Edge, SB; Compton, CC. The American Joint Committee on Cancer, the 7th edition of the AJCC cancer staging manual and the future of TNM. *Ann Surg Oncol*. 17(6), 1471-4.

[43] Shapiro, E. et al. Immunolocalization of estrogen receptor alpha and beta in human fetal prostate. *J Urol*, 2005. 174(5), 2051-3.

[44] Fujimura, T. et al. Differential expression of estrogen receptor beta (ERbeta) and its C-terminal truncated splice variant ERbetacx as prognostic predictors in human prostatic cancer. *Biochem Biophys Res Commun*, 2001. 289(3), 692-9.

[45] Bonkhoff, H. et al. Estrogen receptor expression in prostate cancer and premalignant prostatic lesions. *Am J Pathol*, 1999, 155(2), 641-7.

[46] Linja, MJ; et al. Expression of ERalpha and ERbeta in prostate cancer. *Prostate*, 2003. 55(3), 180-6.

[47] Li, LC. et al. Frequent methylation of estrogen receptor in prostate cancer, correlation with tumor progression. *Cancer Res*, 2000. 60(3), 702-6.

[48] Enmark, E. et al. Human estrogen receptor beta-gene structure, chromosomal localization, and expression pattern. *J Clin Endocrinol Metab*, 1997. 82(12), 4258-65.

[49] Tsurusaki, T. et al. Zone-dependent expression of estrogen receptors alpha and beta in human benign prostatic hyperplasia. *J Clin Endocrinol Metab*, 2003. 88(3), 1333-40.

[50] Leav, I. et al. Comparative studies of the estrogen receptors beta and alpha and the androgen receptor in normal human prostate glands, dysplasia, and in primary and metastatic carcinoma. *Am J Pathol*, 2001. 159(1), 79-92.

[51] Fixemer, T; Remberger, K; Bonkhoff, H. Differential expression of the estrogen receptor beta (ERbeta) in human prostate tissue, premalignant changes, and in primary, metastatic, and recurrent prostatic adenocarcinoma. *Prostate*, 2003. 54(2), 79-87.

[52] Lau, KM. et al. Expression of estrogen receptor (ER)-alpha and ER-beta in normal and malignant prostatic epithelial cells, regulation by methylation and involvement in growth regulation. *Cancer Res*, 2000. 60(12), 3175-82.

[53] Horvath, LG. et al. Frequent loss of estrogen receptor-beta expression in prostate cancer. *Cancer Res*, 2001. 61(14), 5331-5.

[54] Pasquali, D. et al. Loss of estrogen receptor beta expression in malignant human prostate cells in primary cultures and in prostate cancer tissues. *J Clin Endocrinol Metab*, 2001. 86(5), 2051-5.

[55] Zhu, X. et al. Dynamic regulation of estrogen receptor-beta expression by DNA methylation during prostate cancer development and metastasis. *Am J Pathol*, 2004. 164(6), 2003-12.

[56] Cheng, J. et al. Expression of estrogen receptor beta in prostate carcinoma cells inhibits invasion and proliferation and triggers apoptosis. *FEBS Lett*, 2004. 566(1-3), 169-72.

[57] Grandien, K. et al. Estrogen target tissue determines alternative promoter utilization of the human estrogen receptor gene in osteoblasts and tumor cell lines. *Endocrinology*, 1995. 136(5), 2223-9.

[58] Grandien, K. Determination of transcription start sites in the human estrogen receptor gene and identification of a novel, tissue-specific, estrogen receptor-mRNA isoform. *Mol Cell Endocrinol*, 1996. 116(2), 207-12.

[59] Ye, Q. et al. Identification and characterization of estrogen receptor variants in prostate cancer cell lines. *J Steroid Biochem Mol Biol*, 2000. 75(1), 21-31.
[60] Keaveney, M. et al. Evidence for a previously unidentified upstream exon in the human oestrogen receptor gene. *J Mol Endocrinol*, 1991. 6(1), 111-5.
[61] Grandien, KF. et al. Localization of DNase I hypersensitive sites in the human oestrogen receptor gene correlates with the transcriptional activity of two differentially used promoters. *J Mol Endocrinol*, 1993. 10(3), 269-77.
[62] Green, S. et al. Human oestrogen receptor cDNA, sequence, expression and homology to v-erb-A. *Nature*, 1986. 320(6058), 134-9.
[63] White, R. et al. Structural organization and expression of the mouse estrogen receptor. *Mol Endocrinol*, 1987. 1(10), 735-44.
[64] Sasaki, M. et al. Methylation and inactivation of estrogen, progesterone, and androgen receptors in prostate cancer. *J Natl Cancer Inst*, 2002. 94(5), 384-90.
[65] Lewandowski, S; Kalita, K; Kaczmarek, L. Estrogen receptor beta. Potential functional significance of a variety of mRNA isoforms. *FEBS Lett*, 2002. 524(1-3), 1-5.
[66] Leung, YK. et al. Estrogen receptor (ER)-beta isoforms, a key to understanding ER-beta signaling. *Proc Natl Acad Sci U S A*, 2006. 103(35), 13162-7.
[67] Cancel-Tassin, G. et al. Association study of polymorphisms in the human estrogen receptor alpha gene and prostate cancer risk. *Eur Urol*, 2003. 44(4), 487-90.
[68] Suzuki, K. et al. Genetic polymorphisms of estrogen receptor alpha, CYP19, catechol-O-methyltransferase are associated with familial prostate carcinoma risk in a Japanese population. *Cancer*, 2003. 98(7), 1411-6.
[69] Modugno, F. et al. Allelic variants of aromatase and the androgen and estrogen receptors, toward a multigenic model of prostate cancer risk. *Clin Cancer Res*, 2001. 7(10), 3092-6.
[70] Tanaka, Y. et al. Polymorphisms of estrogen receptor alpha in prostate cancer. *Mol Carcinog*, 2003. 37(4), 202-8.
[71] Thellenberg-Karlsson, C; et al. Estrogen receptor beta polymorphism is associated with prostate cancer risk. *Clin Cancer Res*, 2006. 12(6), 1936-41.
[72] Weihua, Z; Warner, M; Gustafsson, JA. Estrogen receptor beta in the prostate. *Mol Cell Endocrinol*, 2002. 193(1-2), 1-5.
[73] Weihua, Z. et al. A role for estrogen receptor beta in the regulation of growth of the ventral prostate. *Proc Natl Acad Sci U S A*, 2001. 98(11), 6330-5.
[74] Cheng, G. et al., A role for the androgen receptor in follicular atresia of estrogen receptor beta knockout mouse ovary. *Biol Reprod*, 2002. 66(1), 77-84.
[75] Ogawa, S. et al. Abolition of male sexual behaviors in mice lacking estrogen receptors alpha and beta (alpha beta ERKO). *Proc Natl Acad Sci U S A*, 2000. 97(26), 14737-41.
[76] McPherson, SJ. et al. Elevated androgens and prolactin in aromatase-deficient mice cause enlargement, but not malignancy, of the prostate gland. *Endocrinology*, 2001. 142(6), 2458-67.
[77] Johnson, JJ. et al. Disruption of androgen and estrogen receptor activity in prostate cancer by a novel dietary diterpene carnosol, implications for chemoprevention. *Cancer Prev Res* (Phila), 2010. 3(9), 1112-23.
[78] Taplin, ME; Ho, SM. Clinical review 134, The endocrinology of prostate cancer. *J Clin Endocrinol Metab*, 2001. 86(8), 3467-77.

[79] Risbridger, GP. et al. Oestrogens and prostate cancer. *Endocr Relat Cancer*, 2003. 10(2), 187-91.
[80] Ho, SM. Estrogens and anti-estrogens, key mediators of prostate carcinogenesis and new therapeutic candidates. *J Cell Biochem*, 2004. 91(3), 491-503.
[81] Ricke, WA; Wang, Y; Cunha, GR. Steroid hormones and carcinogenesis of the prostate, the role of estrogens. *Differentiation*, 2007. 75(9), 871-82.
[82] Merk, FB. et al. Multiple phenotypes of prostatic glandular cells in castrated dogs after individual or combined treatment with androgen and estrogen. Morphometric, ultrastructural, and cytochemical distinctions. *Lab Invest*, 1986. 54(4), 442-56.
[83] Adams, JY. et al. Expression of estrogen receptor beta in the fetal, neonatal, and prepubertal human prostate. *Prostate*, 2002. 52(1), 69-81.
[84] Leav, I. et al. Biochemical alterations in sex hormone-induced hyperplasia and dysplasia of the dorsolateral prostates of Noble rats. *J Natl Cancer Inst*, 1988. 80(13), 1045-53.
[85] Ho, SM. et al. Induction of atypical hyperplasia, apoptosis, and type II estrogen-binding sites in the ventral prostates of Noble rats treated with testosterone and pharmacologic doses of estradiol-17 beta. *Lab Invest*, 1995. 73(3), 356-65.
[86] Ricke, WA. et al. Steroid hormones stimulate human prostate cancer progression and metastasis. *Int J Cancer*, 2006. 118(9), 2123-31.
[87] Carruba, G. et al. Estradiol inhibits growth of hormone-nonresponsive PC3 human prostate cancer cells. *Cancer Res*, 1994. 54(5), 1190-3.
[88] Castagnetta, LA. et al. Growth of LNCaP human prostate cancer cells is stimulated by estradiol via its own receptor. *Endocrinology*, 1995. 136(5), 2309-19.
[89] Kaplan, PJ. et al. Involvement of transforming growth factor alpha (TGFalpha) and epidermal growth factor receptor (EGFR) in sex hormone-induced prostatic dysplasia and the growth of an androgen-independent transplantable carcinoma of the prostate. *Carcinogenesis*, 1996. 17(12), 2571-9.
[90] Wong, YC; Xie, W; Tsao, SW. Structural changes and alteration in expression of TGF-beta1 and its receptors in prostatic intraepithelial neoplasia (PIN) in the ventral prostate of noble rats. *Prostate*, 2000. 45(4), 289-98.
[91] Wang, YZ; Wong, YC. Sex hormone-induced prostatic carcinogenesis in the noble rat, the role of insulin-like growth factor-I (IGF-I) and vascular endothelial growth factor (VEGF) in the development of prostate cancer. *Prostate*, 1998. 35(3), 165-77.
[92] Lau, KM; Leav, I; Ho, SM. Rat estrogen receptor-alpha and -beta, and progesterone receptor mRNA expression in various prostatic lobes and microdissected normal and dysplastic epithelial tissues of the Noble rats. *Endocrinology*, 1998. 139(1), 424-7.
[93] Leav, I. et al. Prolactin receptor expression in the developing human prostate and in hyperplastic, dysplastic, and neoplastic lesions. *Am J Pathol*, 1999. 154(3), 863-70.
[94] Leav, I. et al. Mitogen-activated protein kinase and mitogen-activated kinase phosphatase-1 expression in the Noble rat model of sex hormone-induced prostatic dysplasia and carcinoma. *Lab Invest*, 1996. 75(3), 361-70.
[95] Migliaccio, A. et al. Steroid-induced androgen receptor-oestradiol receptor beta-Src complex triggers prostate cancer cell proliferation. *Embo J*, 2000. 19(20), 5406-17.
[96] Ho, SM. et al. Lack of association between enhanced TRPM-2/clusterin expression and increased apoptotic activity in sex-hormone-induced prostatic dysplasia of the Noble rat. *Am J Pathol*, 1998. 153(1), 131-9.

[97] Ouyang, XS. et al. Up-regulation of TRPM-2, MMP-7 and ID-1 during sex hormone-induced prostate carcinogenesis in the Noble rat. *Carcinogenesis*, 2001. 22(6), 965-73.
[98] Tam, NN. et al. Gene expression profiling identifies lobe-specific and common disruptions of multiple gene networks in testosterone-supported, 17beta-estradiol- or diethylstilbestrol-induced prostate dysplasia in Noble rats. *Neoplasia*, 2008. 10(1), 20-40.
[99] Raghow, S. et al. Toremifene prevents prostate cancer in the transgenic adenocarcinoma of mouse prostate model. *Cancer Res*, 2002. 62(5), 1370-6.
[100] Ricke, WA. et al. Prostatic hormonal carcinogenesis is mediated by in situ estrogen production and estrogen receptor alpha signaling. *Faseb J*, 2008. 22(5), 1512-20.
[101] Ellem, SJ; Risbridger, GP. The dual, opposing roles of estrogen in the prostate. *Ann N Y Acad Sci*, 2009. 1155, 174-86.
[102] Imamov, O. et al. Estrogen receptor beta regulates epithelial cellular differentiation in the mouse ventral prostate. *Proc Natl Acad Sci U S A*, 2004. 101(25), 9375-80.
[103] Krege, JH. et al. Generation and reproductive phenotypes of mice lacking estrogen receptor beta. *Proc Natl Acad Sci U S A*, 1998. 95(26), 15677-82.
[104] Pylkkanen, L; Makela, S; Santti, R, Animal models for the preneoplastic lesions of the prostate. *Eur Urol*, 1996. 30(2), 243-8.
[105] Weihua, Z. et al. Update on estrogen signaling. *FEBS Lett*, 2003. 546(1), 17-24.
[106] Luo, Y, et al. 17beta-estradiol affects proliferation and apoptosis of rat prostatic smooth muscle cells by modulating cell cycle transition and related proteins. *Cell Biol Int*, 2008. 32(8), 899-905.
[107] Hurtado, A. et al. Estrogen receptor beta displays cell cycle-dependent expression and regulates the G1 phase through a non-genomic mechanism in prostate carcinoma cells. *Cell Oncol*, 2008. 30(4), 349-65.
[108] Nakamura, Y. et al. Cyclin D1 (CCND1) expression is involved in estrogen receptor beta (ERbeta) in human prostate cancer. *Prostate*, 2012. 73(6), 590-5.
[109] Pravettoni, A. et al. Estrogen receptor beta (ERbeta) and inhibition of prostate cancer cell proliferation, studies on the possible mechanism of action in DU145 cells. *Mol Cell Endocrinol*, 2007. 263(1-2), 46-54.
[110] Kobayashi, T; Nakata, T; Kuzumaki, T. Effect of flavonoids on cell cycle progression in prostate cancer cells. *Cancer Lett*, 2002. 176(1), 17-23.
[111] Zhang, Z. et al. Membrane association of estrogen receptor alpha mediates estrogen effect on MAPK activation. *Biochem Biophys Res Commun*, 2002. 294(5), 926-33.
[112] Song, RX; Zhang, Z; Santen, RJ. Estrogen rapid action via protein complex formation involving ERalpha and Src. *Trends Endocrinol Metab*, 2005. 16(8), 347-53.
[113] Kampa, M; Pelekanou, V; Castanas, E. Membrane-initiated steroid action in breast and prostate cancer. *Steroids*, 2008. 73(9-10), 953-60.
[114] Maia, CJ. et al. Regucalcin is expressed in rat mammary gland and prostate and down-regulated by 17beta-estradiol. *Mol Cell Biochem*, 2008. 311(1-2), 81-6.
[115] Maia, C. et al. Regucalcin is under-expressed in human breast and prostate cancers, Effect of sex steroid hormones. *J Cell Biochem*, 2009. 107(4), 667-76.
[116] McPherson, SJ. et al. Estrogen receptor-beta activated apoptosis in benign hyperplasia and cancer of the prostate is androgen independent and TNFalpha mediated. *Proc Natl Acad Sci U S A*, 2010. 107(7), 3123-8.

[117] Yan, J. et al. Steroid receptor coactivator-3/AIB1 promotes cell migration and invasiveness through focal adhesion turnover and matrix metalloproteinase expression. *Cancer Res*, 2008. 68(13), 5460-8.
[118] Yu, L. et al. Estrogens promote invasion of prostate cancer cells in a paracrine manner through up-regulation of matrix metalloproteinase 2 in prostatic stromal cells. *Endocrinology*, 2011. 152(3), 773-81.
[119] Leung, YK. et al. Estrogen receptor beta2 and beta5 are associated with poor prognosis in prostate cancer, and promote cancer cell migration and invasion. *Endocr Relat Cancer*, 2010. 17(3), 675-89.
[120] Chan, QK. et al. Activation of GPR30 inhibits the growth of prostate cancer cells through sustained activation of Erk1/2, c-jun/c-fos-dependent upregulation of p21, and induction of G(2) cell-cycle arrest. *Cell Death Differ*, 2010. 17(9), 1511-23.
[121] Kim, IY; et al. Raloxifene, a mixed estrogen agonist/antagonist, induces apoptosis in androgen-independent human prostate cancer cell lines. *Cancer Res*, 2002. 62(18), 5365-9.
[122] Huggins, C; Hodges, CV. Studies on prostatic cancer - I The effect of castration, of estrogen and of androgen injection on serum phosphatases in metastatic carcinoma of the prostate. *Cancer Research*, 1941. 1(4), 293-297.
[123] Huggins, C; Scott, WW; Hodges, CV. Studies on prostatic cancer III The effects of fever, of desoxycorticosterone and of estrogen on clinical patients with metastatic carcinoma of the prostate. *Journal of Urology*, 1941. 46(5), 997-1006.
[124] Huggins, C; Stevens, RE; Hodges, CV. Studies on prostate cancer II The effects of castration on advanced carcinoma of the prostate gland. *Archives of Surgery*, 1941. 43(2), 209-223.
[125] Cox, RL; Crawford, ED. Estrogens in the treatment of prostate cancer. *J Urol*, 1995. 154(6), 1991-8.
[126] Blackard, CE; et al. Incidence of cardiovascular disease and death in patients receiving diethylstilbestrol for carcinoma of the prostate. *Cancer*, 1970. 26(2), 249-56.
[127] Robinson, MR. EORTC protocol 30805, a phase III trial comparing orchidectomy versus orchidectomy and cyproterone acetate and low dose stilboestrol in the management of metastatic carcinoma of the prostate. *Prog Clin Biol Res*, 1988. 260, 101-10.
[128] Farrugia, D. et al. Stilboestrol plus adrenal suppression as salvage treatment for patients failing treatment with luteinizing hormone-releasing hormone analogues and orchidectomy. *BJU Int*, 2000. 85(9), 1069-73.
[129] Smith, DC. et al. A phase II trial of oral diethylstilbesterol as a second-line hormonal agent in advanced prostate cancer. *Urology*, 1998. 52(2), 257-60.
[130] Wilkins, A; et al. Diethylstilbestrol in castration-resistant prostate cancer. *BJU Int*. 110(11 Pt B), E727-35.
[131] Landstrom, M; Damber, JE; Bergh, A. Estrogen treatment postpones the castration-induced dedifferentiation of Dunning R3327-PAP prostatic adenocarcinoma. *Prostate*, 1994. 25(1), 10-8.
[132] Lipsett, MB. et al. Studies on Leydig cell physiology and pathology, secretion and metabolism of testosterone. *Recent Prog Horm Res*, 1966. 22, 245-81.

[133] Baker, HW. et al. Effects of synthetic oral oestrogens in normal men and patients with prostatic carcinoma, lack of gonadotrophin suppression by chlorotrianisene. *Clin Endocrinol* (Oxf), 1973. 2(4), 297-306.
[134] Tomic, R; Bergman, B. Hormonal effects of cessation of estrogen treatment for prostatic carcinoma. *J Urol*, 1987. 138(4), 801-3.
[135] Tomic, R; Bergman, B; Damber, JE. Testicular endocrine function after withdrawal of oestrogen treatment in patients with carcinoma of the prostate. *Br J Urol*, 1983. 55(1), 42-7.
[136] Schulz, P. et al. Evaluation of the cytotoxic activity of diethylstilbestrol and its mono- and diphosphate towards prostatic carcinoma cells. *Cancer Res*, 1988. 48(10), 2867-70.
[137] Geier, R. et al. The synthetic estrogen diethylstilbestrol (DES) inhibits the telomerase activity and gene expression of prostate cancer cells. *Prostate*, 2010. 70(12), 1307-12.
[138] Shimada, K. et al. Requirement of c-jun for testosterone-induced sensitization to N-(4-hydroxyphenyl)retinamide-induced apoptosis. *Mol Carcinog*, 2003. 36(3), 115-22.
[139] Dahllof, B. et al. Estramustine depolymerizes microtubules by binding to tubulin. *Cancer Res*, 1993. 53(19), 4573-81.
[140] Kumar, AP; Garcia, GE; Slaga, TJ. 2-methoxyestradiol blocks cell-cycle progression at G(2)/M phase and inhibits growth of human prostate cancer cells. *Mol Carcinog*, 2001. 31(3), 111-24.
[141] LaVallee, TM. et al. 2-methoxyestradiol up-regulates death receptor 5 and induces apoptosis through activation of the extrinsic pathway. *Cancer Res*, 2003. 63(2), 468-75.
[142] Qadan, LR. et al. 2-Methoxyestradiol induces G2/M arrest and apoptosis in prostate cancer. *Biochem Biophys Res Commun*, 2001. 285(5), 1259-66.
[143] Pickar, JH; MacNeil, T; Ohleth, K. SERMs, progress and future perspectives. *Maturitas*. 67(2), 129-38.
[144] Steiner, MS; Raghow, S. Antiestrogens and selective estrogen receptor modulators reduce prostate cancer risk. *World J Urol*, 2003. 21(1), 31-6.
[145] Neubauer, BL. et al. Endocrine and antiprostatic effects of raloxifene (LY156758) in the male rat. *Prostate*, 1993. 23(3), 245-62.
[146] Glienke, W. et al. Induction of apoptosis in human prostate stromal cells by 4-hydroxytamoxifen, an alternative therapy for benign prostate hyperplasia. *World J Urol*, 2004. 22(6), 452-6.
[147] Mor, G. et al. Regulation of fas ligand expression in breast cancer cells by estrogen, functional differences between estradiol and tamoxifen. *J Steroid Biochem Mol Biol*, 2000. 73(5), 185-94.
[148] Rohlff, C. et al. Prostate cancer cell growth inhibition by tamoxifen is associated with inhibition of protein kinase C and induction of p21(waf1/cip1). *Prostate*, 1998. 37(1), 51-9.
[149] Rossi, V. et al. Raloxifene induces cell death and inhibits proliferation through multiple signaling pathways in prostate cancer cells expressing different levels of estrogen receptor alpha and beta. *J Cell Physiol*, 2011. 226(5), 1334-9.
[150] Kumar, R. et al. Selective estrogen receptor modulators regulate stromal proliferation in human benign prostatic hyperplasia by multiple beneficial mechanisms--action of two new agents. *Invest New Drugs*, 2012. 30(2), 582-93.
[151] Kawashima, H. et al. Effect of anti-estrogens on the androgen receptor activity and cell proliferation in prostate cancer cells. *Urol Res*, 2004. 32(6), 406-10.

[152] Bhattacharyya, RS. et al. Fulvestrant (ICI 182,780) down-regulates androgen receptor expression and diminishes androgenic responses in LNCaP human prostate cancer cells. *Mol Cancer Ther*, 2006. 5(6), 1539-49.
[153] Chadha, MK. et al. Phase II study of fulvestrant (Faslodex) in castration resistant prostate cancer. *Prostate*, 2008. 68(13), 1461-6.
[154] Taneja, SS. et al. Toremifene--a promising therapy for the prevention of prostate cancer and complications of androgen deprivation therapy. *Expert Opin Investig Drugs*, 2006. 15(3), 293-305.
[155] Denis, L; Morton, MS; Griffiths, K. Diet and its preventive role in prostatic disease. *Eur Urol*, 1999. 35(5-6), 377-87.
[156] Sternberg, CN. et al. The medical management of prostate cancer, a multidisciplinary team approach. *BJU Int*, 2007. 99(1), 22-7.
[157] Price, KR; Fenwick, GR. Naturally occurring oestrogens in foods--a review. *Food Addit Contam*, 1985. 2(2), 73-106.
[158] Yan, L; Spitznagel, EL. Meta-analysis of soy food and risk of prostate cancer in men. *Int J Cancer*, 2005. 117(4), 667-9.
[159] Yan, L; Spitznagel, EL. Soy consumption and prostate cancer risk in men, a revisit of a meta-analysis. *Am J Clin Nutr*, 2009. 89(4), 1155-63.
[160] Hwang, YW. et al. Soy food consumption and risk of prostate cancer, a meta-analysis of observational studies. *Nutr Cancer*, 2009. 61(5), 598-606.
[161] Whitten, PL; Patisaul, HB. Cross-species and interassay comparisons of phytoestrogen action. *Environ Health Perspect*, 2001. 109 Suppl 1, 5-20.
[162] An, J. et al. Estrogen receptor beta-selective transcriptional activity and recruitment of coregulators by phytoestrogens. *J Biol Chem*, 2001. 276(21), 17808-14.
[163] Boue, SM. et al. Evaluation of the estrogenic effects of legume extracts containing phytoestrogens. *J Agric Food Chem*, 2003. 51(8), 2193-9.
[164] Molinie, B; Georgel, P. Genetic and epigenetic regulations of prostate cancer by genistein. *Drug News Perspect*, 2009. 22(5), 247-54.
[165] Matsukawa, Y. et al. Genistein arrests cell cycle progression at G2-M. *Cancer Res*, 1993. 53(6), 1328-31.
[166] Misra, RR. et al. Genotoxicity and carcinogenicity studies of soy isoflavones. *Int J Toxicol*, 2002. 21(4), 277-85.
[167] Shen, JC. et al. Low-dose genistein induces cyclin-dependent kinase inhibitors and G(1) cell-cycle arrest in human prostate cancer cells. *Mol Carcinog*, 2000. 29(2), 92-102.
[168] Davis, JN; Kucuk, O; Sarkar, FH. Genistein inhibits NF-kappa B activation in prostate cancer cells. *Nutr Cancer*, 1999. 35(2), 167-74.
[169] Li, Y; Sarkar, FH. Gene expression profiles of genistein-treated PC3 prostate cancer cells. *J Nutr*, 2002. 132(12), 3623-31.
[170] Liu, Y. et al. Focal adhesion kinase (FAK) phosphorylation is not required for genistein-induced FAK-beta-1-integrin complex formation. *Clin Exp Metastasis*, 2000. 18(3), 203-12.
[171] deVere White, RW. et al. Effects of a high dose, aglycone-rich soy extract on prostate-specific antigen and serum isoflavone concentrations in men with localized prostate cancer. *Nutr Cancer*. 62(8), 1036-43.

[172] Hawthorne, S; Gallagher, S. Effects of glycyrrhetinic acid and liquorice extract on cell proliferation and prostate-specific antigen secretion in LNCaP prostate cancer cells. *J Pharm Pharmacol*, 2008. 60(5), 661-6.

[173] Hsu, A. et al. Dietary soy and tea mitigate chronic inflammation and prostate cancer via NFkappaB pathway in the Noble rat model. *J Nutr Biochem*. 22(5), 502-10.

[174] Shenouda, NS. et al. Phytoestrogens in common herbs regulate prostate cancer cell growth in vitro. *Nutr Cancer*, 2004. 49(2), 200-8.

[175] Nakamura, H. et al. Genistein increases epidermal growth factor receptor signaling and promotes tumor progression in advanced human prostate cancer. *PLoS One*. 6(5), e20034.

[176] El Touny, LH; Banerjee, PP. Identification of a biphasic role for genistein in the regulation of prostate cancer growth and metastasis. *Cancer Res*, 2009. 69(8), 3695-703.

[177] Fischer, L. et al. Clinical characteristics and pharmacokinetics of purified soy isoflavones, multiple-dose administration to men with prostate neoplasia. *Nutr Cancer*, 2004. 48(2), 160-70.

[178] Pendleton, JM. et al. Phase II trial of isoflavone in prostate-specific antigen recurrent prostate cancer after previous local therapy. *BMC Cancer*, 2008. 8, 132.

In: Estradiol: Synthesis, Health Effects and Drug Interactions ISBN: 978-1-62808-962-2
Editors: Ricco Palmeri and Sal Grimaudo

Chapter 5

Hydroxyestradiols and Methoxyestradiols as Endogenous Factors Associated to Physiological and Physiopathological Conditions

***Alexis Parada-Bustamante*[1], *Pedro A. Orihuela*[2,3], *Cristián Molina*[1], *Hugo Cardenas*[2,3], *Patricia Reuquén*[2,3], *Cecilia Valencia*[1] *and Ramiro Rincón*[2,3]**

[1]Instituto de Investigaciones Materno-Infantil, Facultad de Medicina, Universidad de Chile
[2]Laboratorio de Inmunología de la Reproducción, Facultad de Química y Biología, Universidad de Santiago de Chile and
[3]Centro para el Desarrollo en Nanociencia y Nanotecnología, Chile

Abstract

Estradiol (E_2) is a steroidal hormone generated by the conversion of testosterone via the p450 aromatase enzymatic complex. The E_2 physiological actions are mainly mediated by its interaction with intracellular receptors known as estrogen receptors (ERs). The E_2-ERs complex is able to alter the gene expression in its target cells binding to specific sequences in the DNA. Besides, estrogens can also activate several intracellular signal transduction cascades (e.g., cAMP-PKA, IP3-Ca^{2+}) by non-genomic mechanisms.

Following to exert its biological effects in their target tissues, E_2 must be inactivated and eliminated by the body through its conversion to soluble compounds with a insignificant or very low estrogenic activity. These reactions are accomplished by several enzymatic processes that involve reactions of oxidations and conjugations. The enzymatic modifications that a molecule of E_2 undergoes to be eliminated include sulfonations, O-methylations, hydroxylations and glucurodinations. Even though the conversion of E_2 to inactive or less active metabolites occurs mainly in the liver, it has been reported that some peripheral tissues, including breast, uterus, placenta and brain, express the enzymes required to inactive E_2.

One of the most studied enzymatic pathways that inactive estradiol in peripheral tissues consists in a C-2 hydroxylation, a reaction catalyzed by the enzyme cytochrome p450, isoform 1A1 (CYP1A1), that generates a molecule of 2-hydroxyestradiol ($2OHE_2$) and the C-4 hydroxylation, a reaction catalyzed by the enzyme CYP1B1 that generates 4-hydroxyestradiol ($4OHE_2$). Then, the hydroxyl group previously added is replaced by a methyl group through a conjugation reaction catalyzed by the enzyme Catechol-O-Methyltransferase (COMT), which originates a molecule of 2- methoxyestradiol ($2ME_2$) from $2OHE_2$ and 4-methoxyestradiol ($4ME_2$) from $4OHE_2$.

Recently, it has been demonstrated that hydroxyestradiols and methoxyestradiols are not inactive molecules since several reports have shown that these estradiol metabolites may exert physiological actions in different organs and tissues, while an unbalanced estradiol metabolization to hydroxyestradiols and methoxyestradiols could be the responsible factor of several diseases including cancer and preeclampsia. In this chapter we will review the available literature concerning to the physiological effects that hydroxyestradiols and methoxyestradiols exert in several organs and how an altered production of hydroxyestradiols or methoxyestradiols could have deleterious effects on several biological functions. We will specially discuss the possible physiological and physiopathological effects of $2ME_2$ in female reproductive tissues, where this estradiol metabolite is able to alter the ovum transport and change the gene expression profile. Particularly, we will describe a group of $2ME_2$-induced genes in the mouse uterus that could be useful as biomarkers to elucidate the role of $2ME_2$ in the female reproductive tract.

Keywords: Hydroxyestradiol, Methoxyestradiol, physiology, physiopathology, reproductive tissues, gene expression

Introduction

Estradiol (E_2) exerts biological actions in several organs, including testis (Carreau et al., 2011), ovary (Drummond and Fuller, 2012), uterus (Groothuis et al., 2007), bone (Khosla et al., 2012), brain (Brown et al., 2009) and in the vascular system (Leung et al., 2007). The mechanisms by which E_2 regulates cell functioning involve its binding to the estrogen receptor α (ERα) and/or β (ERβ), forming a complex that change gene expression (Cheskis et al., 2007). In the last years, it has been also reported that E_2 may alter the functioning of its target cells activating several intracellular signal transduction cascades (e.g., cAMP-PKA, IP3-Ca^{2+}) by non-genomic mechanisms (Raz et al., 2008; Coleman and Smith, 2001).

Following to exert their biological effects, E_2 must be inactivated by its biotransformation to less estrogenic compounds. Four are most known enzymatic modifications that a molecule of E_2 undergoes to be inactivated. These are sulfonations, reactions catalyzed by several estrogen sulfotransferases enzymes; O-methylations, a reaction catalyzed by the enzyme Catechol-O-Methyltransferase; hydroxylations, reactions catalyzed by several cytochrome P450s isoforms enzymes; and glucurodinations, catalyzed by UDP-glucuronosyltransferases enzymes (reviewed in Zhu and Conney, 1998).

Although the conversion of E_2 to inactive metabolites occurs mainly in the liver, some peripheral tissues including breast, uterus, placenta and brain express the enzymes required to inactive estradiol (Tsuchiya et al., 2005). The most studied enzymatic pathways that inactive

E_2 consists in the subsequent conversion of E_2 to hydroxyestradiol and then to methoxyestradiol. These reactions involve a first oxidation in one of the 18 carbons that conforms the aromatic A-ring of estradiol, catalyzed by isoforms of the enzyme Cytochrome p450, which originates a molecule of hydroxyestradiol. Then, the hydroxyl group previously added is replaced by a methyl group (although in some cases, the methyl group may be added in other carbon), through a conjugation reaction catalyzed by the enzyme Catechol-O-Methyltransferase, which originates a molecule of methoxyestradiol (Zhu and Conney, 1998).

According to the literature, in peripheral tissues E_2 is mainly hydroxylated at two specific sites. The C-2 hydroxylation, a reaction catalyzed by the enzyme cytochrome p450, isoform 1A1 (CYP1A1), that generates a molecule of 2-hydroxyestradiol ($2OHE_2$) and the C-4 hydroxylation, a reaction catalyzed by the enzyme CYP1B1 that generates 4-hydroxyestradiol ($4OHE_2$) (Dawling et al., 2004). Due to hydroxyestradiols are highly reactive, they are then transformed to methoxyestradiols in peripheral tissues by the action of the enzyme Catechol-O-Methyltransferase (COMT), which generates 2-methoxyestradiol ($2ME_2$) from $2OHE_2$ and 4-methoxyestradiol ($4ME_2$) from $4OHE_2$. COMT has two active isoforms, a cytoplasmic soluble form (S-COMT) and a membrane-bound form (MB-COMT); this latter is anchored to the cytosolic side of the rough endoplasmic reticulum. Both isoforms are identical, except by an N-terminal extension of 50 amino acids in the amino-terminal in M-COMT, which is responsible to its anchorage to the membrane of the endoplasmic reticulum (Mannisto and Kaakkola, 1999).

When hydroxyestradiols and methoxyestradiols were characterized, they were catalogued as inactive molecules without a biological role; however, in the last years, it has been demonstrated that hydroxyestradiols and methoxyestradiols may exert physiological actions in different organs and tissues, while an unbalanced E_2 metabolization to hydroxyestradiols and methoxyestradiols could be the responsible factor of several diseases including cancer and preeclampsia. In the first part of this chapter, we will review the role of these E_2 metabolites in testis, ovary, placenta, oviduct and vascular system. We will perform a special review of their effects in the uterus, where $2ME_2$ changes the expression of several genes in the mouse, which could be useful as biomarkers to elucidate the role of $2ME_2$ in the female reproductive tract. Finally we will review the reason because high intracellular hydroxyestradiols levels are considered as relevant etiologic factors for different kind of cancers, while 2-methoxyestradiol has emerged as a promissory therapeutic treatment for this disease.

Effects of Hydroxyestradiols and Methoxyestradiols on Gonads and Gametes

Effects on Testis and Spermatozoa

Estradiol is normally produced in the testis from Testosterone by the action of Aromatase enzyme, which is expressed in Leydig, Sertoli, and also in Germ cells (Lardone et al., 2010). Besides to regulate the hypothalamus–pituitary–testis axis, E_2 produced in the testis would exert physiological effects directly in this organ, regulating the expression of steroidogenic enzymes in Leydig cells (Houk et al., 2004), and regulating some spermatogenic processes, such as proliferation of germ cells and differentiation of spermatids (Carreau et al., 2011).

Testicular expression and enzymatic activity of the proteins responsible to produce hydroxyestradiols and methoxyestradiols has been reported in several mammalian species. CYP1B1 expression was reported in human (Sutter et al., 1994; Shimada et al., 1996; Nishimura et al., 2003) and rat (Leung et al., 2009, Deb et al., 2010), while CYP1A1 has been detected at low levels in human (Nishimura et al., 2003), mouse (Choudhary et al., 2003), and rat (Revel et al., 2001). Finally, expression and/or activity of COMT protein have been reported in mouse (Øverbye and Seglen, 2009) and human (Axelrod and Goldzieher, 1962; Vargas et al., 2012).

The biological effects of methoxyestradiols and hydroxyestradiols in mammalian testis reported in the literature are scarce. Although no effects have been described to methoxyestradiols, hydroxyestradiols inhibit the enzymatic activity of soluble adenylate cyclase in germ cells (Braun, 1990) and also inhibit gonadotropin-stimulated testosterone production in Leydig cells (Stammel et al., 1991). On the other hand, it has been reported that certain physiological stimulus affects the expression of CYP1B1 in some testicular cell types. For example, Deb et al. (2011) determined that Luteinizing hormone increased CYP1B1 expression in Leydig cells in a PKA-dependent pathway (Deb et al., 2011), while some agonists of the aryl hydrocarbon receptor (whose activation mediates a significant increase of CYP1B1 expression in different cell systems) were unable to change CYP1B1 expression in Leydig cells (Deb et al., 2010).

Even though is not clear the role of these E_2 metabolites in testicular physiology, studies carried out in animal models and humans indirectly have showed that a disarranged intra-testicular enzymatic pathway that produce hydroxyestradiol and methoxyestradiol, which would favor an increased intra-testicular concentrations of hydroxyestradiols, may be involved in the development of male infertility. For instance, sea urchin spermatozoa (Dendraster excentricus) exposed to $4OH_2$ suffered damage in their DNA by an increased intracellular reactive oxygen species production (Rempel et al., 2009). Moreover, the spermatozoa of this invertebrate incubated with $4OH_2$ had a decreased capability to fertilize, and those spermatozoa that were capable to fertilize an ovum, generated an offspring with a high rate of phenotypical abnormalities (Rempel et al., 2009). In addition, human spermatozoa incubated *in vitro* with $2OHE_2$ or $4OHE_2$ during 15 minutes significantly increased their intracellular levels of reactive oxygen species, while incubation by 2 hours generated a complete loss of spermatozoa motility (Bennetts et al., 2008). In this same study, $2OHE_2$, but not $4OHE_2$ induced damage in DNA spermatozoa (Bennetts et al., 2008). Interestingly, a recent study of our laboratory showed that high doses of both $2OHE_2$ and $2ME_2$ decreased viability of TM4 cells, a non-tumorigenic cell line obtained from mouse Sertoli cells (Molina et al., 2012) by independent cellular mechanisms; given that only $2OHE_2$ generates cell death increasing intracellular reactive oxygen species followed by activation of a caspases-dependent apoptotic process, while $2ME_2$ induces death of TM4 cells by unidentified mechanisms so far (Molina et al., 2012).

Regarding to the possible direct negative effects of hydroxyestradiols in testicular tissue, Seegers et al. (1991) determined that a daily injection to male rats with low doses of $2OHE_2$ or $4OHE_2$ induced a marked damage in the morphology of germ cells, seven days after starting the treatment. Interestingly, the effects induced by $4OHE_2$ and $2OHE_2$ would be attributable to a direct negative effect on Leydig cells more than an effect on hypothalamic-pituitary-gonadal axis, given that these estradiol metabolites decreased serum testosterone levels without alter gonadotropin serum levels. Furthermore, the fact that testis from patients with maturation arrest and Sertoli cell only syndrome have a high level of lipid peroxidation, probably by overproduction of reactive oxygen species (Koksal et al., 2003) may indicate that this damage is mediated by an increased intra-testicular concentration of hydroxyestradiols.

In summary, although the physiological actions of hydroxyestradiols and methoxyestradiols inside the testis are not clear, a disarranged intra-testicular production of hydroxyestradiols and/or methoxyestradiols may be related with the development of the male infertility; however, more studies must be performing in order to elucidate this point.

Effects on Ovary and Oocytes

In the last years, it has been proposed that $2OHE_2$ and $2ME_2$ may have important roles in ovarian physiology. According to the literature, CYP1A1 and COMT are present in the human ovary (Zhu and Conney, 1998). Moreover, the plasma levels of $2ME_2$ and $2OHE_2$ are higher in the luteal than in follicular phase in the menstrual cycle of women (Mueck and Seeger, 2010) and the levels of these estradiol metabolites in follicular fluid is directly correlated with the follicle size in pigs (Bianchi et al., 2007). In contrast to the reported effects of these estradiol metabolites into most other tissues, in ovary $2OHE_2$ would participate in physiological actions, whereas an increased level of $2ME_2$ would be associated with pathological conditions.

Regarding to $2OHE_2$, this E_2 metabolite would have a role during follicular development, mainly in the selection of the dominant follicle (Spicer and Hammond, 1988). As follicle develops, the expression and activity of CYP1A1 is increased, concomitantly with the concentration of $2OHE_2$ (Bianchi et al., 2007). Moreover, $2OHE_2$ stimulates steroidogenesis in pig granulosa cells, showing an additive effect in progesterone synthesis in the presence of gonadotrophins, acting via cyclic AMP-mediated pathway, which is an important regulatory mechanism during follicular development (Spicer and Hammond, 1989).

On the other hand, an excessive intracellular production of $2ME_2$ could be involved in the follicular arrest observed in women with polycystic ovarian syndrome (PCOS), since granulosa cells incubated *in vitro* in a culture medium that mimic a PCOS environment (hyperandrogenism, hyperinsulinism) increased the expression of COMT, whereas these cells increased its proliferation rate and its steroidogenesis capacity in the presence of a COMT inhibitor (Salih et al., 2008). This latter phenomenon is related with the fact that high levels of $2ME_2$ had an inhibitory effect on granulosa cell proliferation (Salih et al., 2008). The mechanisms by which the intra-ovarian levels of $2OHE_2$ or $2ME_2$ could be increased in pathological conditions might involve exposure to environmental pollutants, which increase COMT activity (Karpeta et al., 2012) or CYP1A1 expression (Mizuyachi et al., 2002) in ovarian tissue.

According to the few studies performed so far, oocyte exposure to $2ME_2$ and $2OHE_2$ would have opposite effects on oocyte maturation and early embryo development. While $2ME_2$ would exert negative actions in these processes, $2OHE_2$ would favor oocyte *in vitro* maturation. Regarding to $2ME_2$, Lattanzi et al. (2003) determined that cumulus-enclosed bovine oocytes exposed to high doses of this metabolite (higher than 3 μM) did not affect significantly the cleavage rate, but it was related with an altered embryo development, since the blastocyst formation rate of oocytes exposed to $2ME_2$ and then fertilized *in vitro* was significantly lower compared to control oocytes. Furthermore, Eichenlaub-Ritter et al. (2007) showed that denuded mouse oocytes exposed only to high concentrations of $2ME_2$ (higher than 2.5 μM) during *in vitro* maturation caused hyperploidy of metaphase II oocytes, probably inducing spindle aberrations and chromosome congression failure. In this latter study, the effects on embryo development in oocytes exposed to lower doses of 2ME2 were not explored.

Regarding to $2OHE_2$, the knowledge so far about the effects of this estradiol metabolite on oocyte *in vitro* maturation and early embryo development is limited. Mishra and Joy (2006a and 2006b) determined that $2OHE_2$ induces oocyte maturation in the catfish *Heteropneustes fossilis*. To our understanding, no studies have been performed to explore the role of $2OHE_2$ on oocyte *in vitro* maturation and early embryo development in mammalians.

Effects of Hydroxyestradiols and Methoxyestradiols in Female Reproductive Tissues

Effects on Fallopian Tube

The mammalian oviduct is a tubular organ mainly composed of an intrinsic smooth muscle layer, the myosalpinx and an innermost highly folded mucosa (epithelial and stromal cells), the endosalpynx. Along the oviduct there are differences in the distribution of smooth muscle cells and the degree of folding and cellular composition of the mucosa (reviewed in Croxatto, 1996). This arrangement provides an optimal microenvironment for fertilization, gamete transport and preimplantation embryo development. It is generally accepted that ovarian hormones play a physiological role in the regulation of ovum transport in the rat. Evidence shows that E_2 shortens the passage of the oocytes or embryos along the oviduct from the normal 72-96 hours to only 24 hours (Parada-Bustamante et al., 2007). This phenomenon is known as acceleration of the oviductal egg transport induced by E_2 and the cellular and molecular mechanisms have been widely elucidated in several publications of our group (Reviewed in Orihuela et al., 2013). In this context, we have determined that $2ME_2$ is part of the E_2 nongenomic signaling that accelerates oviductal egg transport only in unmated rats (Parada-Bustamante et al., 2007, 2010), and interestingly $2ME_2$ requires activation of the ER to exerts its effect on the oviduct. On the other hand, Lattanzi et al., (2003) noted that $2ME_2$ inhibits blastocyst development when it is added in the mature oocyte stage showing a role of this metabolite in the regulation of fertilization and embryo development. Thus, $2ME_2$ is able to regulate different biological functions along the oviduct although the physiological relevance of these effects remains undisclosed.

Effects in the Uterus

The uterus is an organ made up of two layers, a thick outer, the myometrium; and an inner and thinner, the endometrium. Myometrium is constituted by smooth muscle cells, while endometrium is composed of luminal epithelium cells and a fibromuscular stroma penetrated by glands. This organ undergoes changes in tissue architecture depending on the cyclic steroid hormones produced by the ovary. For example, ovarian hormones at the preovulatory stage produce endometrial stromal edema in mice, followed by luminal epithelial cell proliferation 16 hours later (Fazleabas, 2007).

The uterus is one of the extrahepatic tissues that express CYP1A1, CYP1B1 and COMT (Desaulniers et al., 2005; Salih et al., 2008; Hevir et al., 2011). In humans, CYP1B1 is more expressed than CYP1A1 (Hevir et al., 2011), whereas COMT is located in myometrial (Wentz et al., 2006) and endometrial tissue (Casey and MacDonald, 1983; Salih et al., 2008). Regarding to human endometrial tissue, both COMT isoforms (S-COMT and M-COMT) are expressed during the menstrual cycle, while S-COMT isoform seems to have a cycle-dependent phase-specific regulation with highest and lowest immunoreactivity during the proliferative and mid secretory phase respectively (Salih et al., 2008) suggesting up regulation by estrogen and down regulation by progesterone.

Although hydroxyestradiols and methoxyestradiols would participate in endometrial shedding (Zhang and Davis, 1992) and uterine vascular tone (Jobe et al., 2013a) regulating prostaglandin secretion in uterus; it is clear that these metabolites would not mediate the classical "estrogenic" actions in this organ. In accordance to this concept, ovariectomized rats exposed to a continuous release of 1 μg/h of $2ME_2$, using a subcutaneously implanted osmotic pump, did not have trophic effects on the uterus (Martucci and Fishman, 1979). Furthermore, Rincón-Rodriguez et al. (2013) have shown that $2ME_2$ 0.1-10 μg/mice injected intraperitoneally during seven days did not change the wet weight and the height of the epithelial cells from endometrium of prepuberal mice. In contrast, Sibonga et al. (2003) observed that doses between 20 - 40 mg/kg/day subcutaneously administered produced uterine hypertrophy and increased uterine epithelial thickness. It is likely that the type of administration or the doses used influences these divergent responses.

Endometriosis affects 10% of premenopausal women (Davis and McMillan, 2003; Bulun, 2009); however, the pathogenesis of this condition is not clearly understood. Singh et al. (2008) reported the expression of CYP1A1 and CYP1B1 in eutopic and ectopic endometrium from women with endometriosis, while $2ME_2$ induces suppression of growth and angiogenesis of endometriotic lesions in a female mice endometriosis model (Becker et al., 2008). These results suggest that an altered local production of hydroxyestradiols and methoxyestradiols in the uterus, which decreases local $2ME_2$ production in ectopic endometrium, may be the factor that promotes the survival of this tissue in women with endometriosis.

$2ME_2$ Changes Gene Expression in Mouse Uterus

Microarray analysis is a useful tool to establish gene expression profiling in several tissues and organs. In order to explore how $2ME_2$ participates in the physiology of the female reproductive tract, we firstly determined whether $2ME_2$ has estrogenic activity in the ovarian and uterus of prepuberal mice. We found that $2ME_2$ did not increase the uterine wet weight and the epithelial cell height of immature mice, while $2ME_2$ mimicked the effect of E_2 on the ovarian weight and on the follicular maturation. This suggests that the differences in the sensitivity between E_2-target organs to $2ME_2$ could reflect different mechanisms of action of this metabolite. Then, we described for the first time a group of genes induced by $2ME_2$ that could be useful to elucidate how $2ME_2$ regulates complex physiological process accomplished by an entire organ composed of diverse cell phenotypes. Since this group of genes only correspond to the 0.23% from the total of analyzed genes it is probable that the effects of $2ME_2$ involve a fine-tuning on the uterine tissues. Interestingly, a group of genes (0.04%) was regulated by $2ME_2$, but not by E_2, suggesting that $2ME_2$ uses intracellular signalling pathways independently of E_2 (Rincón-Rodriguez et al., 2013). These results reinforce the notion that $2ME_2$ uses a novel ER-independent mechanism similar to selective estrogen receptor modulators responsible to confer its tissue selective actions (Maran et al., 2002; Turner et al., 1998). Therefore, $2ME_2$ regulates a group of genes in the mice uterus independently of estrogenic activity, suggesting a functional involvement of $2ME_2$ in the mammalian uterus (Rincón-Rodriguez et al., 2013).

Effects of Methoxyestradiols in Placentation

Preeclampsia is a maternal endothelial dysfunction that generates hypertension, proteinuria and placental hypoxia during pregnancy (Sibai et al., 2005). This condition affects approximately 5% all pregnancies worldwide (Sibai et al., 2005) and it is associated with maternal and perinatal morbidity and mortality (Chesley, 1985; Roberts et al., 1989) perinatal deaths, preterm birth and intrauterine growth foetal restriction (Sibai et al., 2005).

'Angiogenic imbalance' theory postulates that preeclampsia is the result of a disequilibrium between expression and/or actions of pro and anti-angiogenic factors, which generates a poor trophoblastic invasion and incomplete spiral artery remodelling during early pregnancy (Dragun and Haase-Fielitz, 2009; Shenoy et al., 2010). In the latest years, it has been proposed that a decreased $2ME_2$ serum levels during mild pregnancy is one of the main anti-angiogenic factors deregulated in patients with preeclampsia, because of 1) Female mice that do not express COMT (knockout animals) have a similar sintomatology during pregnancy that women with preeclampsia (Kanasaki et al., 2008) and these symptoms are reversed when these mice received a daily dose of $2ME_2$ from day 10 of the pregnancy until labor (Kanasaki et al., 2008); 2) $2ME_2$ is a potent anti-angiogenic factor (Pribluda et al., 2000) and 3) E_2, $2OHE_2$ and $2ME_2$ serum levels in women with mild or severe preeclampsia are significantly lower in comparison to those found in normotensive pregnant women (Jobe et al., 2013b).

Even though the mechanisms by which $2ME_2$ mediates a correct placentation process have not been completely elucidated, it is postulated that $2ME_2$ would mediate mainly their effects down-regulating hypoxia-inducible factor 1 alpha (HIF-1α) protein expression in placental tissue, a hypothesis supported by the elegant experiments of Lee et al., using the human cytotrophoblast cell line HTR-8 (Lee et al., 2010). HIF-1α is a transcription factor whose expression is normally increased under hypoxic conditions and it would have an important role during early placentation (Caniggia et al., 2000), when their levels are highly increased by the hypoxic environment at this stage (Lee et al., 2010); however, the HIF-1α levels must be then down-regulated during mild placentation process. This latter is supported by the fact of HIF-1α overexpression in pregnant mice was associated with fetal intrauterine growth restriction, decreased placental weights, and histopathological placental abnormalities similar to those found in women with preeclampsia (Tal et al., 2010). Moreover, HIF-1α protein levels are highly increased in the placenta of preeclamptic women compared to normotensive pregnant women (Nishi et al., 2004). The mechanisms by which abnormally high HIF-1α expression levels are associated with preeclampsia would involve increased production of transforming growth factor β3 (TGF β3), followed by increased synthesis of soluble receptor-1 VEGF (sVEGFR1), which blocks VEGF signal transduction and consequently worsen placental perfusion (Vuorela et al., 2000).

The mechanisms by which women with preeclampsia generate lower $2ME_2$ levels may involve a decrease in the expression and or activity of M-COMT and S-COMT in the placenta (Kanasaki et al., 2008, Pérez-Sepúlveda et al., 2013). According to several reports, one of the pathways by which some individuals may generate lower $2ME_2$ levels may involve intrinsic genetic differences in COMT gene. The human COMT gene is located on chromosome 22, where it codes to S-COMT and M-COMT (Mannisto and Kaakkola, 1999). It has been reported that human COMT gene have several polymorphic sites, which are associated with higher or lesser COMT protein expression and/or COMT enzymatic activity. For instance, COMT gene contains several single nucleotide polymorphisms (SNPs), being one of the most studied the SNPs rs4680, which determines a G/A transition (codon 158 in M-COMT and codon 108 in MB-COMT gene sequence), resulting in valine to methionine substitution. It has been determined that methionine substitution generate a lesser thermostable COMT enzyme, which exhibits a 3-fold reduction in protein activity compared to those enzyme with valine aminoacid in that position (reviewed in Mannisto and Kaakkola, 1999). Some studies have found that women with preeclampsia have a high prevalence of Val158met substitution compared to normotensive pregnant women (Lim et al., 2010; Liang et al., 2012) suggesting that a lower $2ME_2$ production rate in these women is due to the presence of this polymorphism; however, other studies have not found this correlation (Hill et al., 2011). On the other hand, it has been shown that some women with preeclampsia also have lesser COMT protein levels in their placental tissue (Kanasaki et al., 2008); however, the mechanisms involved in this particular COMT protein pattern have not been elucidated.

Effects of Hydroxyestradiols and Methoxyestradiols on Vascular system

It is broadly known that E_2 exerts different protective effects on vascular system (Tostes et al., 2003); however, the fact of E_2 was capable to inhibit the growth of vascular smooth muscle cells in mice that do not express estrogen receptors (Iafrati et al., 1997; Karas et al., 1999) suggested that the antitmitogenic actions on vascular system previously attributable to E_2 could be exerted by estradiol metabolites more than estradiol itself. Indeed, the study performed by Zacharia and collaborators (2003) clearly showed that conversion of E_2 to $2OHE_2$ and then to $2ME_2$ would mediate the antimitogenic effects attributable to E_2. In this latter study, these investigators compared the antitmitogenic effects of E_2 and $2OHE_2$ on aortic smooth muscle cells obtained from mice that do not express the enzyme COMT (COMT-KO) and in those from wild type mice (COMT-WT). Their results showed that E_2 and $2OHE_2$ inhibited serum-induced DNA synthesis, cell numbers, and collagen synthesis in

COMT-WT cells, but not in COMT-KO cells, while $2ME_2$ induced these effects in both COMT-WT and COMT-KO cells. The antitmitogenic actions of hydroxyestradiols and methoxyestradiols have been also reported in cardiac fibroblasts (Dubey et al., 2005a), coronary arteries (Dubey et al., 2005b) and glomerular mesangial cells (Dubey et al., 2002) obtained from humans.

The cellular mechanisms by which these E_2 metabolites generate these effects involve several direct and indirect actions. Barchiesi and collaborators (2006) determined that in human aortic smooth muscle cells, $2ME_2$ would exert its antimitogenic effect inducing inhibition of cyclin D1 and cyclin B1 expression, inhibition of CDK1 and CDK2 activity, and block of retinoblastoma protein hyperphosphorylation. These effects may be mediated by inhibition of protein extracellular signal-regulated kinase (ERK) 1/2, and Akt phosphorylation and/or by prostaglandin formation, increasing COX-2 expression (Barchiesi et al., 2006). Moreover, these actions may also induced by inhibition of cAMP production, a phenomenon observed in cultured preglomerular vascular smooth muscle cells (Tofovic et al., 2009).

On the other hand, $2OHE_2$ and $2ME_2$ may exert direct effects on vascular system functioning; for instance, it has been shown that $2OHE_2$ and $2ME_2$ are capable to inhibit KCl-induced contraction of rat coronary arterial *in vitro* by non-genomic and estrogen receptor-independent mechanisms, given that cycloheximide (a protein synthesis inhibitor) and ICI 182780 (an estrogen receptor antagonist) did not block this effect (Hill et al., 2010). Moreover, $2OHE_2$ and $2ME_2$ inhibited endothelin 1 synthesis in porcine coronary artery endothelial cells, acting by estrogen receptor-independent mechanisms and probably inhibiting MAP kinase activity by non-genomic actions (Dubey et al., 2001). Besides, $2ME_2$ is also capable of down-regulating the expression of Angiotensin type I receptor by ERK1/2 activation in primary rat aortic smooth muscle cells (Koganti et al., 2012), indicating that $2ME_2$ may be an important factor to prevent or delay cardiovascular events, since a chronic Angiotensin type I receptor activation is related to several pathologic cardiovascular and inflammatory conditions (Stegbauer and Coffman, 2011).

Participation of Hydroxyestradiols and Methoxyestradiols in Cancer

Hydroxyestradiols as Etiologic Factors of Cancer

The association between some kind of cancers, such as breast cancer, and high endogenous estrogen levels has been clearly established (Adlercreutz et al., 1994; Toniolo et al., 1995, Khan et al., 1998). In the last years, it has been postulated that biotransformation of E_2 to hydroxyestradiols is also an important etiological factor for cancer (Singh et al., 2005; Crooke et al., 2006; Wang et al., 2011). When hydroxyestradiols levels are increased, these E_2 metabolites would act as genotoxic compounds, given that they are converted to estradiol quinones (an estradiol molecule with two molecules of oxygen bound by a double bond in two different molecules of carbon located on its aromatic ring). $2OHE_2$ is mainly transformed to E_2-2-3-Q, while $4OHE_2$ is transformed to E_2-3-4-Q (Parl et al., 2009). These estradiol quinones forms adducts with the molecule of DNA (a direct attach between estradiol quinone and a DNA molecule) that potentially may cause genetic mutations (Cavalieri et al., 2000). In addition, reactive oxygen species are produced when hydroxyestradiols are converted to estradiol quinones (Liehrand Roy, 1990; Chen et al., 2005; Fussell et al., 2011). These reactive oxygen species induce extra damage to the molecule of DNA (Cerda and Weitzman, 1997; Hurh et al., 2004) and they also activate several redox-sensitive signaling pathways that favor the development of cancer (Yager and Liehr, 1996; Okoh et al., 2011). Moreover, there are mathematical models that use the kinetic parameters of biotransformation of E_2 to hydroxyestradiols and methoxyestradiols in patients, in order to evaluate the risk to suffer cancer (Crooke et al., 2006; Crooke et al., 2011).

The mechanisms by which hydroxyestradiols levels are increased in cancer involve an increase in the expression and/or activity of the enzymes CYPs and/or a decrease in the expression and/or activity of COMT, a condition that has been found in some cancer tissues (Singh et al., 2005; Crooke et al., 2006; Wang et al., 2011). For instance, Vinothini and Nagini (2010) found a significant increased expression of CYP1A1 and CYP1B1 in breast tumor tissues compared to adjacent uninvolved tissues. Moreover, Rodriguez and Potter (2013) recently showed that a biological or a pharmacological decrease of CYP1A1 expression in two different cell lines obtained from breast cancer, induced a decrease in cell proliferation rate, a decrease in colony formation and it blocked the cell cycle at G0/G1 in these cells, indicating that CYP1A1, perhaps increasing hydroxyestradiols levels, may promote breast cancer proliferation and survival.

Finally, some natural antioxidants found in fruits, vegetables and/or red wine, (such as resveratrol and Lycopene) may decrease the risk to suffer cancer, because they prevent hydroxyestradiols quinones-DNA adduct formation *in vitro* (Muzandu et al., 2005; Zahid et al., 2007; Zahid et al., 2008), suggesting that a diet rich in these compounds could be used to cancer prevention.

2-Methoxyestradiol as a Drug for Cancer Treatment

Inversely to the effects of hydroxyestradiols, several studies have demonstrated that $2ME_2$ can inhibit cell growth and also induce cell death in a variety of malignant cell lines, such as lung carcinoma, colon carcinoma, tumors of the nervous system, melanoma, ovarian carcinoma, renal carcinoma, prostate carcinoma, pancreatic cancer cells, tumors of the musculature, tumor of the eye, cervical carcinoma, endometrial cancer, vascular tumors, esophageal cancer, stomach cancer, pancreatic cancer and breast cancer (Schumacher et al., 1999; Arbiser et al., 1999; Dubey et al., 2002; Fotsis et al., 1994; Lakhani et al., 2003; Zhu and Conney, 1998; Mueck and Seeger, 2010).

The cellular mechanisms by which $2ME_2$ decreases cell viability and/or inhibit cancer proliferation are diverse. For example, this estradiol metabolite is capable to suppress cancer cell growth by inhibiting angiogenesis (Fotsis et al., 1994; Klauber et al., 1997; Pribluda et al., 2000), inducing apoptosis by caspases-dependent mechanisms (LaVallee et al., 2003) and independent-caspases mechanisms (Lambert et al., 2004) and also inhibiting cell proliferation interacting at the colchicine site in tubulin protein, blocking its polymerization (D'Amato et al., 1994; Klauber et al., 1997; Pribluda et al., 2000). According to the literature, these effects do not require a functional estrogen receptor (LaVallee et al., 2002), similarly to the biological effects previously described in this chapter.

The clinical application of $2ME_2$ is limited, due to its poor water solubility and resulting low bioavailability (Cho et al., 2011). In fact, a clinical trial of $2ME_2$ was closed as a result of extremely low plasma concentrations relative to the administered dose (Dahut et al., 2006). To better understand the bioavalability and absorption of $2ME_2$, Guo et al. (2009) used an *in situ* rat intestinal recirculation perfusion technique. They demonstrated that concentrations had no influence on the absorption rate constant. Furthermore, with the exception of the duodenum, $2ME_2$ absorbed at each intestinal segment and showed the best absorption at the ileum (Guo et al., 2009). From collections of urine from cancer patients the metabolism of $2ME_2$ has been assessed and revealed that <0.01% of the administered dose is excreted in the urine unchanged and approximately 1% is excreted as glucuronides, suggesting that glucuronidation and subsequent urinary excretion are elimination pathways for $2ME_2$ (Lakhani et al., 2007).

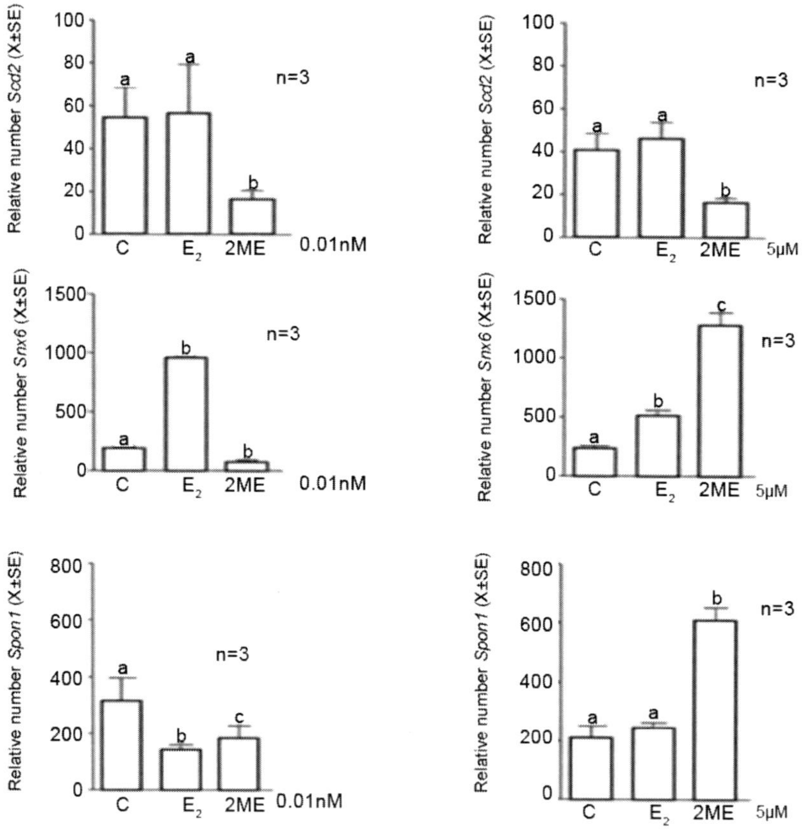

Figure 1. Expression of *spon1*, *scd2* or *snx6* in the cell line Ishikawa treated with E_2 or $2ME_2$. Real-time PCR analysis was done 12 hours after treatment with a non anti-tumoral concentration of $2ME_2$ (0.01 nM) or an anti-tumoral concentration of $2ME_2$ (5 μM). Furthermore, E_2 that do not induce anti-tumoral activity was added as comparison of the specific effects of $2ME_2$. Different letters are significantly different from each other within each graph. $a \neq b \neq c$, $p<0.05$.

Attempts to overcome the limitation of low bioavailability have been made by developing other formulations. The formulation of $2ME_2$ as a nano-suspension has been reported (Du et al., 2010) along with the formulation of poly-(organophosphazenes) that act as injectable carriers for this metabolite. In the latter example, the hydrogel containing a relatively low concentration of $2ME_2$ demonstrated improved antitumor and antiangiogenic activity in a mouse orthotopic breast tumor model relative to the original delivery method (Cho et al., 2011). A further approach to overcome the problem of low plasma availability was to engineer modifications into the structure of $2ME_2$ to increase half-life and lower excretion.

On the other hand, in the context of searching molecular marker that could be useful as a prognostic of the anticancer effects of $2ME_2$ we have performed a quantitative analysis of 3 genes whose expression is regulated by $2ME_2$ in the mouse uterus (Rincon-Rodriguez et al., 2013). Thus, we compared the effect of an antitumoral or non-antitumoral concentration of $2ME_2$ on the mRNA level of stearoyl-coenzyme Adesaturase 2 (*scd2*, Miyazaki et al., 2002), sorting nexin 6 (*snx6*, Parks et al., 2001) and F-spondin (*spon1*, Hoe et al., 2005) in Ishikawa cell line. Figure 1 shows that *Spon1* and *scd2* were increased following treatment with an anti-tumoral concentration of $2ME_2$, indicating that *spon1* and *scd2* could participate in the signaling pathway by which $2ME_2$ exerts apoptotic activity in tumoral cell lines. Furthermore, both transcripts could be used as biomarkers in the diagnostic of cancer patients with potential probabilities for treatment with $2ME_2$.

In summary, even though it is not possible to discard that $2ME_2$ does not have negative effects in different organs or biological processes, this estradiol metabolite is a promising drug to treat different kind of cancers.

Acknowledgments

This work was funded by Program U-Apoya, University of Chile and FONDECYT 11110457 to Alexis Parada-Bustamante and FONDECYT 1110662 and Proyecto BASAL FBO-07 to Pedro Orihuela.

References

Adlercreutz H, Gorbach SL, Goldin BR, Woods MN, Dwyer JT, Hämäläinen E. Estrogen metabolism and excretion in Oriental and Caucasian women. *J. Natl. Cancer Inst.* 1994;86(14):1076-82.

Arbiser JL, Panigrathy D, Klauber N, Rupnick M, Flynn E, Udagawa T, D'Amato RJ. The antiangiogenic agents TNP-470 and 2-methoxyestradiol inhibit the growth of angiosarcoma in mice. *J. Am. Acad. Dermatol.* 1999;40(6 Pt 1):925-9.

Axelrod LR, Goldzieher JW. Formation of 2-methoxyestradiol-17beta in human steroid-producing tissues by a transmethylation reaction. *Endocrinology*. 1962;70:943-5.

Barchiesi F, Jackson EK, Fingerle J, Gillespie DG, Odermatt B, Dubey RK. 2-Methoxyestradiol, an estradiol metabolite, inhibits neointima formation and smooth muscle cell growth via double blockade of the cell cycle. *Circ. Res*. 2006;99(3):266-74.

Becker CM, Rohwer N, Funakoshi T, Cramer T, Bernhardt W, Birsner A, Folkman J, D'Amato RJ. 2-methoxyestradiol inhibits hypoxia-inducible factor-1{alpha} and suppresses growth of lesions in a mouse model of endometriosis. *Am. J. Pathol.* 2008;172(2):534-44.

Bennetts LE, De Iuliis GN, Nixon B, Kime M, Zelski K, McVicar CM, Lewis SE, Aitken RJ. Impact of estrogenic compounds on DNA integrity in human spermatozoa: evidence for cross-linking and redox cycling activities. *Mutat Res.* 2008;641(1-2):1-11.

Bianchi F, Careri M, Mangia A, Musci M, Santini SE, Basini G. Porcine follicular fluids: comparison of solid-phase extraction and matrix solid-phase dispersion for the GC-MS determination of hormones during follicular growth. *J. Pharm. Biomed. Anal.* 2007;44:711-7.

Braun T. Inhibition of the soluble form of testis adenylate cyclase by catechol estrogens and other catechols. *Proc. Soc. Exp. Biol. Med.* 1990;194(1):58-63.

Brown CM, Suzuki S, Jelks KA, Wise PM. Estradiol is a potent protective, restorative, and trophic factor after brain injury. *SeminReprod Med.* 2009;27(3):240-9.

Bulun SE. Endometriosis. *N. Engl. J. Med.* 2009;360(3):268-79.

Caniggia I, Mostachfi H, Winter J, Gassmann M, Lye SJ, Kuliszewski M, Post M. Hypoxia-inducible factor-1 mediates the biological effects of oxygen on human trophoblast differentiation through TGFbeta(3) *J. Clin. Invest.* 2000;105(5):577-87.

Carreau S, Bouraima-Lelong H, Delalande C. Estrogens: new players in spermatogenesis. *Reprod. Biol.* 2011;11(3):174-93.

Casey ML, MacDonald PC. Characterization of catechol-O-methyltransferase activity in human uterine decidua vera tissue. *Am. J. Obstet Gynecol.* 1983;145(4):453-7.

Cavalieri E, Frenkel K, Liehr JG, Rogan E, Roy D. Estrogens as endogenous genotoxic agents--DNA adducts and mutations. *J. Natl. Cancer Inst. Monogr.* 2000;(27):75-93.

Cerda S, Weitzman SA. Influence of oxygen radical injury on DNA methylation.*Mutat Res.* 1997;386(2):141-52.

Chen ZH, Na HK, Hurh YJ, Surh YJ. 4-Hydroxyestradiol induces oxidative stress and apoptosis in human mammary epithelial cells: possible protection by NF-kappaB and ERK/MAPK. *ToxicolApplPharmacol.* 2005;208(1):46-56.

Cheskis BJ, Greger JG, Nagpal S, Freedman LP. Signaling by estrogens. *J. Cell Physiol.* 2007;213(3):610-7.

Chesley LC. Hypertensive disorders in pregnancy. *J. Nurse Midwifery.* 1985;30(2):99-104.

Cho JK, Hong KY, Park JW, Yang HK, Song SC. Injectable delivery system of 2-methoxyestradiol for breast cancer therapy using biodegradable thermosensitivepoly(organophosphazene) hydrogel. *J. Drug Target.* 2011;19(4):270-80.

Choudhary D, Jansson I, Schenkman JB, Sarfarazi M, Stoilov I. Comparative expression profiling of 40 mouse cytochrome P450 genes in embryonic and adult tissues. *Arch. Biochem. Biophys.* 2003;414(1):91-100.

Coleman KM, Smith CL. Intracellular signaling pathways: nongenomic actions of estrogens and ligand-independent activation of estrogen receptors. *Front Biosci.* 2001;6:D1379-91.

Crooke PS, Ritchie MD, Hachey DL, Dawling S, Roodi N, Parl FF. Estrogens, enzyme variants, and breast cancer: a risk model. *Cancer Epidemiol. Biomarkers Prev.* 2006;15(9):1620-9.

Crooke PS, Justenhoven C, Brauch H; GENICA Consortium, Dawling S, Roodi N, Higginbotham KS, Plummer WD, Schuyler PA, Sanders ME, Page DL, Smith JR, Dupont WD, Parl FF. Estrogen metabolism and exposure in a genotypic-phenotypic model for breast cancer risk prediction. *Cancer Epidemiol. Biomarkers Prev.* 2011;20(7):1502-15.

Croxatto HB 1996. Gamete transport. In: Reproductive Endocrinology, Surgery and Technology, edn 3, pp 385-402. Eds EY Adashi, JA Rock, and Z Rosenwaks Z. Lippincott-Raven Publishers, Philadelphia.

Dawling S, Hachey DL, Roodi N, Parl FF. In vitro model of mammary estrogen metabolism: structural and kinetic differences between catechol estrogens 2- and 4-hydroxyestradiol. *Chem. Res. Toxicol.* 2004;17(9):1258-64.

D'Amato RJ, Lin CM, Flynn E, Folkman J, Hamel E. 2-Methoxyestradiol, an endogenous mammalian metabolite, inhibits tubulin polymerization by interacting at the colchicine site. *Proc. Natl. Acad. Sci. USA*. 1994;91(9):3964-8.

Dahut WL, Lakhani NJ, Gulley JL, Arlen PM, Kohn EC, Kotz H, McNally D, Parr A, Nguyen D, Yang SX, Steinberg SM, Venitz J, Sparreboom A, FiggWD. Phase I clinical trial of oral 2-methoxyestradiol, an antiangiogenic and apoptotic agent, in patients with solid tumors. *Cancer Biol. Ther.* 2006;5(1):22-7.

Davis CJ, McMillan L. Pain in endometriosis: effectiveness of medical and surgical management. *Curr. Opin. Obstet. Gynecol.* 2003;15(6):507-12.

Desaulniers D, Xiao GH, Leingartner K, Chu I, Musicki B, Tsang BK. Comparisons of brain, uterus, and liver mRNA expression for cytochrome p450s, DNA methyltransferase-1, and catechol-o-methyltransferase in prepubertal female Sprague-Dawley rats exposed to a mixture of aryl hydrocarbon receptor agonists. *Toxicol. Sci.* 2005;86(1):175-84.

Deb S, Kawai M, Chang TK, Bandiera SM. CYP1B1 expression in rat testis and Leydig cells is not inducible by aryl hydrocarbon receptor agonists. *Xenobiotica* 2010;40:447-57.

Deb S, Bandiera SM. Regulation of cytochrome P450 1B1 expression by luteinizing hormone in mouse MA-10 and rat R2C Leydig cells: role of protein kinase A. *Biol. Reprod.* 2011;85:89-96.

Dragun D, Haase-Fielitz A. Low catechol-O-methyltransferase and 2-methoxyestradiol in preeclampsia: more than a unifying hypothesis. *Nephrol. Dial Transplant.* 2009;24(1):31-3.

Drummond AE, Fuller PJ. Ovarian actions of estrogen receptor-β: an update. *Semin Reprod Med.* 2012;30(1):32-8.

Du B, Li XT, Zhao Y, A YM, Zhang ZZ. Preparation and characterization of freeze-dried 2-methoxyestradiol nanoparticle powders. *Pharmazie.* 2010;65(7):471-6.

Dubey RK, Jackson EK, Keller PJ, Imthurn B, Rosselli M. Estradiol metabolites inhibit endothelin synthesis by an estrogen receptor-independent mechanism. *Hypertension.* 2001;37(2 Pt 2):640-4.

Dubey RK, Gillespie DG, Keller PJ, Imthurn B, Zacharia LC, Jackson EK. Role of methoxyestradiols in the growth inhibitory effects of estradiol on human glomerular mesangial cells. *Hypertension.* 2002;39(2 Pt 2):418-24.

Dubey RK, Jackson EK, Gillespie DG, Rosselli M, Barchiesi F, Krust A, Keller H, Zacharia LC, Imthurn B. Cytochromes 1A1/1B1- and catechol-O-methyltransferase-derived metabolites mediate estradiol-induced antimitogenesis in human cardiac fibroblast. *J Clin. Endocrinol. Metab. 2005a;90(1):247-55.*

Dubey RK, Jackson EK, Gillespie DG, Rosselli M, Barchiesi F, Krust A, Keller H, Zacharia LC, Imthurn B. Cytochromes 1A1/1B1- and catechol-O-methyltransferase-derived metabolites mediate estradiol-induced antimitogenesis in human cardiac fibroblast. *J Clin. Endocrinol. Metab.* 2005b;90(1):247-55.

Eichenlaub-Ritter U, Winterscheidt U, Vogt E, Shen Y, Tinneberg HR, Sorensen R. 2-methoxyestradiol induces spindle aberrations, chromosome congression failure, and nondisjunction in mouse oocytes. *Biol. Reprod.* 2007;76(5):784-93.

Fazleabas AT. Physiology and pathology of implantation in the human and nonhuman primate.*Semin. Reprod. Med.* 2007;25(6):405-9.

Fotsis T, Zhang Y, Pepper MS, Adlercreutz H, Montesano R, Nawroth PP, Schweigerer L. The endogenous oestrogen metabolite 2-methoxyoestradiol inhibits angiogenesis and suppresses tumour growth. *Nature.* 1994;368(6468):237-9.

Fussell KC, Udasin RG, Smith PJ, Gallo MA, Laskin JD. Catechol metabolites of endogenous estrogens induce redox cycling and generate reactive oxygen species in breast epithelial cells. *Carcinogenesis.* 2011;32(8):1285-93.

Groothuis PG, Dassen HH, Romano A, Punyadeera C. Estrogen and the endometrium: lessons learned from gene expression profiling in rodents and human. *Hum. Reprod. Update.* 2007;13(4):405-17.

Guo XH, Zhang N, Cui FD, Du B, Zhang ZZ.An investigation on intestinal absorption of a new anticancer drug, 2-methoxyestradiol. *Pharmazie.* 2009;64(11):748-51.

Hevir N, Sinkovec J, Rižner TL. Disturbed expression of phase I and phase II estrogen-metabolizing enzymes in endometrial cancer: lower levels of CYP1B1 and increased expression of S-COMT. *Mol. Cell Endocrinol.* 2011;331(1):158-67.

Hill BJ, Gebre S, Schlicker B, Jordan R, Necessary S. Nongenomic inhibition of coronary constriction by 17ß-estradiol, 2-hydroxyestradiol, and 2-methoxyestradiol. *Can. J. Physiol. Pharmacol.* 2010;88(2):147-52.

Hill LD, York TP, Kusanovic JP, Gomez R, Eaves LJ, Romero R, Strauss JF 3rd. Epistasis between COMT and MTHFR in maternal-fetal dyads increases risk for preeclampsia. *PLoS One.* 2011;6(1):e16681.

Hoe HS, Wessner D, Beffert U, Becker AG, Matsuoka Y, Rebeck GW. F-spondin interaction with the apolipoprotein E receptor ApoEr2 affects processing of amyloid precursor protein. *Mol. Cell Biol.* 2005;25(21):9259-68.

Houk CP, Pearson EJ, Martinelle N, Donahoe PK, Teixeira J. Feedback inhibition of steroidogenic acute regulatory protein expression in vitro and in vivo by androgens. *Endocrinology.* 2004;145(3):1269-75.

Hurh YJ, Chen ZH, Na HK, Han SY, Surh YJ. 2-Hydroxyestradiol induces oxidative DNA damage and apoptosis in human mammary epithelial cells. *J. Toxicol. Environ. Health A.* 2004;67(23-24):1939-53.

Iafrati MD, Karas RH, Aronovitz M, Kim S, Sullivan TR Jr, Lubahn DB, O'Donnell TF Jr, Korach KS, Mendelsohn ME. Estrogen inhibits the vascular injury response in estrogen receptor alpha-deficient mice. *Nat. Med.* 1997;3(5):545-8.

Jobe SO, Ramadoss J, Wargin AJ, Magness RR. Estradiol-17β and its cytochrome P450- and catechol-O-methyltransferase-derived metabolites selectively stimulate production of prostacyclin in uterine artery endothelial cells: role of estrogen receptor-α versus estrogen receptor-β. *Hypertension.* 2013a;61(2):509-18.

Jobe SO, Tyler CT, Magness RR.Aberrant synthesis, metabolism, and plasma accumulation of circulating estrogens and estrogen metabolites in preeclampsia implications for vascular dysfunction. *Hypertension.* 2013b;61(2):480-7.

Kanasaki K, Palmsten K, Sugimoto H, Ahmad S, Hamano Y, Xie L, Parry S, Augustin HG, Gattone VH, Folkman J, Strauss JF, Kalluri R. Deficiency in catechol-O-methyltransferase and 2-methoxyoestradiol is associated with pre-eclampsia. *Nature.* 2008;453(7198):1117-21.

Karpeta A, Warzecha K, Jerzak J, Ptak A, Gregoraszczuk EL. Activation of the enzymes of phase I (CYP2B1/2) and phase II (SULT1A and COMT) metabolism by 2,2',4,4'-tetrabromodiphenyl ether (BDE47) in the pig ovary. *Reprod. Toxicol.* 2012;34(3):436-42.

Karas RH, Hodgin JB, Kwoun M, Krege JH, Aronovitz M, Mackey W, Gustafsson JA, Korach KS, Smithies O, Mendelsohn ME. Estrogen inhibits the vascular injury response in estrogen receptor beta-deficient female mice. *Proc. Natl. Acad. Sci. USA.* 1999;96(26):15133-6.

Khan SA, Rogers MA, Khurana KK, Meguid MM, Numann PJ.Estrogen receptor expression in benign breast epithelium and breast cancer risk. *J. Natl. Cancer Inst.* 1998;90(1):37-42.

Khosla S, Oursler MJ, Monroe DG.Estrogen and the skeleton. *Trends Endocrinol. Metab.* 2012;23(11):576-81.

Klauber N, Parangi S, Flynn E, Hamel E, D'Amato RJ. Inhibition of angiogenesis and breast cancer in mice by the microtubule inhibitors 2-methoxyestradiol and taxol. *Cancer Res.* 1997;57(1):81-6.

Koganti S, Snyder R, Thekkumkara T. Pharmacologic effects of 2-methoxyestradiol on angiotensin type 1 receptor down-regulation in rat liver epithelial and aortic smooth muscle cells. *Gend. Med.* 2012;9(2):76-93.

Koksal IT, Usta M, Orhan I, Abbasoglu S, Kadioglu A. Potential role of reactive oxygen species on testicular pathology associated with infertility. *Asian J. Androl.* 2003; 5(2):95-9.

Lakhani NJ, Sarkar MA, Venitz J, Figg WD. 2-Methoxyestradiol, a promising anticancer agent. *Pharmacotherapy.* 2003;23(2):165-72.

Lakhani NJ, Sparreboom A, Xu X, Veenstra TD, Venitz J, Dahut WL, Figg WD. Characterization of in vitro and in vivo metabolic pathways of the investigational anticancer agent, 2-methoxyestradiol. *J. Pharm. Sci.* 2007;96(7):1821-31.

Lambert C, Apel K, Biesalski HK, Frank J. 2-methoxyestradiol induces caspase-independent, mitochondria-centered apoptosis in DS-sarcoma cells. *Int. J. Cancer.* 2004;108(4):493-501.

Lardone MC, Castillo P, Valdevenito R, Ebensperger M, Ronco AM, Pommer R, Piottante A, Castro A. P450-aromatase activity and expression in human testicular tissues with severe spermatogenic failure. *Int. J. Androl.* 2010;33(4):650-60.

Lattanzi ML, Santos CB, Mudry MD, Baranao JL. Exposure of bovine oocytes to the endogenous metabolite 2-methoxyestradiol during in vitro maturation inhibits early embryonic development. *Biol. Reprod.* 2003;69(6):1793-800.

LaVallee TM, Zhan XH, Herbstritt CJ, Kough EC, Green SJ, Pribluda VS. 2-Methoxyestradiol inhibits proliferation and induces apoptosis independently of estrogen receptors alpha and beta. *Cancer Res.* 2002;62(13):3691-7.

LaVallee TM, Zhan XH, Johnson MS, Herbstritt CJ, Swartz G, Williams MS, Hembrough WA, Green SJ, Pribluda VS. 2-methoxyestradiol up-regulates death receptor 5 and induces apoptosis through activation of the extrinsic pathway. *Cancer Res.* 2003;63(2):468-75.

Lee SB, Wong AP, Kanasaki K, Xu Y, Shenoy VK, McElrath TF, Whitesides GM, Kalluri R. Preeclampsia: 2-methoxyestradiol induces cytotrophoblast invasion and vascular development specifically under hypoxic conditions. *Am. J. Pathol.* 2010;176(2):710-20.

Leung SW, Teoh H, Keung W, Man RY. Non-genomic vascular actions of female sex hormones: physiological implications and signalling pathways. *Clin. Exp. Pharmacol. Physiol.* 2007;34(8):822-6.

Leung GS, Kawai M, Tai JK, Chen J, Bandiera SM, Chang TK. Developmental expression and endocrine regulation of CYP1B1 in rat testis.*Drug MetabDispos.* 2009;37(3):523-8.

Liang S, Liu X, Fan P, Liu R, Zhang J, He G, Liu Y, Bai H. Association between Val158Met functional polymorphism in the COMT gene and risk of preeclampsia in a Chinese population. *Arch. Med. Res.* 2012;43(2):154-8.

Liehr JG, Roy D. Free radical generation by redox cycling of estrogens. *Free Radic. Biol. Med.* 1990;8(4):415-23.

Lim JH, Kim SY, Kim do J, Park SY, Han HW, Han JY, Lee SW, Yang JH, Ryu HM. Genetic polymorphism of catechol-O-methyltransferase and cytochrome P450c17α in preeclampsia. *Pharmacogenet Genomics.* 2010;20(10):605-10.

Ma W, Tan J, Matsumoto H, Robert B, Abrahamson DR, Das SK, Dey SK. MolEndocrinol. 2001;15(11):1983-92. Adult tissue angiogenesis: evidence for negative regulation by estrogen in the uterus.

Maran A, Zhang M, Kennedy AM, Sibonga JD, Rickard DJ, Spelsberg TC, Turner RT. 2-methoxyestradiol induces interferon gene expression and apoptosis in osteosarcoma cells. *Bone.* 2002;30(2):393-8.

Martucci CP, Fishman J. Impact of continuously administered catechol estrogens on uterine growth and luteinizing hormone secretion. *Endocrinology.* 1979;105(6):1288-92.

Mannisto PT, Kaakkola S. Catechol-O-methyltransferase (COMT): biochemistry, molecular biology, pharmacology, and clinical efficacy of the new selective COMT inhibitors. *Pharmacol. Rev.* 1999;51:593–628.

Mishra A, Joy KP. 2-Hydroxyestradiol-17beta-induced oocyte maturation: involvement of cAMP-protein kinase A and okadaic acid-sensitive protein phosphatases, and their interplay in oocyte maturation in the catfish Heteropneustesfossilis. *J. Exp. Biol.* 2006a;209:2567-75.

Mishra A, Joy KP. 2-Hydroxyestradiol-17beta-induced oocyte maturation in catfish (Heteropneustesfossilis) involves protein kinase C and its interaction with protein phosphatases. *Comp. Biochem. Physiol. A. MolIntegr. Physiol.* 2006b;144(4):416-22.

Miyazaki M, Gomez FE, Ntambi JM. Lack of stearoyl-CoA desaturase-1 function induces a palmitoyl-CoA Delta6 desaturase and represses the stearoyl-CoA desaturase-3 gene in the preputial glands of the mouse. *J. Lipid Res.* 2002;43(12):2146-54.

Mizuyachi K, Son DS, Rozman KK, Terranova PF. Alteration in ovarian gene expression in response to 2,3,7,8-tetrachlorodibenzo-p-dioxin: reduction of cyclooxygenase-2 in the blockage of ovulation. *Reprod. Toxicol.* 2002;16(3):299-307.

Molina C, Vargas C, Tapia-Pizarro A, Castro A, Parada-Bustamante A. Effects of Hydroxyestradiols and Methoxyestradiols on viability of cultured Sertoli cells. XXIII annual meeting Chilean Society of reproduction and development. Page 56.

Mueck AO, Seeger H. 2-Methoxyestradiol--biology and mechanism of action. *Steroids.* 2010;75(10):625-31.

Muzandu K, El Bohi K, Shaban Z, Ishizuka M, Kazusaka A, Fujita S. Lycopene and beta-carotene ameliorate catechol estrogen-mediated DNA damage. *Jpn J. Vet. Res.* 2005;52(4):173-84.

Nishi H, Nakada T, Kyo S, Inoue M, Shay JW, Isaka K. Hypoxia-inducible factor 1 mediates upregulation of telomerase (hTERT). *Mol. Cell Biol.* 2004;24(13):6076-83.

Nishimura M, Yaguti H, Yoshitsugu H, Naito S, Satoh T. Tissue distribution of mRNA expression of human cytochrome P450 isoforms assessed by high-sensitivity real-time reverse transcription PCR. *YakugakuZasshi.* 2003;123(5):369-75.

Okoh V, Deoraj A, Roy D. Estrogen-induced reactive oxygen species-mediated signalings contribute to breast cancer. *Biochim. Biophys. Acta.* 2011;1815(1):115-33.

Orihuela PA, Parada-Bustamante A, Cárdenas H, Tapia-Pizarro A, Oróstica L, Reuquén P. Mating effects on female reproductive organs. In. Human and Animal Mating: Strategies, Gender differences and Environmental Influences, edn 1, pp 1-30. Eds. M Nakamura and T Ito. Nova Publishers, New York.

Øverbye A, Seglen PO. Phosphorylated and non-phosphorylated forms of catechol O-methyltransferase in rat liver, brain and other tissues. *Biochem. J.* 2009;417(2):535-45.

Parada-Bustamante A, Orihuela PA, Ríos M, Navarrete-Gómez PA, Cuevas CA, Velásquez LA, Villalón MJ, Croxatto HB. Catechol-o-methyltransferase and methoxyestradiols participate in the intraoviductal nongenomic pathway through which estradiol accelerates egg transport in cycling rats. *Biol. Reprod.* 2007;77(6):934-41.

Parada-Bustamante A, Orihuela PA, Ríos M, Cuevas CA, Oróstica ML, Velásquez LA, Villalón MJ, Croxatto HB. A non-genomic signaling pathway shut down by mating changes the estradiol-induced gene expression profile in the rat oviduct. *Reproduction.* 2010;139(3):631-44.

Parks WT, Frank DB, Huff C, Renfrew Haft C, Martin J, Meng X, de Caestecker MP, McNally JG, Reddi A, Taylor SI, Roberts AB, Wang T, Lechleider RJ. Sorting nexin 6, a novel SNX, interacts with the transforming growth factor-beta family of receptor serine-threonine kinases. *J. Biol. Chem.* 2001;276(22):19332-9.

Parl FF, Dawling S, Roodi N, Crooke PS. Estrogen metabolism and breast cancer: a risk model. *Ann. N. Y. Acad. Sci. 2009*;1155:68-75.

Pérez-Sepúlveda A, España-Perrot PP, Norwitz ER, Illanes SE. Metabolic Pathways Involved in 2-Methoxyestradiol Synthesis and Their Role in Preeclampsia. *Reprod. Sci.* 2013 (In press)

Pribluda VS, Gubish ER Jr, Lavallee TM, Treston A, Swartz GM, Green SJ. 2-Methoxyestradiol: an endogenous antiangiogenic and antiproliferative drug candidate. *Cancer Metastasis Rev.* 2000;19:173-9.

Raz L, Khan MM, Mahesh VB, Vadlamudi RK, Brann DW. Rapid estrogen signaling in the brain. *Neurosignals.* 2008;16(2-3):140-53.

Rempel MA, Hester B, Deharo H, Hong H, Wang Y, Schlenk D. Effects of 17beta-estradiol, and its metabolite, 4-hydroxyestradiol on fertilization, embryo development and oxidative DNA damage in sand dollar (Dendrasterexcentricus) sperm. *Sci. Total Environ.* 2009;407(7):2209-15.

Revel A, Raanani H, Younglai E, Xu J, Han R, Savouret JF, Casper RF. Resveratrol, a natural aryl hydrocarbon receptor antagonist, protects sperm from DNA damage and apoptosis caused by benzo(a)pyrene. *Reprod. Toxicol.* 2001;15(5):479-86.

Rincón-Rodríguez RJ, Oróstica ML, Díaz P, Reuquén P, Cárdenas H, Orihuela PA. Changes in the gene expression pattern induced by 2-methoxyestradiol in the mouse uterus. *Endocrine.* 2013 (In press).

Roberts JM, Taylor RN, Musci TJ, Rodgers GM, Hubel CA, McLaughlin MK. Preeclampsia: an endothelial cell disorder. *Am. J. Obstet. Gynecol.* 1989;161(5):1200-4.

Rodriguez M, Potter DA. Cytochrome P450 1A1 Regulates Breast Cancer Cell Proliferation *and Survival. Mol. Cancer Res.* 2013 (In press).

Salih SM, Salama SA, Fadl AA, Nagamani M, Al-Hendy A. Expression and cyclic variations of catechol-O-methyl transferase in human endometrial stroma. *Fertil. Steril.* 2008;90(3):789-97.

Schumacher G, Kataoka M, Roth JA, Mukhopadhyay T. Potent antitumor activity of 2-methoxyestradiol in human pancreatic cancer cell lines. *Clin. Cancer Res.* 1999; 5(3):493-9.

Seegers JC, van Aswegen CH, Nieuwoudt BL, Joubert WS. Morphological effects of the catecholestrogens on cells of the seminiferous tubules of Sprague-Dawley rats. *Andrologia.* 1991;23(5):339-45.

Shenoy V, Kanasaki K, Kalluri R. Pre-eclampsia: connecting angiogenic and metabolic pathways. *Trends Endocrinol. Metab.* 2010;21(9):529-36.

Shimada T, Hayes CL, Yamazaki H, Amin S, Hecht SS, Guengerich FP, Sutter TR. Activation of chemically diverse procarcinogens by human cytochrome P-450 1B1. *Cancer Res.* 1996;56(13):2979-84.

Sibai B, Dekker G, Kupferminc M. Pre-eclampsia. *Lancet.* 2005;365(9461):785-99.

Sibonga JD, Lotinun S, Evans GL, Pribluda VS, Green SJ, Turner RT. Dose-response effects of 2-methoxyestradiol on estrogen target tissues in the ovariectomized rat. *Endocrinology.* 2003;144(3):785-92.

Singh S, Chakravarti D, Edney JA, Hollins RR, Johnson PJ, West WW, Higginbotham SM, Cavalieri EL, Rogan EG. Relative imbalances in the expression of estrogen-metabolizing enzymes in the breast tissue of women with breast carcinoma. *Oncol. Rep.* 2005;14(4):1091-6.

Singh MN, Stringfellow HF, Taylor SE, Ashton KM, Ahmad M, Abdo KR, El-Agnaf OM, Martin-Hirsch PL, Martin FL. Elevated expression of CYP1A1 and gamma-SYNUCLEIN in human ectopic (ovarian) endometriosis compared with eutopic endometrium. *Mol. Hum. Reprod.* 2008;14(11):655-63.

Spicer LJ, Hammond JM. Catecholestrogens inhibit proliferation and DNA synthesis of porcine granulosa cells in vitro: comparison with estradiol, 5 alpha-dihydrotestosterone, gonadotropins and catecholamines. *Mol. Cell Endocrinol.* 1989;64:119-26.

Spicer LJ, Hammond JM. Regulation of ovarian function by catecholestrogens: Current concepts. *J. Steroid Biochem.* 1989;33:489-501.

Stammel W, Thomas H, Staib W, Kühn-Velten WN. Tetrahydroisoquinoline alkaloids mimic direct but not receptor-mediated inhibitory effects of estrogens and phytoestrogens on testicular endocrine function. Possible significance for Leydig cell insufficiency in alcohol addiction. *Life Sci.* 1991;49(18):1319-29.

Stegbauer J, Coffman TM. New insights into angiotensin receptor actions: from blood pressure to aging. *Curr. Opin. Nephrol. Hypertens.* 2011;20(1):84-8.

Sutter TR, Tang YM, Hayes CL, Wo YY, Jabs EW, Li X, Yin H, Cody CW, Greenlee WF. Complete cDNA sequence of a human dioxin-inducible mRNA identifies a new gene subfamily of cytochrome P450 that maps to chromosome 2. *J. Biol. Chem.* 1994;269(18):13092-9.

Tal R, Shaish A, Barshack I, Polak-Charcon S, Afek A, Volkov A, Feldman B, Avivi C, Harats D. Effects of hypoxia-inducible factor-1alpha overexpression in pregnant mice: possible implications for preeclampsia and intrauterine growth restriction. *Am. J. Pathol.* 2010;177(6):2950-62.

Tofovic PS, Rosado BM, Dubey KR, Mi Z, Jackson EK. Effects of estradiol metabolites on cAMP production and degradation. *Prilozi.* 2009;30(1):5-24.

Toniolo PG, Levitz M, Zeleniuch-Jacquotte A, Banerjee S, Koenig KL, Shore RE, Strax P, Pasternack BS. A prospective study of endogenous estrogens and breast cancer in postmenopausal women. *J. Natl. Cancer Inst. 1995*;87(3):190-7.

Tostes RC, Nigro D, Fortes ZB, Carvalho MH. Effects of estrogen on the vascular system. *Braz J. Med. Biol. Res.* 2003;36(9):1143-58.

Tsuchiya Y, Nakajima M, Yokoi T. Cytochrome P450-mediated metabolism of estrogens and its regulation in human. *Cancer Lett.* 2005;227(2):115-24.

Turner CD, in General Endocrinology, 3rd edn. (WB Saunders Company, Philadelphia, 1961) pp. 365–409.

Vargas C, Molina C, Ebensperger M, Valdevenito R, Lardone MC, Piottante A, Florez M, Castro A, Parada-Bustamante A. Expression of the enzymes CYP1A1, CYP1B1 and COMT in human testicular tissue with conserved spermatogenesis. XXIII annual meeting Chilean Society of reproduction and development. Page 67.

Vinothini G, Nagini S. Correlation of xenobiotic-metabolizing enzymes, oxidative stress and NFkappaB signaling with histological grade and menopausal status in patients with adenocarcinoma of the breast. *Clin. Chim. Acta.* 2010;411(5-6):368-74.

Vuorela P, Helske S, Hornig C, Alitalo K, Weich H, Halmesmäki E. Amniotic fluid--soluble vascular endothelial growth factor receptor-1 in preeclampsia. *Obstet. Gynecol.* 2000;95(3):353-7.

Wang Q, Li H, Tao P, Wang YP, Yuan P, Yang CX, Li JY, Yang F, Lee H, Huang Y. Soy isoflavones, CYP1A1, CYP1B1, and COMT polymorphisms, and breast cancer: a case-control study in southwestern China. *DNA Cell Biol.* 2011;30(8):585-95.

Wentz MJ, Jamaluddin M, Garfield RE, Al-Hendy A. Regulation of catechol-O-methyltransferase expression in human myometrial cells. *Obstet Gynecol.* 2006;108(6):1439-47.

Yager JD, Liehr JG. Molecular mechanisms of estrogen carcinogenesis. *Annu. Rev. Pharmacol. Toxicol.* 1996;36:203-32.

Zacharia LC, Gogos JA, Karayiorgou M, Jackson EK, Gillespie DG, Barchiesi F, Dubey RK. Methoxyestradiols mediate the antimitogenic effects of 17beta-estradiol: direct evidence from catechol-O-methyltransferase-knockout mice. *Circulation.* 2003;108(24):2974-8.

Zahid M, Gaikwad NW, Rogan EG, Cavalieri EL. Inhibition of depurinating estrogen-DNA adduct formation by natural compounds. *Chem. Res. Toxicol.* 2007;20(12):1947-53.

Zahid M, Gaikwad NW, Ali MF, Lu F, Saeed M, Yang L, Rogan EG, Cavalieri EL. Prevention of estrogen-DNA adduct formation in MCF-10F cells by resveratrol. *Free Radic. Biol. Med.* 2008;45(2):136-45.

Zhang Z, Davis DL. Cell-type specific responses in prostaglandin secretion by glandular and stromal cells from pig endometrium treated with catecholestrogens, methoxyestrogens and progesterone. *Prostaglandins.* 1992;44(1):53-64.

Zhu BT, Conney AH. Is 2-methoxyestradiol an endogenous estrogen metabolite that inhibits mammary carcinogenesis? *Cancer Res.* 1998;58(11):2269-77.

In: Estradiol: Synthesis, Health Effects and Drug Interactions ISBN: 978-1-62808-962-2
Editors: Ricco Palmeri and Sal Grimaudo

Chapter 6

Estrogen and Functional Gastrointestinal Disorders

Gengqing Song[1], Sunny Joseph[1], M. Showkat Ali[2] and Richard W. McCallum[1,*]

[1]Department of Internal Medicine, Texas Tech University Health Sciences Center, Paul L. Foster School of Medicine, El Paso, TX, US

[2]Department of Clinical Investigation, William Beaumont Army Medical Center, El Paso, TX, US

Abstract

This chapter will review: 1) the pathophysiological mechanisms of functional gastrointestinal disorders (FGIDs); 2) the effects of estrogen on motor dysfunction, visceral pain, gastrointestinal (GI) symptoms and some FGIDs such as gastroesophageal reflux disease (GERD), functional dyspepsia (FD), gastroparesis, irritable bowel syndrome (IBS) and constipation.

Keywords: Estrogen, functional gastroenterology disorders, GI motor dysfunction, visceral pain, GI symptoms, gastroesophageal reflux disease, functional dyspepsia, gastroparesis, iritable bowel syndrome, constipation

Introduction

FGIDs represent common conditions affecting up to 25% of the US population [1-6]. These are syndromes causing chronic or recurrent symptoms attributable to the GI tract, unexplained by any structural or biochemical abnormalities [4]. Approximately 50% of

* Correspondence: Richard W. McCallum, Department of Internal Medicine,Texas Tech University Health Sciences Center, Paul L. Foster School of Medicine,4800 Alberta Avenue, El Paso, TX 79905. E-mail: Richard.mccallum@ttuhsc.edu.

patients seen in GI subspecialty practices have functional complaints [7]. Abdominal pain and/or discomfort is one of the major complaints in FGIDs such as IBS and FD. IBS is typically characterized by low abdominal pain that is associated with alteration in stool form and/or frequency. FD constitutes a constellation of symptoms believed to arise from the upper GI tract. Both conditions exclude evidence of structural disease to explain symptoms. In IBS and FD, the abdominal discomfort or pain is worsened by meals as are the additional symptoms of bloating, early satiety, fullness, belching, nausea, ect [4, 7]. Various pathophysiological mechanisms may account for the symptoms, including GI motility abnormalities, visceral hypersensitivity to distension, autonomic dysfunction, as well as disturbed central nervous function [8, 9]. However, FGIDs is still poorly understood and there is a lack of an effective therapy.

Interestingly, a number of FGIDs such as IBS and FD are seen more often and appear more severe in women than in men [10-15]. In Australia, a population-based study showed that female adults substanstially outnumbered males in most FGIDs [16]. For instance, in IBS, approximately 70 to 80% of the IBS population was female. Also, several studies noted a consistent female preponderance (up to 87%) with dyspepsia [16-20]. In addition, symptoms such as nausea, vomiting, abdominal pain, distension, satiety, bloating, diarrhea, or constipation, are frequently related to pregnancy, menstrual cycle or perimenopausal and menopausal states. Furthermore, motility disorders, such as reflux of GI contents and delayed GI transit, are frequently reported in patients who maintain serum estrogen concentrations at high levels, for example, through the use of oral contraceptive drugs and during gestation. These phenomena indicate that sex hormones, e.g., estrogen, may be involved in many GI physiological processes, including but not limited to motor function, visceral sensitivity and autonomic and central nerves. Given this widespread role for estrogen in the gut, it is not surprising that estrogen may be also implicated in the development or progression of many FGIDs. In many of these diseases, estrogen may mediate its effects through the estrogen receptors (ER), which can serve as the basis to understand the pathophysiological roles of estrogen in these diseases.

Pathophysiological Mechanisms of FGIDs

GI tract is a complex system. Coordinated movements of each compartment such as stomach and intestines are required to digest and propel intraluminal contents along the digestive tract. The complex patterns of contraction and relaxation are necessary for proper motility of the GI tract. Each segment of the GI tract is separated by a dedicated muscular sphincter that controls the entry of contents from one into another. For example, relaxation of the lower esophageal sphincter allows passage of ingested contents into the stomach. Each part serves its own particular set of functions, and together with the liver, gallbladder, and pancreas, form the complex human digestive system.

Motor Function Abnormalities

Esophagus

Gastroesophageal reflux (GER) may cause heartburn that is common and occurs in 18% of the adult population in the United State [21]. The development of GER is a multifactorial process and main motor dysfunctions include:

1) Decreased lower esophageal sphincter (LES) pressure. There is a positive pressure gradient between the stomach and the esophagus that tends to promote the reflux from the stomach into the esophagus. LES normally can counteract this pressure gradient and effectively prevent reflux by maintenance of a basal resting pressure at gastroesophageal junction (GEJ) between 10-40 mmHg. Resting LES pressure represents a combination of the intrinsic sphincter which is a 3 cm apart of tonically contracting smooth muscle at the GEJ as well as the contribution by the left crus of diaphragm - sometimes referred to the external LES. Low resting LES pressure (<10 mm Hg) usually leads to episodes of GER particularly at night during sleep when the benefits of upright posture and gravity are lost. This has been frequently observed in patients with severe GERD [22, 23]. The LES pressure is a significant predictor of erosive esophagitis [24].
2) Increased Transient LES Relaxations (TLESRs). This has been considered as the major LES mechanisms for reflux, especially in patients with normal resting LESP [25, 26]. Under normal conditions, the LES relaxes for 3-10 seconds to allow the swallowed bolus to enter the stomach. Brief episodes of GER can occur during this transient opening in normal individuals [27]; while in patients, pathological TLESRs occur spontaneously unrelated to swallowing and esophageal peristaltic contractions, and can last longer (up to 45 seconds) [25, 26]. There is a propensity for TLESRs to occur in greater numbers after specific precipitating events e.g., gastric distension from eating and episodes of belching. It has been reported that in patients with GERD, approximately 55-80% of reflux episodes are the result of TLESRs [25, 27].
3) Inadequate LES response. This deficiency in response to increased abdominal pressure also contributes to GER. Normally, LES pressure rises rapidly with a sudden abdominal pressure elevation, and the increased LES response is the result of diaphragmatic contraction augmenting internal LES pressure during abdominal compression events e.g., coughing, sneezing, straining, valsalva or lifting. In some patients, particularly those with lower resting LES pressure, this rapid increase in the LES pressure may be absent because of the presence of hiatal hernia which changes the anatomy. The intrinsic LES is not juxtaposed with the diaphragm because the intrinsic LES is now above the diaphragm due to the hiatal hernia. GER ensues when the sudden increase in abdominal pressure is not accompanied by a commensurate rise in the LES pressure, and the gastric content is propelled into the esophagus.
4) Decreased esophageal clearance capacity. Normally, most of the refluxed caustic material can be cleared from the esophagus by the combined effect of gravity and secondary peristaltic contractions, and the residues are further neutralized by saliva and bicarbonate produced by the esophageal submucosal glands as well as saliva and bicarbonate been swallowed after secretion by the salivary glands. Impaired esophageal clearance prolongs the exposure of the esophagus to caustic materials.

5) Delayed gastric emptying. This has been observed in about 30% of GERD patients [28]. A delay in gastric emptying results from prolonged presence of food inside the stomach and sustained gastric distention leading to increased TLESRs and hence more exposure to GER, because of more episodes of TLESRs after meals.

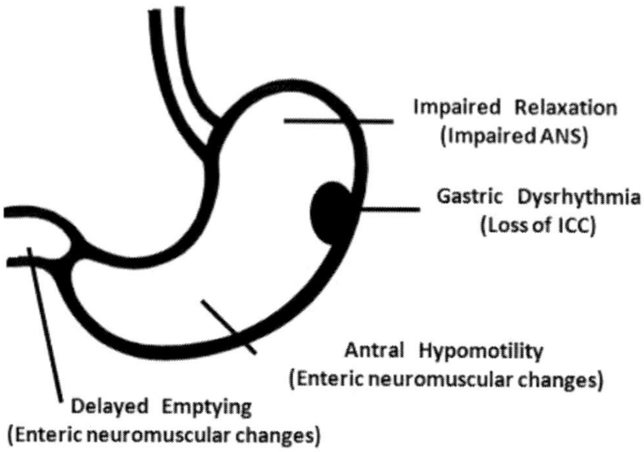

Figure 1. Pathophysiological factors of FD and gastroparesis: impaired fundic relaxation (impaired autonomic nervous system, ANS), gastric dysrhythmia (Loss of interstitial cell of cajal (ICC), antral hypomotility and delayed gastric emptying (Enteric neuromuscular changes).

Stomach

Gastric dysmotility may cause secondary abdominal discomfort or pain in FGIDs. For gastroparesis or FD patients, major gastric motor dysfunctions include (Figure 1):

1) Impaired gastric fundic relaxation has been frequently reported in patients with gastroparesis [29] and FD. In healthy subjects, the stomach relaxes upon food ingestion to accommodate food without an increase in gastric pressure (no feeling of fullness or bloating). This accommodation reflex is mediated by the vagal pathway: the sensory neurons detect food ingestion and send a signal to the brain via the vagal afferent; the brain sends a signal to the stomach via the vagal efferent, leading to a release of nitric oxide and causing the stomach to relax. This accommodation reflex is impaired in diabetes due to the impairment of the autonomic nervous system and also in post-vagotomy settings. A relationship between impaired gastric accommodation and dyspeptic symptoms has been reported in the subgroup of FD patients where meal induced symptoms are dominant.
2) Gastric dysrhythmias or abnormalities in gastric pacemaking activities. Gastric slow waves are abnormal in about 50-75% of patients with gastroparesis, often reflected as tachygastria (slow waves with a frequency higher than 4 cycles/min) and attributed to ectopic tachygastria located in the distal antrum, as a result of loss of interstitial cell of cajal (ICC). About 36% of FD patients display gastric dysrhythmias which have been linked to delayed gastric emptying, but not to symptoms [30].
3) Antral hypomotility (absence of contractions or contractions with low amplitude and loss of coordination with pylorus and duodendum) is common in gastroparesis and FD. This has been attributed to damage to vagal nerves and myoenteric plexus. But

in FD patients, the lack of a consistent correlation between symptoms and the detected abnormalities casts doubts on their primary role in symptom production [31].

4) Delayed gastric emptying is a feature of gastroparesis as explained by the abnormalities described above and is present in 30-40% FD patients [31]. In healthy humans, more than 90% of ingested food is emptied from the stomach 4 hours after the meal. In patients with gastroparesis or some FD patients, however, the ingested meal remains in the stomach for a much longer time.

Small Intestine

Abnormalities of neuromuscular regulation of intestinal muscle may lead to intestinal dysmotility. In chronic intestinal pseudo-obstruction, neuropathy and myopathy induce ineffective intestinal contractions and propulsion, which may mimic the presentation of intestinal obstruction, e.g., dilation of the bowel, in the absence of an occluding lesion of the intestinal lumen hence the term "pseudo-obstruction". The major disease associations of intestinal pseudo obstruction are diabetes, connective tissue diseases, and CNS disorders, e.g., Parkinson's, multiple sclerosis, and females dominated GI manifestations.

Colon and Anorectum

In IBS, the dysmotility only occur in some of the patients. IBS patients show an exaggerated response in the colon, rectum and small intestine to a variety of provocative stimuli including meals, distention, stress, cholecystokinin, neostigmine, and corticotropin-releasing hormone injection [32]. Also, dysmotility may interact with low sensory thresholds to generate symptoms: delayed transit of gas produces greater abdominal perception in IBS than healthy controls [33].

For constipation, colon motility, pelvic floor function and visceral sensation are important pathophysiological factors. Colon motility constitutes rhythmic phasic contractions, giant migrating contractions and tonic contractions. Pelvic floor function includes contractions of pelvic floor muscles, anorectctal motility and anal sphincter contractions. Impaired colon contractions may lead to slow colon transit, while paradoxical contractions of the external anal sphincter, loss of internal sphincter relaxation and decreased rectal sensation may cause functional outlet obstruction.

Biliary Tract, Gall Bladder and Oddi's Spincter

Biliary tract pressure, gall bladder contraction and sphincter of oddi (SO) activity are important factors in controlling bile flow. Dysmotility at either site is a potential cause of biliary type colicky pain in the absence of stones [34]. The biliary tract is a low pressure system undergoing minimal pressure changes despite substantial changes in bile flow during fasting and postprandial state. Increased pressure in the biliary tract results in decreased bile secretion. Gallbladder emptying and the activity of the SO are complex processes and both involves autonomic nervous system and hormonal mechanism such as cholecystokinin (CCK) [35-38] and motilin [39]. Diminished gallbladder emptying measured by biliary scintigraphy is an indication for cholecystectomy, although some controversies persist regarding clinical benefit. It is likely that patients who benefit from cholecystectomy may be identified by careful selection for cholescintigraphic testing, as many of patients have had missed stones or sludge [34]. The role of SO is to regulate bile flow into the duodenum, prevent reflux from it, and divert hepatic bile into the gall bladder. Increased basal SO pressure is predictive of clinical response to sphincterotomy in patients with postcholecystectomy pain [34]. However, patients with suspected SO dysfunction have the highest complication rate from endoscopic retrograde cholangiogram and sphincterotomy, and, therefore, careful patient selection is mandatory.

Visceral Hypersensitivity

Altered gut perception is a unifying feature of FGIDs. Patients often present a heightened sensitivity to experimental gut stimulation, termed visceral hypersensitivity. This is highly prevalent in FGIDs and its possible mechanisms may involve abnormalities in the periphery, the spinal cord, the brain, autonomic nervous system, or a combination of these. Visceral hypersensitivity is frequently found in patients with FD and IBS and plays a major role in pain perceptions. Data are based on studies of balloon and barostat in the rectum, sigmoid colon, stomach and esophagus demonstrating a decreased threshold to perceive pain and heightened responses to each degree of volume expansion. In FD patients, the experiments performed utilized rapid drinking water or caloric liquids to induce gastric distension, pain and/or satiety.

1) The Periphery

Peripheral release of several inflammatory mediators may cause peripheral sensitization of nociceptive afferent nerves by reducing their transduction thresholds or by inducing the expression and recruitment of previously silent nociceptors. These mediators include adenosine triphosphate, 5-hydroxytryptamine (5-HT), bradykinins, prostaglandins, the transient receptor potential vallinoid (TRPV) receptors 1 and 4, the protease activated receptor 2 (PAR(2)), nitric oxide (NO), mast cells, etc [40-45]. Other factors such as a number of ion channels (e.g., voltage-gated sodium channels), neurotransmitter receptors and trophic factors have also been involved in the development of peripheral sensitization [46]. These mediators and factors may result in an increase in pain sensitivity at the site of injury known as primary hyperalgesia [47].

2) The Spinal Cord

Prostaglandin E2 (PGE2) and the n-methyl d-aspartate (NMDA) receptor are the two major molecular factors in the development of spinal sensitization at the spinal dorsal horn [48, 49]. Pharmacological studies have showed that antagonism of the PGE2 or the NMDA receptor prevents the development of spinal sensitization. In addition, some antagonisms of the NMDA receptor (e.g., ketamine) may even reverse established visceral hypersensitivity [49, 50]. Spinal sensitization may appear after a noxious stimulus is applied locally to an anatomical site or similar observation may be seen after applying the stimulus to a distant location. Hobson et al. reported that application of a noxious stimulus to the duodenum resulted in esophageal sensitization and balloon distension in the left colon led to rectal sensitization [51]. In patients with IBS, spinal sensitization may ensue as manifested by rectal hyperalgesia following repetitive sigmoid colon distension, and increased viscerosomatic referral through experimental rectal distension [52].

3) The Brain

Peripheral and spinal sensitizations are not exclusive entities in explaining visceral hypersensitivity in humans. Central processing of nociceptive input involves a number of cortical and subcortical brain structures. Noxious affterent signals from the dorsal horn may activate in the thalamus and anterior cingulate. The thalamus relays the signal to the anterior cingulate which is an intergrative brain center involved in emotion, attention and pain [53]. Functional neuroimaging, such as functional magnetic resonance imaging (fMRI), positron emission tomography (PET), magnetoencephalography (MEG), electroencephalography (EEG) and cortical evoked potentials (CEPs) have facilitated the examination of the complete neural axis implicated in central areas. In human studies, increase of blood flow detected by functional brain imaging correlated well with sensory rating activated by noxious intestinal distension [54, 55]. Mayer et al. found in an fMRI study, that in response to experimental rectosigmoid distension, IBS patients have inadequate activation in the subcortical brain regions involved with affective-emotional aspects of pain perception such as the limbic system, the periaqueductal grey (PAG) matter and thalamic regions [56]. Abnormal areas of activation have been observed in other areas such as the anterior cingulate cortex [57], amygdala and brainstem in IBS patients, suggesting that the aberrant visceral nociception observed in this group may be, in part, due to central mechanisms [58, 59]. Future studies using a combination of these functional imaging techniques, in conjunction with improvements in study design, will no doubt further advance our understanding of the mechanisms involved.

4) Autonomic Nervous System (ANS)

ANS communicates between central nerves and the GI tract through its branches, parasympathetic nervous system (PNS) and sympathetic nervous system (SNS). Autonomic dysfunction may co-exist in a number of syndromes where chronic pain is a feature, such as IBS [60]. Heart rate variability (HRV) is an important methodological consideration in the interpretation of results from ANS studies. It may serve as a surrogate marker of ANS parameters reflecting specific gut autonomic innervation. Although a number of studies reported no difference in HRV by comparison of IBS population with healthy controls, changes may be found by dividing the IBS sample into subgroups--based on their predominant bowel symptoms, the severity of clinical course, the presence of depressive symptoms, or a history of abuse in the past--revealed changes in autonomic functioning [60].

The Effects of Estrogen on Motor Dysfunction and Visceral Pain

Estrogen and GI Motor Function

Fluctuation of female sex hormones such as estrogen and progesterone may cause alterations in motility throughout GI tract, including a decrease in LES pressure, changes in gastric motor function, a reduction in small intestine and colon transit rate, and stasis of bile flow.

Esophagus

Symptomatic heartburn is highly prevalent in pregnant women as the progressive rise in plasma estrogen and progesterone during pregnancy has long been thought to be responsible for decreased LES pressure [61-64]. Recently, exogenous estrogen therapy was related to symptomatic GER [65] but no association was found in other studies [66, 67]. An interaction between estrogen use and obesity on the risk of symptomatic GER was also noted in one study [65]. LES pressure and tone may be impaired by smooth muscle relaxing agents such as estrogen and progesterone. During pregnancy, levels of estrogen and progesterone are elevated. Eight women were studied during early pregnancy regarding their LES function. The basal LES pressure was normal; however, the LES pressure responses to hormonal, pharmacological and physiological stimulation were reduced. The serum concentration of gastrin was noted to be unchanged during pregnancy [68].

In an animal study, Fisher and colleagues [61] examined strips of circular smooth muscle from LES of opossums and found that dose-response curves to gastrin and acetylcholine were blocked by 17-β-estradiol, progesterone, or the combination of sex hormones added to the system. The combination of progesterone and estradiol, however, were more potent blockers than either hormone alone, while dihydrotestosterone had no effect [61].

Van Thiel and colleagues studied normal menstruating women who took sequential oral contraceptives. They reported a significant reduction of LES pressure during administration of estrogen and progesterone [69]. Similar story was found by Filipone and colleagues. They showed that the resting LES pressure was significantly reduced with administration of estrogen, progesterone or both in five transsexual patients.

Stomach

A demographic analysis of gastroparesis patients shows that 82% are females and 68% of patients are less than 40 years old [70]. One major etiology (30-40% of all gastroparesis) is diabetes mellitus. Despite a normal gender distribution in diabetes, those diabetic developing gastroparesis are 70-80% female. Unlike the established etiologies of diabetes mellitus and post gastric surgery or vagotomy, idiopathic gastroparesis does not have a known cause. 88% of idiopathic gastroparesis patients are female. They had 7% higher gastric retention of an isotope labeled meal at four hours compared to their male counterparts. Female patients had higher symptom severity scores than males for nausea, bloating, visible stomach distension, and constipation [71]. In addition, idiopathic gastroparesis patients have a higher abdominal pain index than other etiologies and it was reported that physical and sexual abuse occurred in 62% of female patients with idiopathic gastroparesis [70].

The menstrual cycle can be divided into the follicular phase and the luteal phase. The follicular phase includes menses and then the proliferative phase. Ovulation occurs in the middle of the 28 day cycle and marks the beginning of the luteal phase. Gastroparesis patients not taking oral contraceptive pills showed worsening symptoms during the luteal phase. However, gastroparesis patients taking oral contraceptive pills did not have variations in symptoms [72].

Among the normal volunteers enrolled in the protocol that was utilized to create the standard four hour gastric emptying test meal, differences were noted between women and men. Women had a significantly higher percent retention of food than men at 1 and 2 hours. However, by four hours, women and men had no significant differences in retention [70].

This observation of slower gastric emptying rates in women compared to men was previously reported in a study of 20 men and 40 women. Pre- and postmenopausal women and postmenopausal women taking oral estrogens had slower gastric emptying than men [73]. Antral motility was also measured during this study, and there was no difference between men and women [73]. Also, a study of nine women in the first ten days of their menstrual cycle (the luteal phase - estrogen dominated) and 13 men of similar ages showed an increased gastric emptying scintigraphy T ½ time and lower mid-antrum contractility measured by dynamic antral scintigraphy for women [74]. In addition, Hutson and colleagues evaluated mixed liquid and solid meal gastric emptying in men and women and they found premenopausal and postmenopausal women being treated with sex hormone replacement had a decreased rate of gastric emptying of solids compared to men and those without hormone replacement [73].

The wireless motility capsule measures intraluminal pH and pressure. The device can be used to record transit time and contractile activity throughout the gastrointestinal tract. In a wireless motility capsule study, healthy women volunteers had slower gastric emptying time than healthy men [75]. Normal females had higher rates of contraction compared to normal males in the stomach and also higher rates in the proximal small bowel but there was no correlation with gastric emptying or small bowel transit. The study lacked the power to examine gender based differences among gastroparetic patients [76].

Several animal studies have shown that estradiol-17 β delays gastric emptying [77-79]. Chen and colleagues studied effects of sex steroid hormones on gastric emptying in rats and the data showed that estradiol and a mixture of estradiol and progesterone inhibit gastric emptying whereas testosterone had no effects [77]. Ali and McCallum examined female diabetic, gastroparetic rats and demonstrated that gender and estrogens may be leading factors for the slowed gastric emptying of solids, possibly through molecular changes involved in nitric oxide synthesis down-regulation within the antrum and pylorus [80].

Female sex hormone may affect gastric myoelectrical activity. An increased prevalence of gastric dysrhythmias in nauseated pregnant women was found by Koch and colleagues who evaluated gastric myoelectrical activity in 32 pregnant women by using electrogastrogram [81]: Gastric dysrhythmias were demonstrated in all 26 women with nausea; normal gastric rhythms were found in 6 women with minimal to no nausea.

Small Intestine

Gender differences have been noted in diseases of the small intestine. Small-bowel transit can be safely determined using the lactulose hydrogen breath test. Using this technique, Wald and colleagues measured GI transit and sex hormone levels during the 3rd trimester of pregnancy and 4 to 6 weeks after delivery. Small bowel transit time was significantly greater during pregnancy when progesterone and estradiol levels were substantially increased compared to the postpartum period [82]. It has been postulated that estrogen and progesterone may suppress motilin release, thereby contributing to the delayed motility [83].

Colon and Anorectum

Ryan and Bhojwani [84] studied the effect of female sex hormones on colonic transit using radiolabeled markers. A significant slower colon transit time, as measured by geometric mean, was observed in rats with a high estrogen-progesterone cycle stage compared with those with a low hormonal stage. Overariectomized rats pretreated with estrogen and progesterone had significantly slower transit times than untreated ovariectomized animals. There were no significant differences of colonic transit times between pregnant rats and those of animals pretreaated with hormone.

Gastrointestinal transit time was noted to be significantly prolonged in healthy women during the luteal phase when progesterone levels are elevated [85]. In the wireless motility capsule study examining normal and constipated patients, healthy women had slower colonic transit times than men. Whole gut transit time occurs between ingestion of the capsule and its exit from the body, and this time was significantly slower in healthy women compared to healthy men [75]. However, among constipated patients there was no gender difference this study [75].

Although limited data are available on the relationship between sex hormones and chronic constipation, patient with severe chronic idiopathic constipation (CIC) are almost exclusively women of reproductive age. CIC is a condition that individuals have a healthy bowel and suffer from chronic constipation, but their symptoms are not relieved through standard treatment. Kamm et al. investigated 26 patients with CIC and found that CIC was associated with a reduced level of ovarian and adrenal steroid hormones [86]. One in vitro study explored the possible mechanisms for slow-transit constipation (STC) and demonstrated that the over-expression of progesterone receptors may down-regulate contractile G-proteins and up-regulate inhibitory G-proteins in colonic circular muscle cells, which leads to STC in women [87].

As we mentioned before, IBS is more prevalent among women where approximately 70 to 80% of the IBS population are female. IBS is also a very common entity being reported in approximately 15% of the US population. IBS patients are generally divided into three categories as far as their clinical presentation: IBS-diarrhea, IBS-constipation, and IBS-fluctuating. A review of North American data showed about twice as many women than men had constipated IBS [88]. A French study showed a female to male ratio of 2.3 [89]. Also, women with IBS were more likely to report gas, diarrhea, or constipation during menses [90]. A meta-analysis of IBS patients showed women were more likely to report abdominal pain and constipation than men; however, men were more likely to report diarrhea [91]. In this review, both IBS and healthy women reported increased IBS symptoms during menses versus other phases [91]. When measured by balloon dilation, rectal sensitivity increased at menses compared to all other phases of the menstrual cycle. Also, stool consistency was firmer during the luteal phase (progesterone dominated) in this study of 29 patients with IBS [92]. According to an Iceland postal based 10-year follow up survey, in the year 2006, 74% of women had dysmenorrhea and 26% of women with dysmenorrhea had IBS according to Rome III criteria [93].

Gallbladder and Oddi's Spincter

The gallbladder and biliary system are another area of interest regarding female sex hormones where effects have been demonstrated both in normal function and in disease. Female sex hormones are known to affect cholesterol metabolism and gallbladder motility. The liver, which produces bile, has estrogen receptors present. Estrogens act on these receptors to inhibit gallbladder contraction, decrease the gallbladders response to CCK, induce cholesterol levels in bile to spike, and thus cause bile stasis and increase gallstone formation. A number of animal and human studies have demonstrated that estrogen increases the chances for gall stone formation. Uhler and colleagues [94] examined the role of estrgen replacement therapy on the development of gallbladder disease in postmenopausal women and they found estrogen replacement therapy in postmenopausal women increased the rate of gallstone formation.

With ultrasound imaging, gallbladder volume was noted to increase during the duration of pregnancy [95]. Compared to nonpregnant women, pregnant women had increased gallbladder residual volume and a 30% decreased rate of emptying. Women using oral contraceptives did not have changes in function [96]. Looking at the menstrual cycle, women in the luteal phase had higher fasting gallbladder volume and higher ejection fractions than women in the follicular phase [97].

Among people over age 50, 25% of women have gallstones compared to 10 to 15% of men [98]. The relative risk of developing gallbladder disease was 2.0 between women using oral contraceptive pills and non-users [99]. A meta-analysis showed an odds ratio of 1.36 for gallbladder disease between ever and never users of oral contraceptive pills [100]. Among twenty two healthy women studied during oral contraceptive pills and regular menstrual cycles, gallbladder bile was more saturated with cholesterol during contraceptive use [101]. Postmenopausal women using estrogen replacement therapy had a 2.2 relative risk of cholecystectomy compared to never-users [102]. Among male patients randomized to receive estrogen or orchiectomy for prostate cancer, ultrasound imaging one year later showed 5 of 28 patients receiving estrogen developed gallstones compared to 0 of 26 orchidectomized patients.

Estrogen therapy also increased the relative concentration of cholesterol and cholesterol saturation of bile by approximately 30% [103]. Two estrogen receptors have been identified in the body, alpha and beta. In a mouse model, an estrogen receptor alpha agonist increased hepatic cholesterol output leading to cholesterol supersaturated bile and gallstones. The estrogen beta receptor agonist did not have this effect [104].

Tierney and colleagues examined SO phasic wave frequency, amplitude, and motility index during intravenous infusions of different doses of beta-estradiol in male prairie dogs [105]. The results showed SO motility was significantly reduced during estrogen infusion at the higher dose of 10 mg but not the lower doses of 0.1 mg or 1 mg, mainly due to decreased phasic wave frequency. Females dominate the entity termed "sphincter of oddi spasm" or "SO dysfunction" linked to unexlained upper qudrant pain. It is possible that estrogen effects on the SO contributes to the higher incidence of gallstones and sphincter dysfunction seen in premenopausal women [105].

Estrogen and Visceral Hypersensitivity

Many forms of chronic pain or functional pain are more often seen in women and this may be attributed to a direct role of estrogens in the modulation of pain perception by hormonal variations e.g., the menstrual cycle. Hypersensitivity of visceral nociceptive pathways, either of the sensory afferents from peripheral organs or of the central neurons, is the most frequent symptom of conditions such as IBS and FD [106-109].

In FD patients [110], Tack Y et al. examined seventy-four FD patients and 87% of the patients are females. These patients underwent a nutrient drinking test to assess the relationship of sex with maximal tolerated nutrient volume. They found women had a lower tolerated threshold with nutrient drinking than men for induction of early satiety and generation of symptoms e.g., pain in FD patients as well as in healthy controls. They repeated the test which was reproducible.

Similarly, in IBS, patients have been shown to have heightened visceral sensitivity using sigmoid colon and rectal stimulation in comparison of healthy control subjects. Chang et al. [111] found that female IBS patients had a lower discomfort threshold with sigmoid stimulation, compared with their male counterparts. However, a Korean study [112] reported no differences in colorectal perception between male and female in IBS patients and thus they concluded that the increased prevalence of IBS in women was not attributed to gender-related differences in visceroperception. One thing needs to be pointed out in the Korean study is that measurements were made during "nonmenses" days only and some of the women were postmenopausal. It is unclear whether the controversies in visceral sensitivity data are due to menstrual cycle phase or to inherent genetic or cultural variations across groups.

A number of studies have been shown that menstruation status -linked differences in both visceral and somatic sensitivity [92, 113, 114]. One study showed decreased perceptual thresholds in response to rectal distension during the menses phase compared to other cycle (i.e., follicular, ovulatory, luteal) phases by using the barostat to measure visceral sensitivity [92]. In other words, pain sensitivity is elevated at menses relative to other menstrul cycle phases. It is known that estrogen and progesterone is decreased at the menses phase indicating that estrogen or progesterone may act as a protective factor in pain perception.

Similar results were found in animal studies. A number of animal studies investigated the roles of sex hormone in pain sensitivity. These studies used different animal models which included ovariectomy or orchiectomy with and without hormone replacement and pregnancy, as well as measurements made during specific estrus cycle phases. Most of these studies showed that estrogen and progesterone were involved in the regulation of sensitivity to stimuli such as pain and temperature [115-118]. For example, some studies found that ovariectomy improved stress-induced visceral hypersensitivity produced by colorectal distension [119], while others reported that somatic and visceral pain sensitivity was suppressed during pregnancy, a time of high ovarian hormone levels [120].

Both estrogen and progesterone influence nociceptive pathways, either of the sensory afferents from peripheral organs or of the central neurons. At the menses phase or with low estrogen levels, several of the pain conditions that overlap with IBS e,g., migraine headache are more likely to be intense [121]. Cong et al. reported that progesterone and estrogen might work by affecting serotonin and GI and uterine prostaglandins pathways. They found that plasma serotonin levels were lower during menses than during the luteal phase in women with IBS-diarrhea [122]. In another study, the estradiol effects on modulation of pain sensitivity was demonstrated at least partially via the μ-opioid system by using PET with healthy women [123].

Estrogen and Autonomic Nervous System

In addition to the intrinsic enteric nervous system, the extrinsic sympathetic and parasympathetic nerves also play important roles in the regulation of gut function [124-128]. The ANS provides the major linkage between the gut and the brain. However, our understanding of how estrogen and ANS play roles in motility and visceral sensitivity in FGIDs is very limited.

Cowan et al. have demonstrated significant differences of ANS function markers e.g., HRV between men and women in healthy age-matched controls [129]. In IBS, greater sympathetic modulation was found in men than women by measuring HRV and skin conductance at baseline and in response to rectosigmoid balloon distension [130]. Jarret et al. recorded 24-h HRV and noted that vagal activity was decreased in women with IBS as well as healthy control women who had a history of depression and/or anxiety. This indicates that additional factors need to be considered when studing peripheral markers of ANS function between genders [131]. Also, impaired vagal activity has been found in other conditions e.g., women with fibromyalgia [132] and patients with post traumatic stress disorder [133]. In addition, Matsumoto et al. demonstrated a menstrual cycle-linked difference in ANS activity particularly in symptomatic women [134]. However, limited data is available to asertain whether these differences are due to gonadal hormones.

Conclusion

This review attempts to capture some of the historical perspectives as well as highlights of a large body of literature and to understand the roles of estrogen in neurogastroenterology and gastointestinal motility. In many ways, as reflected in the article, it is clear that women dominant conditions ranging from esophagus to colon. We provide evidence to explain these worldwide observations.

One important area that we have not addressed in this article is treatment responses. One hypothysis is that female patients may respond differently to therapies than their male counterparts with "functional" bowel disease. Most of the clinical trials for these "functional disorders" are dominanted by females. Hence investigating the real difference, if any in the female and male responses to pharmacologic agents and therapies has been difficult. The development of new medications to treat the clinical problems discussed in this review article can really be viewed as the development of new drugs that may help females since they are the majority in all the entities we have discussed. The possibility that the remaining minority of patients, who are males, may be as or less responsive or not responsive to these medications, is hard to determine. Future clinical trials will require stratification of females and males for these individual diseases in order to expose both genders equally to new agents versus placebo to ascertain whether gender may play in the efficacy of new therapies.

References

[1] Lydiard, R. B., Increased prevalence of functional gastrointestinal disorders in panic disorder: clinical and theoretical implications. *CNS Spectr,* 2005. 10(11): p. 899-908.

[2] Wu, W., et al. The prevalence of functional gastrointestinal disorders in the chinese air force population. *Gastroenterol Res Pract.* 2013: p. 497585.

[3] Lopez-Colombo, A. et al., The epidemiology of functional gastrointestinal disorders in Mexico: a population-based study. *Gastroenterol Res Pract.* 2012: p. 606174.

[4] Talley, N. J., Functional gastrointestinal disorders as a public health problem. *Neurogastroenterol Motil,* 2008. 20 Suppl 1: p. 121-9.

[5] Uc, A., Hyman P. E., and Walker L. S., Functional gastrointestinal disorders in African American children in primary care. *J Pediatr Gastroenterol Nutr,* 2006. 42(3): p. 270-4.
[6] Xu, J. R. et al., *A population-based study of associations between functional gastrointestinal disorders and psychosocial characteristics in Xi'an,* China. Neurogastroenterol Motil.
[7] Drossman, D. A. et al., U. S. householder survey of functional gastrointestinal disorders. Prevalence, sociodemography, and health impact. *Dig Dis Sci,* 1993. 38(9): p. 1569-80.
[8] Mertz, H. R., Overview of functional gastrointestinal disorders: dysfunction of the brain-gut axis. *Gastroenterol Clin North Am,* 2003. 32(2): p. 463-76, v.
[9] Ouyang, A. and Locke G. R., 3rd, Overview of neurogastroenterology-gastrointestinal motility and functional GI disorders: classification, prevalence, and epidemiology. *Gastroenterol Clin North Am,* 2007. 36(3): p. 485-98, vii.
[10] Ahlawat, S. K., Cuddihy M. T., and Locke G. R., 3rd, Gender-related differences in dyspepsia: a qualitative systematic review. *Gend Med,* 2006. 3(1): p. 31-42.
[11] Blanchard, E. B., et al., Gender differences in psychological distress among patients with irritable bowel syndrome. *J Psychosom Res,* 2001. 50(5): p. 271-5.
[12] Chang, L., et al., Gender, age, society, culture, and the patient's perspective in the functional gastrointestinal disorders. *Gastroenterology,* 2006. 130(5): p. 1435-46.
[13] Flier, S. N. and Rose S., Is functional dyspepsia of particular concern in women? A review of gender differences in epidemiology, pathophysiologic mechanisms, clinical presentation, and management. *Am J Gastroenterol,* 2006. 101(12 Suppl): p. S644-53.
[14] Tang, Y. R., et al., Sex differences in the symptoms and psychological factors that influence quality of life in patients with irritable bowel syndrome. *Eur J Gastroenterol Hepatol.* 24(6): p. 702-7.
[15] Welen, K., Faresjo A. and Faresjo T., Functional dyspepsia affects women more than men in daily life: a case-control study in primary care. *Gend Med,* 2008. 5(1): p. 62-73.
[16] Koloski, N. A., Talley N. J., and Boyce P. M., Epidemiology and health care seeking in the functional GI disorders: a population-based study. *Am J Gastroenterol,* 2002. 97(9): p. 2290-9.
[17] Caballero-Plasencia, A. M., et al., Irritable bowel syndrome in patients with dyspepsia: a community-based study in southern Europe. *Eur J Gastroenterol Hepatol,* 1999. 11 (5): p. 517-22.
[18] Kay, L. and Jorgensen T., Epidemiology of upper dyspepsia in a random population. Prevalence, incidence, natural history, and risk factors. *Scand J Gastroenterol,* 1994. 29 (1): p. 2-6.
[19] Lu, C. L. et al., Prevalence and health/social impacts of functional dyspepsia in Taiwan: a study based on the Rome criteria questionnaire survey assisted by endoscopic exclusion among a physical check-up population. *Scand J Gastroenterol,* 2005. 40(4): p. 402-11.
[20] Shaib, Y. and El-Serag H. B., The prevalence and risk factors of functional dyspepsia in a multiethnic population in the United States. *Am J Gastroenterol,* 2004. 99(11): p. 2210-6.
[21] Zheng, Z. et al., Effects of estrogen with and without progestin and obesity on symptomatic gastroesophageal reflux. *Gastroenterology,* 2008. 135(1): p. 72-81.

[22] Jones, M. P. et al., Hiatal hernia size is the dominant determinant of esophagitis presence and severity in gastroesophageal reflux disease. *Am J Gastroenterol,* 2001. 96 (6): p. 1711-7.

[23] Kahrilas, P. J. et al., Esophageal peristaltic dysfunction in peptic esophagitis. *Gastroenterology,* 1986. 91(4): p. 897-904.

[24] Dodds, W. J. et al., Mechanisms of gastroesophageal reflux in patients with reflux esophagitis. *N Engl J Med,* 1982. 307(25): p. 1547-52.

[25] Holloway, R. H., Penagini R., and Ireland A. C., Criteria for objective definition of transient lower esophageal sphincter relaxation. *Am J Physiol,* 1995. 268(1 Pt 1): p. G1 28-33.

[26] Kahrilas, P. J., The role of hiatus hernia in GERD. *Yale J Biol Med,* 1999. 72(2-3): p. 101-11.

[27] Mittal, R. K. et al., Transient lower esophageal sphincter relaxation. *Gastroenterology,* 1995. 109(2): p. 601-10.

[28] McCallum, R. W., Berkowitz D. M., and Lerner E., Gastric emptying in patients with gastroesophageal reflux. *Gastroenterology,* 1981. 80(2): p. 285-91.

[29] Tack, J. et al., Role of impaired gastric accommodation to a meal in functional dyspepsia. *Gastroenterology,* 1998. 115(6): p. 1346-52.

[30] Leahy, A. et al., Abnormalities of the electrogastrogram in functional gastrointestinal disorders. *Am J Gastroenterol,* 1999. 94(4): p. 1023-8.

[31] Timmons, S., Liston R., and Moriarty K. J., Functional dyspepsia: motor abnormalities, sensory dysfunction, and therapeutic options. *Am J Gastroenterol,* 2004. 99(4): p. 739-49.

[32] Drossman, D. A. et al., AGA technical review on irritable bowel syndrome. *Gastroenterology,* 2002. 123(6): p. 2108-31.

[33] Mayer, E. A. and Raybould H. E., Role of visceral afferent mechanisms in functional bowel disorders. *Gastroenterology,* 1990. 99(6): p. 1688-704.

[34] Chathadi, K. V. and Elta G. H., Motility and dysmotility of the biliary tract. *Semin Gastrointest Dis,* 2003. 14(4): p. 199-207.

[35] Behar, J. and Biancani P., Effect of cholecystokinin and the octapeptide of cholecystokinin on the feline sphincter of Oddi and gallbladder. *Mechanisms of action. J Clin Invest,* 1980. 66(6): p. 1231-9.

[36] Geenen, J. E., et al., Intraluminal pressure recording from the human sphincter of Oddi. *Gastroenterology,* 1980. 78(2): p. 317-24.

[37] LaMorte, W. W. et al., Choledochal sphincter relaxation in response to histamine in the primate. *J Surg Res,* 1980. 28(4): p. 373-8.

[38] Sarles, J. C. et al., Action of cholecystokinin and caerulein on the rabbit sphincter of Oddi. *Digestion,* 1976. 14(5-6): p. 415-23.

[39] Muller, E. L. et al., Influence of motilin and cholecystokinin on sphincter of Oddi and duodenal mobility. *Am J Physiol,* 1987. 253(5 Pt 1): p. G679-83.

[40] Yu, S. et al., TRPA1 in mast cell activation-induced long-lasting mechanical hypersensitivity of vagal afferent C-fibers in guinea pig esophagus. *Am J Physiol Gastrointest Liver Physiol,* 2009. 297(1): p. G34-42.

[41] Jones, R. C., 3rd, Xu L., and Gebhart G. F., The mechanosensitivity of mouse colon afferent fibers and their sensitization by inflammatory mediators require transient

receptor potential vanilloid 1 and acid-sensing ion channel 3. *J Neurosci,* 2005. 25(47): p. 10981-9.

[42] Sipe, W. E. et al., Transient receptor potential vanilloid 4 mediates protease activated receptor 2-induced sensitization of colonic afferent nerves and visceral hyperalgesia. *Am J Physiol Gastrointest Liver Physiol,* 2008. 294(5): p. G1288-98.

[43] Bueno, L., Protease activated receptor 2: a new target for IBS treatment. *Eur Rev Med Pharmacol Sci,* 2008. 12 Suppl 1: p. 95-102.

[44] Toda, N. et al., Modulation of opioid actions by nitric oxide signaling. *Anesthesiology,* 2009. 110(1): p. 166-81.

[45] Ohashi, K. et al., Colonic mast cell infiltration in rats with TNBS-induced visceral hypersensitivity. *J Vet Med Sci,* 2007. 69(12): p. 1223-8.

[46] Liu, M. and Wood J. N., The roles of sodium channels in nociception: implications for mechanisms of neuropathic pain. *Pain Med,* 2011. 12 Suppl 3: p. S93-9.

[47] Knowles, C. H. and Aziz Q., Visceral hypersensitivity in non-erosive reflux disease. *Gut,* 2008. 57(5): p. 674-83.

[48] Grundy, D. et al., Fundamentals of neurogastroenterology: basic science. *Gastroentero-logy,* 2006. 130(5): p. 1391-411.

[49] Sarkar, S. et al., The prostaglandin E2 receptor-1 (EP-1) mediates acid-induced visceral pain hypersensitivity in humans. *Gastroenterology,* 2003. 124(1): p. 18-25.

[50] Willert, R. P. et al., The development and maintenance of human visceral pain hypersensitivity is dependent on the N-methyl-D-aspartate receptor. *Gastroenterology,* 2004. 126(3): p. 683-92.

[51] Hobson, A. R. et al., Development of esophageal hypersensitivity following experimen-tal duodenal acidification. *Am J Gastroenterol,* 2004. 99(5): p. 813-20.

[52] Munakata, J. et al., Repetitive sigmoid stimulation induces rectal hyperalgesia in patients with irritable bowel syndrome. *Gastroenterology,* 1997. 112(1): p. 55-63.

[53] Devinsky, O., Morrell M. J. and Vogt B. A., Contributions of anterior cingulate cortex to behaviour. *Brain,* 1995. 118 (Pt 1): p. 279-306.

[54] Mertz, H. et al., Regional cerebral activation in irritable bowel syndrome and control subjects with painful and nonpainful rectal distention. *Gastroenterology,* 2000. 118(5): p. 842-8.

[55] Silverman, D. H. et al., Regional cerebral activity in normal and pathological perception of visceral pain. *Gastroenterology,* 1997. 112(1): p. 64-72.

[56] Mayer, E. A., Spinal and supraspinal modulation of visceral sensation. *Gut,* 2000. 47 Suppl 4: p. iv69-72; discussion iv76.

[57] Sabbatini, M. et al., The pattern of c-Fos immunoreactivity in the hindbrain of the rat following stomach distension. *Exp Brain Res,* 2004. 157(3): p. 315-23.

[58] Chang, L. et al., Brain responses to visceral and somatic stimuli in patients with irritable bowel syndrome with and without fibromyalgia. *Am J Gastroenterol,* 2003. 98(6): p. 1354-61.

[59] Coen, S. J. et al., Effects of attention on visceral stimulus intensity encoding in the male human brain. *Gastroenterology,* 2008. 135(6): p. 2065-74, 2074 e1.

[60] Mazurak, N. et al., Heart rate variability in the irritable bowel syndrome: a review of the literature. *Neurogastroenterol Motil,* 2012. 24(3): p. 206-16.

[61] Fisher, R. S. et al., Inhibition of lower esophageal sphincter circular muscle by female sex hormones. *Am J Physiol,* 1978. 234(3): p. E243-7.

[62] Marrero, J. M. et al., Determinants of pregnancy heartburn. *Br J Obstet Gynaecol,* 1992. 99(9): p. 731-4.
[63] Schulze, K. and Christensen J., Lower sphincter of the opossum esophagus in pseudopregnancy. *Gastroenterology,* 1977. 73(5): p. 1082-5.
[64] van Thiel, D. H. et al., Heartburn of pregnancy. *Gastroenterology,* 1977. 72(4 Pt 1): p. 666-8.
[65] Nilsson, M. et al., Obesity and estrogen as risk factors for gastroesophageal reflux symptoms. *JAMA,* 2003. 290(1): p. 66-72.
[66] Jacobson, B. C. et al., Body-mass index and symptoms of gastroesophageal reflux in women. *N Engl J Med,* 2006. 354(22): p. 2340-8.
[67] Mohammed, I. et al., Genetic influences in gastro-oesophageal reflux disease: a twin study. *Gut,* 2003. 52(8): p. 1085-9.
[68] Fisher, R. S. et al., Altered lower esophageal sphincter function during early pregnancy. *Gastroenterology,* 1978. 74(6): p. 1233-7.
[69] van Thiel, D. H., Gavaler J.S. and Stremple J., Lower esophageal sphincter pressure in women using sequential oral contraceptives. *Gastroenterology,* 1976. 71(2): p. 232-4.
[70] Soykan, I. et al., Demography, clinical characteristics, psychological and abuse profiles, treatment, and long-term follow-up of patients with gastroparesis. *Dig Dis Sci,* 1998. 43 (11): p. 2398-404.
[71] Parkman, H. P. et al., Clinical features of idiopathic gastroparesis vary with sex, body mass, symptom onset, delay in gastric emptying, and gastroparesis severity. *Gastro-enterology.* 140(1): p. 101-15.
[72] Verrengia, M. et al., Variation of symptoms during the menstrual cycle in female patients with gastroparesis. *Neurogastroenterol Motil.* 23(7): p. 625-e254.
[73] Hutson, W. R., Roehrkasse R. L. and Wald A., Influence of gender and menopause on gastric emptying and motility. *Gastroenterology,* 1989. 96(1): p. 11-7.
[74] Knight, L. C. et al., Delayed gastric emptying and decreased antral contractility in normal premenopausal women compared with men. *Am J Gastroenterol,* 1997. 92(6): p. 968-75.
[75] Rao, S. S. et al., Investigation of colonic and whole-gut transit with wireless motility capsule and radiopaque markers in constipation. *Clin Gastroenterol Hepatol,* 2009. 7 (5): p. 537-44.
[76] Kloetzer, L. et al., Motility of the antroduodenum in healthy and gastroparetics characterized by wireless motility capsule. *Neurogastroenterol Motil.* 22(5): p. 527-33, e117.
[77] Chen, T. S. et al., Effects of sex steroid hormones on gastric emptying and gastrointestinal transit in rats. *Am J Physiol,* 1995. 268(1 Pt 1): p. G171-6.
[78] Gonenne, J. et al., Effect of female sex hormone supplementation and withdrawal on gastrointestinal and colonic transit in postmenopausal women. *Neurogastroenterol Motil,* 2006. 18(10): p. 911-8.
[79] Walsh, J. W. et al., Progesterone and estrogen are potential mediators of gastric slow-wave dysrhythmias in nausea of pregnancy. *Am J Physiol,* 1996. 270(3 Pt 1): p. G506-14.
[80] Showkat Ali, M. et al., Gender and estradiol as major factors in the expression and dimerization of nNOSalpha in rats with experimental diabetic gastroparesis. *Dig Dis Sci.* 57(11): p. 2814-25.

[81] Koch, K. L. et al., Gastric dysrhythmias and nausea of pregnancy. *Dig Dis Sci,* 1990. 35 (8): p. 961-8.
[82] Wald, A. et al., Effect of pregnancy on gastrointestinal transit. *Dig Dis Sci,* 1982. 27 (11): p. 1015-8.
[83] Christofides, N. D. et al., Decreased plasma motilin concentrations in pregnancy. *Br Med J (Clin Res Ed),* 1982. 285(6353): p. 1453-4.
[84] Ryan, J. P. and Bhojwani A., Colonic transit in rats: effect of ovariectomy, sex steroid hormones, and pregnancy. *Am J Physiol,* 1986. 251(1 Pt 1): p. G46-50.
[85] Wald, A. et al., Gastrointestinal transit: the effect of the menstrual cycle. *Gastroenterology,* 1981. 80(6): p. 1497-500.
[86] Kamm, M. A. et al., Steroid hormone abnormalities in women with severe idiopathic constipation. *Gut,* 1991. 32(1): p. 80-4.
[87] Xiao, Z. L. et al., Role of progesterone signaling in the regulation of G-protein levels in female chronic constipation. *Gastroenterology,* 2005. 128(3): p. 667-75.
[88] Saito, Y. A., Schoenfeld P., and Locke G. R., 3rd, The epidemiology of irritable bowel syndrome in North America: a systematic review. *Am J Gastroenterol,* 2002. 97(8): p. 1910-5.
[89] Bommelaer, G. et al., Prevalence of irritable bowel syndrome in the French population according to the Rome I criteria. *Gastroenterol Clin Biol,* 2002. 26(12): p. 1118-23.
[90] Whitehead, W. E. et al., Evidence for exacerbation of irritable bowel syndrome during menses. *Gastroenterology,* 1990. 98(6): p. 1485-9.
[91] Adeyemo, M. A., Spiegel B. M., and Chang L., Meta-analysis: do irritable bowel syndrome symptoms vary between men and women? *Aliment Pharmacol Ther.* 32(6): p. 738-55.
[92] Houghton, L. A. et al., The menstrual cycle affects rectal sensitivity in patients with irritable bowel syndrome but not healthy volunteers. *Gut,* 2002. 50(4): p. 471-4.
[93] Olafsdottir, L. B. et al., Natural history of irritable bowel syndrome in women and dysmenorrhea: a 10-year follow-up study. *Gastroenterol Res Pract.* 2012: p. 534204.
[94] Uhler, M. L., Marks J. W., and Judd H. L., Estrogen replacement therapy and gallbladder disease in postmenopausal women. *Menopause,* 2000. 7(3): p. 162-7.
[95] Stauffer, R. A. et al., Gallbladder disease in pregnancy. *Am J Obstet Gynecol,* 1982. 144(6): p. 661-4.
[96] Braverman, D. Z., Johnson M. L. and Kern, F. Jr., Effects of pregnancy and contraceptive steroids on gallbladder function. *N Engl J Med,* 1980. 302(7): p. 362-4.
[97] Xynos, E. et al., Effect of the menstrual cycle on gallbladder fasting volume and postprandial emptying in nulliparous young females. *Invest Radiol,* 1997. 32(6): p. 330-4.
[98] Diehl, A. K., Epidemiology and natural history of gallstone disease. *Gastroenterol Clin North Am,* 1991. 20(1): p. 1-19.
[99] Oral contraceptives and venous thromboembolic disease, surgically confirmed gallbladder disease, and breast tumours. Report from the Boston Collaborative Drug Surveillance Programme. *Lancet,* 1973. 1(7817): p. 1399-404.
[100] Thijs, C. and Knipschild P., Oral contraceptives and the risk of gallbladder disease: a meta-analysis. *Am J Public Health,* 1993. 83(8): p. 1113-20.
[101] Bennion, L. J. et al., Effects of oral contraceptives on the gallbladder bile of normal women. *N Engl J Med,* 1976. 294(4): p. 189-92.

[102] Grodstein, F., Colditz G. A., and Stampfer M. J., Postmenopausal hormone use and cholecystectomy in a large prospective study. *Obstet Gynecol,* 1994. 83(1): p. 5-11.

[103] Henriksson, P. et al., Estrogen-induced gallstone formation in males. Relation to changes in serum and biliary lipids during hormonal treatment of prostatic carcinoma. *J Clin Invest,* 1989. 84(3): p. 811-6.

[104] Wang, H. H., Afdhal N. H., and Wang D. Q., Estrogen receptor alpha, but not beta, plays a major role in 17beta-estradiol-induced murine cholesterol gallstones. *Gastroenterology,* 2004. 127(1): p. 239-49.

[105] Tierney, S., et al., Estrogen inhibits sphincter of Oddi motility. *J Surg Res,* 1994. 57(1): p. 69-73.

[106] Anand, P. et al., Peripheral and central mechanisms of visceral sensitization in man. *Neurogastroenterol Motil,* 2007. 19(1 Suppl): p. 29-46.

[107] Cervero, F. and Laird J. M., Role of ion channels in mechanisms controlling gastrointestinal pain pathways. *Curr Opin Pharmacol,* 2003. 3(6): p. 608-12.

[108] Eckler, S. A., Kuehn R., and Gautam M., Deletion of N-terminal rapsyn domains disrupts clustering and has dominant negative effects on clustering of full-length rapsyn. *Neuroscience,* 2005. 131(3): p. 661-70.

[109] Triadafilopoulos, G., Finlayson M. and Grellet C., Bowel dysfunction in postmenopausal women. *Women Health,* 1998. 27(4): p. 55-66.

[110] Kindt, S. et al., Reproducibility and symptomatic predictors of a slow nutrient drinking test in health and in functional dyspepsia. *Neurogastroenterol Motil,* 2008. 20(4): p. 320-9.

[111] Chang, L. et al., Effect of sex on perception of rectosigmoid stimuli in irritable bowel syndrome. *Am J Physiol Regul Integr Comp Physiol,* 2006. 291(2): p. R277-84.

[112] Kim, H. S. et al., Gender-related differences in visceral perception in health and irritable bowel syndrome. *J Gastroenterol Hepatol,* 2006. 21(2): p. 468-73.

[113] Jackson, N. A. et al., Does the menstrual cycle affect anorectal physiology? *Dig Dis Sci,* 1994. 39(12): p. 2607-11.

[114] Robbins, A., Berkley K. J., and Sato Y., Estrous cycle variation of afferent fibers supplying reproductive organs in the female rat. *Brain Res,* 1992. 596(1-2): p. 353-6.

[115] Bradshaw, H. B. et al., Estrous variations in behavioral responses to vaginal and uterine distention in the rat. *Pain,* 1999. 82(2): p. 187-97.

[116] Fillingim, R. B., Sex, gender, and pain: women and men really are different. *Curr Rev Pain,* 2000. 4(1): p. 24-30.

[117] Giamberardino, M. A. et al., Changes in visceral pain reactivity as a function of estrous cycle in female rats with artificial ureteral calculosis. *Brain Res,* 1997. 774(1-2): p. 234-8.

[118] Sanoja, R. and Cervero F., Estrogen-dependent abdominal hyperalgesia induced by ovariectomy in adult mice: a model of functional abdominal pain. *Pain,* 2005. 118(1-2): p. 243-53.

[119] Bradesi, S. et al., Stress-induced visceral hypersensitivity in female rats is estrogen-dependent and involves tachykinin NK1 receptors. *Pain,* 2003. 102(3): p. 227-34.

[120] Cogan, R. and Spinnato J. A., Pain and discomfort thresholds in late pregnancy. *Pain,* 1986. 27(1): p. 63-8.

[121] le Resche, L. et al., Changes in temporomandibular pain and other symptoms across the menstrual cycle. *Pain,* 2003. 106(3): p. 253-61.

[122] Cong, P. et al., Abnormalities of prostaglandins and cyclooxygenase enzymes in female patients with slow-transit constipation. *Gastroenterology,* 2007. 133(2): p. 445-53.
[123] Smith, Y. R. et al., Pronociceptive and antinociceptive effects of estradiol through endogenous opioid neurotransmission in women. *J Neurosci,* 2006. 26(21): p. 5777-85.
[124] Appenzeller, O., Vinken P., and Bruyn G., *The Autonomic Nervous System.* 1999: Elsevier Health Sciences.
[125] Costanzo, L., *Physiology.* 4th ed. 2006: Lippincott Williams & Wilkins. 334.
[126] Goldstein, D., *The Autonomic Nervous System in Health and Disease.* 2000: Informa Health Care. 618.
[127] Jänig, W., *The Integrative Action of the Autonomic Nervous System: Neurobiology of Homeostasis.* 2006: Cambridge University Press. 610.
[128] Robertson, D., *Primer on the Autonomic Nervous System.* 2nd ed. Gastrointestinal Function, ed. M. Camilleri. 2004: Academic Press. 488.
[129] Cowan, M. J., Pike K., and Burr R. L., Effects of gender and age on heart rate variability in healthy individuals and in persons after sudden cardiac arrest. *J Electrocardiol,* 1994. 27 Suppl: p. 1-9.
[130] Tillisch, K. et al., Sex specific alterations in autonomic function among patients with irritable bowel syndrome. *Gut,* 2005. 54(10): p. 1396-401.
[131] Jarrett, M. E. et al., Anxiety and depression are related to autonomic nervous system function in women with irritable bowel syndrome. *Dig Dis Sci,* 2003. 48(2): p. 386-94.
[132] Stein, P. K. et al., Sex effects on heart rate variability in fibromyalgia and Gulf War illness. *Arthritis Rheum,* 2004. 51(5): p. 700-8.
[133] Bryant, R. A., Longitudinal psychophysiological studies of heart rate: mediating effects and implications for treatment. *Ann N Y Acad Sci,* 2006. 1071: p. 19-26.
[134] Matsumoto, T. et al. Autonomic nervous system activity in the late luteal phase of eumenorrheic women with premenstrual symptomatology. *J Psychosom Obstet Gynaecol,* 2006. 27(3): p. 131-9.

In: Estradiol: Synthesis, Health Effects and Drug Interactions ISBN: 978-1-62808-962-2
Editors: Ricco Palmeri and Sal Grimaudo

Chapter 7

Estradiol and Memory: Morphological and Behavioural Implications

Brianne C. Wartman ***and Matthew R. Holahan***
Carleton University, Department of Neuroscience, Ottawa, Ontario, Canada

Abstract

The role of estradiol as a sex hormone is well-established. However, estradiol also exerts actions in the central nervous system that extend beyond basic sexual and reproductive functions. In this respect, estradiol exerts pronounced effects on the morphology and function of brain regions not typically considered for their contribution to reproductive function. As such, circulating levels of estradiol have been shown to produce marked effects on both reproductive and non-reproductive behaviors. The well-documented effects of estradiol on dendritic spine density in hippocampal pyramidal cells, an area critical to learning and memory, indicate an important role for estradiol in memory function. These "non-reproductive" behavioural effects remain unclear and the precise actions of estradiol on memory function are yet to be fully elucidated. The effects of estradiol on the brain throughout the lifespan are of particular interest due to the therapeutic implications which may be derived. While this is of particular interest during aging, it is also important to examine the effects of estradiol on the young adult and adolescent brain to determine the functional implications of estradiol's effects. A review of the pertinent literature concerning estradiol's morphological consequences in the brain, in particular, the hippocampus, and effects on memory function will be examined.

Keywords: Estradiol; Memory; Hippocampus

* Corresponding author: Carleton University 1125 Colonel By Drive, 325 Life Sciences Research Building, Ottawa, ON, Canada, K1S 5B6, Tele: 613-520-2600 ext 1543, Fax: 613-520-3667, Email: briannewartman@cmail.carleton.ca.

Introduction

Overview

Historically, estrogens have been considered sex hormones associated with reproductive behaviours. The focus of this chapter, however, is on the non-reproductive effects of estradiol, specifically the effects of estradiol on cognitive processes such as learning and memory. A number of findings in the last few decades have highlighted a potentially causal link between estradiol and cognition. Estrogen receptors are expressed within brain areas related to learning and memory such as the prefrontal cortex and hippocampus (Shughrue & Merchenthaler, 2000; Shughrue et al. 1997a, b; Milner 2001, 2005; Osterlund et al. 2000) and research has discovered morphological changes within these structures in response to estradiol (Woolley et al. 1990; Gould et al. 1990). This has led to an interest in estradiol's functional role in learning and memory. As such, cognitive decline has been noted following menopause after which estradiol levels drop drastically (Sherwin, 2006; Sherwin & Henry, 2008; Wolf & Kirschbaum, 2002). There is also a putative connection between estradiol and neurodegenerative diseases such as Alzheimer's (Hogervorst et al. 2000; Launer et al. 1999; Sherwin, 1999; Wolf & Kirschbaum, 2002; Zandi et al. 2002). Although the non-reproductive roles of estradiol have been gaining attention, a concrete role for estradiol in learning and memory remains elusive. A number of variables appear to play a role in determining estradiol's effects on learning and memory processes and special attention must be paid to details including duration of estradiol administration, timing of administration, dose of estradiol administered, and age of the animal. These factors are discussed below.

Estradiol

Estrogens comprise a class of steroid hormones including estradiol-17β (estradiol or E), estriol, and estrone. Estradiol is considered the most biologically active form of estrogen (Srivastava & Penzes, 2011). The primary sources of estrogens in females are the ovaries. However, estradiol may also be synthesized *de novo* within the brain (Srivastava & Penzes, 2011; Konkle & McCarthy, 2011; Hojo et al. 2008). With the onset of puberty, hormone signals from the brain elicit a cyclic manner of estrogen production. In rodents, estradiol levels fluctuate naturally across a 4 day cycle. During the estrous cycle, estradiol levels reach their peak during the proestrus phase then rapidly decline over approximately 24 hours reaching their lowest levels during the estrus phase (Butcher et al., 1974). Estradiol levels can be manipulated experimentally, through exogenous administration of estradiol or via ovariectomy (OVX), an effective and commonly used surgical method. Following OVX, estradiol levels decrease significantly compared to intact, cycling rats (Davidge et al., 2001).

Estrogen Receptors

Estradiol binds to estrogen receptors alpha (ERα), beta (ERβ) and the newly termed GPER (previously GPR30) (Barton, 2012). ERα and ERβ have been identified throughout the brain in regions including the hippocampus, cortex and amygdala (Shughrue & Merchenthaler, 2000; Shughrue et al. 1997a, b; Milner 2001, 2005; Osterlund et al. 2000). These receptors are located in nuclear, cytoplasmic and membrane compartments (McEwen et al. 2001; Spencer et al. 2008). Historically, ERα and ERβ were considered genomic receptors. These receptors were believed to be located intracellularly, where once bound by estradiol, receptors would dimerize and act as transcription factors. The complex would bind to the estrogen response element on DNA (see McEwen & Alves, 1999) and exert a slow mechanism of action via transcriptional processes. More recently, non-genomic mechanisms of action have been attributed to estrogen receptors. Estrogen receptors have been found on cell membranes (Milner 2001, 2005) and rapid actions of estradiol have been identified through their role in intracellular signalling cascades.

Learning and Memory Effects of Estradiol

The role of estradiol in learning and memory function, although not a novel research area, merits continued investigation. Brain areas typically linked to learning and memory function, most notably the hippocampus, are sensitive to estradiol manipulation and warrant exploration into potential functional effects. A number of studies have examined the cognitive effects of estradiol manipulation, producing a great deal of data, but many questions remain. Studies have reported improved place memory (Zurkovsky et al. 2007; Zurkovsky et al. 2006), working memory on spatial tasks (Daniel et al. 1997; Daniel et al. 2006), improved memory retention on a delayed matching-to-place water maze task (Sandstrom & Williams, 2001), improved place-learning on an inhibitory avoidance task (Frye & Rhodes, 2002) and improved object and place recognition (Scharfman et al., 2007) associated with elevated levels of circulating estrogens. Others have reported no effect of elevated estrogens on working memory (Galea et al., 2001; Stackman et al. 1997) or spatial task performance (Berry et al. 1997) and some have found impaired working memory (Holmes et al. 2002; Wide et al. 2004) following elevated levels of estrogens. Attention must be paid to methodological details when sorting through estradiol research. An overview of recent and relevant research is described below, with an emphasis on hippocampal-dependent learning and memory.

Chronic Effects of Estradiol on Learning and Memory

Largely due to the classic belief that activation of ERs have only a genomic mode of action, many estradiol studies have examined the long-term effects of estradiol manipulation. Although not all studies are in agreement, a wealth of research supports the finding that chronic estradiol treatment enhances learning and memory function, indicating estradiol has long-term effects on cognitive function. Daniel et al. (1997) showed a positive effect of chronic estradiol treatment (via silastic capsule) on radial arm maze performance in OVX rats. Korol & Kolo (2002) demonstrated enhanced performance on a place task in OVX rats administered two subcutaneous estradiol treatments 48 and 24hours prior to testing. Li et al.

(2004) reported that performance on an object placement task was significantly enhanced in OVX rats administered estradiol for 5 days, when testing took place two days following cessation of treatment. Wallace et al. (2006) examined the effect of OVX on performance in an object placement and object recognition task. Both tasks showed a significant decline in performance in OVX rats compared to intact rats. This decline was significant at 4 weeks post OVX in the object placement task and 1 week post OVX in the object recognition task, indicating task-specific differences. More recently, Lipatova and Toufexis (2013) examined the effect of long-term estradiol treatment in OVX rats. Results showed that estradiol-treated and control rats acquired a spatial reference memory task at the same rate, performing the task similarly. However, when memory was tested following at a 21-day retention interval, estradiol treated rats performed significantly better than control rats. These studies suggest a positive effect of chronic estradiol treatment in mediating cognitive function which falls in line with the genomic actions of nuclear ERα and ERβ receptors.

Acute Effects of Estradiol on Learning and Memory

The discovery of non-nuclear ERs motivated a change in the way research examined estradiol's effects on brain and behavioral function (Milner 2001; Milner 2005). Instead of only a slow acting method mediating estradiol's cognitive effects, a rapid method of mediation became known and acute and immediate effects of estradiol were examined in learning and memory procedures. For example, Luine et al. (2003) examined whether OVX rats that received subcutaneous acute injections of estradiol 30 minutes prior to, or immediately following, learning would show memory enhancements. Rats that received injections of estradiol and were tested 4 hours later on an object or place recognition test, showed enhancements on both tasks compared to vehicle-treated controls. Interestingly, a two hour delay in the injection of estradiol following learning did not result in an enhancement of memory on these tasks. These results indicated a rapid enhancement of memory by estradiol, which implicated the involvement of non-genomic, non-nuclear estrogen receptors. Estradiol manipulation leading to rapid enhancements in memory has spurred research delving into the time course of estradiol's actions. A number of studies have been published which show that estradiol administration peripherally (Packard & Teather, 1997; Packard, 1998; Walf et al. 2006; Fernandez et al. 2008) or centrally (Fan et al. 2010; Fernandez et al. 2008) enhanced memory on a water maze retention test (spatial) (Packard et al. 1997; Packard 1998) and an object recognition test (non-spatial) (Walf et al. 2006; Fan et al. 2010; Fernandez et al. 2008) when given directly after training, but not when injections were delayed by 1-2 hours post training, suggesting a window of opportunity for estradiol to exert it's positive effects on memory. MacLusky et al. (2005) examined whether morphological changes induced by estradiol would occur rapidly enough to account for the behavioural effects. They found that post synaptic spine density was increased within 30 minutes of estradiol administration and persisted for at least 4.5 hours after estradiol administration. These findings suggested morphological changes could contribute to the behavioural effects noted with acute estradiol administration. This window of opportunity is consistent with the time line of consolidation processes (McGaugh, 1989; McGaugh, 2000) indicating post-training infusions of estradiol may be beneficial to consolidation processes and mediated through signalling cascades which result in memory enhancements (Fan et al. 2010; Fernandez et al. 2008).

Estradiol Dosage on Learning and Memory

An important consideration in estradiol research is the dose of estradiol administered and the method through which this administration occurs. Estradiol is often administered through injection, allowing the experimenter to manipulate not only the dose, but the timing of administration. This method allows the researcher to mimic cyclic variations of estradiol if desired, producing an estradiol profile more similar to that seen naturally. Alternatively, estradiol may be administered via implanted capsule or pellet. This method also allows for the choice of dose, however, cyclic variations in estradiol levels are not possible.

The dose at which estradiol is delivered has important implications on both the behavioural and morphological effects seen. Inagaki et al. (2010) provided a useful dose-response report on both 17-α and 17-β estradiol. These investigators provide strong evidence corroborating earlier reports (Luine et al. 2003) of an inverted U dose-response relationship for estradiol. Findings suggested 17-α estradiol acts more potently to elicit behavioural effects compared to 17-β estradiol, as lower doses of 17-α estradiol resulted in enhancements in memory consolidation on both object placement and object recognition tasks. Higher doses of both isomers were required to produce enhancements in object place compared to object recognition tasks (Luine et al. 2003; Inagaki et al. 2010). The most effective dose for enhancement in memory consolidation on the object placement task was 5ug/kg of 17-α estradiol and 20ug/kg of 17-β estradiol (Inagaki et al., 2010). The most effective dose for enhancement in memory consolidation on the object recognition task was 1-2ug/kg of 17-α estradiol and 5ug/kg of 17-β estradiol (Inagaki et al., 2010). McLaughlin and colleagues (2008) examined the effect of estradiol dose on the performance of three behavioural tasks: object placement, water maze and Y maze. Performance on the object placement task was enhanced by a dose of 10ug of 17-β estradiol (the highest dose used in this experiment), while performance on the water maze task was enhanced by a dose of 5ug of 17-β estradiol. Y maze performance was not enhanced by either dose. Evidence also suggests there is a dose-age interaction. Foster et al. (2003) showed that aged rats performed best when implanted with a high dose silastic capsule filled with estradiol benzoate, middle-aged rats performed best when implanted with a low dose silastic capsule and young rats performed best with no estradiol administration. These results indicate the effects of estradiol dose are task-specific and intricate, highlighting the complexity of estradiol's functional consequences. MacLusky et al. (2005) provided information on the post synaptic spine density response in reaction to different doses and isomers of estradiol. Findings indicated that a 45ug/kg dose of 17- β estradiol was sufficient to cause a significant increase in post synaptic spine density at 30 minutes and 4.5 hours following administration (a 15ug/kg dose was ineffective). Similar to Inagaki et al., 17- α estradiol was found to have more potent effects compared to 17- β estradiol, resulting in a larger increase in post synaptic spine density. The findings discussed above suggest important differences in behavioural and morphological outcomes due to different methods, doses and isomers of estradiol administration, a factor which should be taken into consideration when examining literature regarding estradiol's effects on cognitive processes such as memory.

Strategy Bias

A discussion of estradiol's cognitive effects would not be complete without at least a brief discussion of cognitive bias (see Korol 2004 for review). Briefly, estradiol levels play a role in biasing the learning strategy used to perform a task: high levels of estradiol seem to favour the use of hippocampal-based strategies, while low levels of estradiol seem to favour striatal-based strategies. Therefore, it seems that estradiol can act to both enhance and impair certain aspects of cognition depending on the task demands being tapped. These data help to address some discrepancies in the literature as to whether estradiol is cognitive enhancing or cognitive impairing. Estradiol does not necessarily convey an overall enhancement or impairment in terms of cognition, but rather, estradiol's effects seem to depend on the specific task demands.

One of the most convincing demonstrations of this cognitive bias comes from Korol & Kolo (2002). Rats were OVX and trained on a place or a response task. Prior to training on the tasks, rats were given injections of estradiol or vehicle, such that cytological examination of vaginal smears demonstrated that estradiol-treated rats displayed proestrus profiles while vehicle-treated rats displayed diestrus profiles. Rats administered estradiol performed better on the place task compared to vehicle-treated rats. Rats administered vehicle performed better on the response task compared to estradiol-treated rats. These findings suggested estradiol's actions in the brain may be task-specific and dependent upon the strategy used to solve the task. Korol et al. (2004) examined whether natural fluctuations across the estrous cycle resulted in the same strategy biases that were seen with exogenously administered estradiol. Findings showed that intact female rats were more likely to choose place strategies during the proestrous phase and response strategies during the estrus phase, indicating this strategy bias is present in normally cycling rats. Daniel & Lee (2004) examined the strategy selection bias on a water maze task using OVX rats with silastic estradiol or cholesterol implants. Results indicated estradiol-treated rats were biased against using a landmark /visible cue, suggesting they were biased toward using a hippocampal-based strategy to solve the task, supporting the findings gathered by Korol & Kolo (2002), Korol et al. (2004) and other studies (Walf et al. 2006; Zurkovsky et al. 2007).

Morphological Effects of Estradiol

Synaptic Plasticity and Spines

Synaptic plasticity is a process representing a change in the strength and number of connections between neurons due to experience. These changes in the strength and number of connections are believed to underlie learning and memory processes at the systems and behavioral levels. Dendrites and dendritic spines are specialized structures which represent the postsynaptic point of contact in a synapse and receive synaptic input. Changes in spine number and/ or morphology represent potential functional variations that are considered important in learning and memory. For example, increases in dendritic density have been associated with memory formation (Restivo et al. 2009; Restivo et al. 2006; Knafo et al. 2004; Leuner et al., 2003). Dendritic spine size and type undergo changes in response to neuronal stimulation (Matsuzaki et al. 2004; 2001; Okamoto et al. 2004; Zhou et al. 2004) and a difference in function between spine types has been suggested. Mushroom spines, spines with constricted necks and heads exceeding 0.6 microns in diameter (Harris et al. 1992) are considered "memory spines" and are involved in long-term memory storage. Mushroom spines can form strong synapses due to large postsynaptic densities that accommodate greater numbers of AMPA receptors (Bourne & Harris, 2007; Ashby et al. 2006; Ganeshina et al. 2004; Harris et al., 1992). Thin spines, spines with a constricted neck and small head (Harris et al., 1992) are considered "learning spines" and are involved in transient events. Thin spines are flexible, responsive to changes in synaptic activity levels and have smaller postsynaptic densities that contain fewer AMPA receptors but many NMDA receptors (Hubener & Bonhoeffer, 2010; Bourne & Harris 2008; 2007; Ashby et al., 2006; Ganeshina et al., 2004; Farris et al. 2001; Harris et al., 1992). Research has identified a relationship between hippocampal spine density and type (Leuner & Shors 2004; Restivo et al., 2009; Restivo et al. 2006; Knafo et al. 2004; Leuner et al. 2003) as well as NMDA receptor activation and number (Bashir et al. 1990; Morris, 1989; Coan et al. 1987; Morris et al., 1986; Collingridge et al1983) in modulating learning and memory function. These observations lead to the question of whether estradiol modulates functional aspects of learning and memory through these changes in spine type or density.

Estrogen and Dendritic Spines

The first seminal studies demonstrating a role for estrogen in mediating morphological changes in the hippocampus came from the laboratory of Bruce McEwen in the early 1990's. Gould et al. (1990) demonstrated a striking effect of OVX on dendritic spine density, whereby adult female OVX rats showed a dramatic decrease in spine density in CA1 pyramidal cells of the hippocampus. This decrease was prevented by estradiol replacement and augmented by progesterone administration. The effects due to this estradiol manipulation came about rapidly, and led experimenters to determine whether CA1 pyramidal cell spine density fluctuated naturally, across the rat estrous cycle. Woolley et al. (1990) examined the effect of the naturally occurring estrous cycle on spine density in the hippocampus. A 30% decrease in apical spine density was found between proestrus (when estradiol levels reach their peak) to estrus (when estradiol levels reach their lowest) phases of the cycle, corresponding to a 24hr time period. This fluctuation in spine density was specific to the apical region of the CA1 hippocampal pyramidal cell dendritic tree. Further research (Woolley & McEwen, 1992) demonstrated that the density of synapses in the hippocampal CA1 region correlated with spine density and fluctuated naturally across the estrous cycle. Importantly, similar morphological findings in response to estradiol treatment were found in nonhuman primates (Leranth et al. 2002) and other brain areas such as the hypothalamus (Frankfurt et al. 1990) and prefrontal cortex (Tang et al. 2004; Srivastava et al. 2008).

Although the mechanisms underlying estradiol's morphological manifestations are still under investigation, research has provided some answers. Woolley and McEwen (1994) provided evidence suggesting the effects of estradiol on dendritic spine density on CA1 pyramidal cells was regulated via an NMDA receptor mechanism. Estradiol's effects on spine density in the CA1 were blocked by treatment using NMDA receptor antagonists (MK-801 and CGP 43487) but not by antagonists of AMPA or muscarinic receptors. Further research also demonstrated an estradiol-induced increase in binding to NMDA receptors, increasing the sensitivity of CA1 pyramidal cells (Woolley et al., 1997). These findings indicated the importance of estradiol in modulating mechanisms involved in learning and memory function. The connection between estradiol's effects on memory tasks and its dramatic morphological effects on the hippocampus, a structure linked to learning and memory, makes for an interesting correlation to examine.

It is challenging to determine whether the morphological manifestations attributed to estradiol's effects relate to the behavioural effects noted in the literature. It becomes difficult to examine both the morphological and behavioural consequences of estradiol treatment as it is often the case that behavioural training and testing procedures used for assessment cause confounding morphological changes. For example, Frick and colleagues (2004) showed that estradiol administration to behaviourally naïve rats resulted in an increase in CA1 spine synapse density compared to vehicle controls. However, CA1 spine synapse density did not differ between control-treated water-maze tested rats and estradiol-treated behaviourally naïve rats, suggesting that the water maze protocol masked estradiol-induced changes in CA1 synaptic plasticity. A study by Bohacek & Daniel (2007) demonstrated that the potential memory enhancing effects of estradiol administration become masked by handling procedures used in experimental protocols. Findings such as these may help explain why the literature regarding estradiol's effects (both morphological and behavioral) is conflicting.

An interesting study by Sandstrom and Williams (2001) investigated the memory retention effects of estradiol administration using identical doses, timing, routes of administration, and strains of rats as previous studies (Woolley et al., 1990; Woolley & McEwen, 1992). Results from this study found that enhancements in working memory retention were temporally related to increases in CA1 spine density resulting from estradiol treatment in OVX rats, suggesting changes in hippocampal connectivity moderated by estradiol may bring about the memory enhancing effects observed. Wallace et al. (2006) carried out a study that examined both behavioural and morphological endpoints in relation to changes in estradiol levels. In this study, OVX and intact rats were tested on a spatial and non-spatial memory task. OVX rats displayed a deficit in performance on both tasks compared to intact rats. Additionally, the deficit in performance seen in OVX animals was associated with a decrease in dendritic spine density in the CA1 region of the hippocampus and prefrontal cortex. Results from this study suggested a connection between memory impairments associated with OVX (i.e. lower estradiol levels) and morphological manifestations resulting from lower levels of estradiol. Findings using mice differed slightly from those found with rats. Mice treated with estradiol did not show an increase in dendritic spine density in the CA1 (Li et al. 2004). However, estradiol treatment led to an increase in the number of mushroom-shaped spines and an up-regulation of presynaptic (syntaxin) and postsynaptic (PSD95, spinophilin) proteins in the hippocampus. This study highlights the importance of examining spine type in dendritic analyses regarding estradiol.

Although methodological concerns make it difficult to directly relate morphological consequences of estradiol levels to behavioural consequences of estradiol levels, the findings discussed above suggest the two may be connected. Temporal patterns of behavioural enhancements correlate well with patterns of increased dendritic density in regions related to behavioural function (i.e. the hippocampus; prefrontal cortex), and this connection will benefit from future studies investigating the particulars of morphological changes and their correlations to functional effects.

Estradiol across the Lifespan

To fully understand the potential therapeutic uses of estradiol, an understanding of estradiol's effects throughout the lifespan is necessary. Evidence suggests that the onset of menopause, associated with a decrease in estradiol levels, is associated with cognitive decline (Sherwin, 2006; Sherwin & Henry, 2008; Wolf & Kirschbaum, 2002). Despite negative findings regarding estradiol's potential for therapeutic use (Espeland et al., 2004; Rapp et al., 2003b; Shumaker et al., 2004, 2003), recent research has suggested estradiol therapy may be beneficial. Reports have indicated that estradiol replacement, in the form of hormone therapy, has helped to alleviate these cognitive issues (Sherwin, 2006; Sherwin & Henry, 2008; Wolf & Kirschbaum, 2002; Hogervorst *et al.,* 2000; LeBlanc *et al.,* 2001; Yaffe *et al.,* 1998b). A number of rodent studies have examined the effect of estradiol administration throughout the lifespan (Diz Chaves et al. 2012; Foster et al. 2003; Kiss et al. 2013; McLauglin et al. 2008; Meyer & Korz, 2013; Pleil & Williams, 2010; Wang et al. 2009; Wang et al. 2011). Diz Chaves et al. (2012) published a recent study examining age-dependent effects of estradiol administration. Rats were OVX at 2 or 20 months of age and administered estradiol for 10 weeks. Estradiol treatment in aged rats improved object recognition memory compared to vehicle treated controls. Object recognition memory was not improved in young rats. These findings indicate the age at which estradiol administration takes place influences treatment outcomes. Foster et al. (2003) examined the effect of estradiol treatment on OVX young, middle-aged and aged rats on performance of a water maze task. Young animals exhibited their best performance with no estradiol administration, middle-aged animals benefited the greatest with low doses of estradiol and aged animals benefited the most from high doses of estradiol. These results suggest estradiol elicits dose-dependent effects based on age. Talboom et al. (2008) also showed effects of estradiol to depend on age. This group used estradiol pellets (or vehicle) to elicit a tonic release of estradiol (many other studies use injection of estradiol to create a cyclic release pattern of estradiol). Talboom and colleagues showed that young rats were behaviourally sensitive to OVX as well as estradiol administration, while middle-aged rats were not behaviourally sensitive to OVX, but were sensitive to estradiol administration. Importantly, in this study, it was found that higher serum levels of estradiol replacement were correlated with enhanced spatial reference memory performance but estradiol levels in intact animals did not correlate with enhanced performance. Aged rats were not found to be behaviourally sensitive to either OVX or estradiol administration at the dose given, indicating varying effects of estradiol across the lifespan.

The juvenile period is an interesting time point to examine in terms of the effect of estradiol on learning and memory processes. A great deal of research on estradiol's function has been done in young adult rodents, but few investigations examine time points before and just after the onset of puberty. It is quite reasonable to expect that estradiol would exert learning and memory effects at these early time points as ERα hippocampal expression is first visible on postnatal day 4, increases to maximum expression by postnatal day 10 and decreases to steady adult levels by postnatal day 15 (Solum & Handa, 2001). ERβ appears slightly later in development compared to ERα, around postnatal day 14 (Perez et al. 2003), still well before the onset of puberty in most rodent species.

As discussed previously, high levels of estradiol bias rats to use a place strategy while low levels of estradiol bias rats to use a response strategy (Korol & Kolo, 2002; Korol et al. 2004; Korol, 2004). Pleil & Williams found that estradiol administration biased prepubertal rats (postnatal day 26) to use a place strategy. This effect was not found when rats were given estradiol on postnatal days 16 or 21. Additionally, it was of interest to determine if prepubertal rats would show a bias for response strategies, as they have low estradiol levels. No such bias was found. Wartman et al. (2012) also investigated the effect of estradiol administration in juvenile rats. Prepubertal rats were given estradiol (or vehicle) for 4 consecutive days (postnatal day 19-22). Half of these rats then received juvenile training on a water maze task. No group differences between estradiol or vehicle treatment were observed during juvenile water maze training. All rats then received water maze training during adolescence. Not surprisingly, on day 1 of adolescent training, rats that had received juvenile training outperformed those that did not. Interestingly, rats that received estradiol administration in conjunction with, or without, juvenile training outperformed those treated with vehicle on measures of memory retention. Additionally, significant group differences were found in the number of pERK1/2 (a kinase implicated in memory formation and involved in dendritic spine plasticity following activity dependent processes) positive cells. The estradiol-treated group showed fewer pERK1/2 positive cells in the CA1 compared to vehicle-treated controls and more pERK1/2 positive cells in the CA3 region of the hippocampus. These results suggested a latent beneficial effect of juvenile estradiol treatment on adolescent spatial performance and suggest an organizational effect of prepubertal exogenously applied estradiol. In support of a beneficial effect of estradiol extending beyond the period of exposure, are findings reported by Rodgers et al. (2010). Estradiol was administered to middle-aged rats for 40 days following OVX. Enhanced spatial memory performance was reported for up to 7 months after the period of estradiol treatment. The suggested mechanism driving this effect was increased levels of ERα in the hippocampus. Additionally, results from a study conducted in women by Bagger and colleagues (2005) suggested that short-term use (2-3 years) of hormone therapy during the early stages of menopause may convey long-term (5-15 years) protection against cognitive impairment.

Morphological examination has corroborated the age-dependent effects of estradiol. Adams et al. (2001) examined spine density in young and aged rats treated with estradiol. Findings indicated estradiol given to young rats (3-4 months) resulted in the typical spine density elevation seen in the hippocampus, while the same dose of estradiol given to aged rats (23-24 months) did not result in this spine density elevation. Interestingly, aged rats treated with estradiol demonstrated an increase in NMDA receptor density per spine synapse, which was not found in young rats treated with estradiol. These findings indicate age-related differences in synaptic plasticity resulting from estradiol treatment.

Estrogen receptor efficacy and number represent potential mechanisms through which age may alter the effect of estradiol treatment. Research has shown that the number of synapses that contain ERα decreases in aged animals compared to young animals (Adams et al., 2002). Bohacek & Daniel (2009) demonstrated that chronic estradiol treatment influenced the quantity of ERα in the hippocampus and prefrontal cortex of OVX rats. Results indicated that age, timing of estradiol administration, and brain area examined were all factors in ERα number. Estradiol administration to young OVX rats resulted in an increase in ERα levels in both the hippocampus and prefrontal cortex. When estradiol administration to middle-aged rats began at the time of OVX, ERα levels in the hippocampus, but not in the prefrontal cortex, were increased. If administration of estradiol was delayed significantly (5 months), the increase in the hippocampus was diminished, while a significant increase was noted in the prefrontal cortex.

Behavioural and morphological research suggests the effects of estradiol are age-dependent. This is an important consideration pertaining to the potential therapeutic uses of estradiol. The varying effects of estradiol administration across the lifespan may indicate different therapeutic uses at different ages and prompts an evaluation of age-appropriate dosage. Also of interest is the long-lasting effect of terminated estradiol treatment noted in some studies indicating potential long-term effects resulting from acute treatment.

Estradiol Replacement and Learning and Memory

The Bohacek & Daniel study discussed above highlights an important consideration when examining the age-dependent effects of estradiol treatment: the length of time of hormone deprivation (either naturally in aged animals or via surgical procedures i.e. OVX) before estradiol administration begins, sometimes called the critical period hypothesis. Gibbs (2000) presented a study suggestive of a critical period during which estradiol replacement can prevent impairments in cognitive function. Rats received estradiol replacement immediately, 3 months or 10 months following OVX. Testing on a spatial memory task occurred 8-12 months following OVX. Rats treated with estradiol immediately or 3 months following OVX showed enhanced performance on the task. Rats treated with estradiol 10 months following OVX did not show enhanced performance. These results suggest a window of opportunity following loss of ovarian function whereby estradiol treatment can protect against cognitive decline. Daniel et al. (2006) reported similar findings concluding that estradiol administration had positive outcomes on a working memory task when administered immediately following hormone deprivation (i.e. OVX) but was not effective when administered after a sustained period (5 months) of hormone deprivation. Walf et al. (2009) examined performance on an object placement task. Estradiol administration began at the time of OVX or after a 5 month delay. In agreement with other studies, results indicated performance was enhanced when estradiol treatment began immediately following OVX, but not following a 5 month delay.

Findings corroborating the above behavioural studies come from a study done by McLaughlin et al. (2008) who examined the morphological effects of a delay in estradiol administration. This group examined differences in spine density in animals that were OVX and given intermittent injections of estradiol over a 10 week period compared to those that were OVX and not administered estradiol until 72 hours before sacrifice. In agreement with most literature, intermittent injections of estradiol throughout the 10 week time period following OVX resulted in an increase in CA1spine density. Interestingly, animals not given estradiol until 72 hours before sacrifice (i.e. no estradiol administered during the 10 week period following OVX) showed an increase in CA1 spine density, but not to the same extent as those given estradiol administration throughout the 10-week period. These results suggest an optimal time frame following OVX for estradiol administration to exert its morphological effects, indicating long periods of estradiol deprivation may result in reduced sensitivity to exogenous estradiol treatment.

Conclusion

Behavioural and morphological findings present a convincing case for the involvement of estradiol in memory processes. Although estradiol's precise role is still unclear, it has become apparent that estradiol plays a role in memory function. Conflicts in the literature regarding estradiol's effects are abundant, underlining the importance of considering variables which may change from one study to the next. Finally, the link between the behavioural and morphological consequences of estradiol treatment highlights important brain areas to examine (i.e. hippocampus, prefrontal cortex) and potential mechanisms which may underlie memory enhancement.

References

Adams, M. M., Fink, S. E., Shah, R. A., Janssen, W. G. M., Hayashi, S., Milner, T. A., McEwen, B. S. & Morrison, J. H. (2002). Estrogen and aging affect the subcellular distribution of estrogen receptor-α in the hippocampus of female rats. *J. Neurosci*, *22*, 3609-3614.

Adams, M. M., Shah, R. A., Janssen, W. G. M., & Morrison, J. H. (2001). Different modes of hippocampal plasticity in response to estrogen in young and aged female rats. *PNAS*, *98*, 8071-8076

Ashby, M. C., Maier, S. R., Nishimune, A. & Henley, J. M. (2006). Lateral diffusion drives constitutive exchange of AMPA receptors at dendritic spines and is regulated by spine morphology. *J Neurosci.*, *26*, 7046-7055.

Bagger, Y. Z., Tanko, L. B., Alexandersen, P., Qin, G., & Christiansen, C. (2005). Early postmenopausal hormone therapy may prevent cognitive impairment later in life. *Menopause*, *12*, 12-17.

Barton, M. (2012). Position paper: The membrane estrogen receptor GPER-Clues and questions. *Steroids*, *77*, 935-942.

Bashir, Z. I., Tam, B. & Collingridge, G. L. (1990). Activation of the glycine site in the NMDA receptor is necessary for the induction of LTP. *Neurosci. Lett.*, *108*, 261-266.

Berry, B., McMahan, R. & Gallagher, M. (1997). Spatial learning and memory at defined points of the estrous cycle: effects on performance of a hippocampal-dependent task. *Behavioral Neuroscience*, *111*(2), 267-274.

Bohacek, J. & Daniel, J. M. (2007). Increased daily handling of ovariectomized rats enhances performance on a radial-maze task and obscured effects of estradiol replacement. *Hormones and Behavior*, *52*, 237-243.

Bohacek, J. & Daniel, J. M. (2009). The ability of oestradiol administration to regulate protein levels of oestrogen receptor alpha in the hippocampus and prefrontal cortex of middle-aged rats is altered following long-term ovarian hormone deprivation. *J Neuroendo.*, *21*, 640-647.

Bourne, J. & Harris, K. M. (2007). Do thin spines learn to be mushroom spines that remember? *Curr. Opin. Neurobiol.*, *17*, 381-386.

Bourne, J. & Harris, K. M. (2008). Balancing structure and function at hippocampal dendritic spines. *Annu. Rev. Neurosci.*, *31*, 47-67.

Butcher, R. L., Collins, W. E. & Fugo, N. W. (1974). Plasma concentration of LH, FSH, Prolactin, Progesterone and Estradiol-17β throughout the 4-day estrous cycle of the rat. *Endocrinology*, *94*, 1704-1708.

Coan, E. J., Saywood, W. & Collingridge, G. L. (1987). MK-801 blocks NMDA receptor-mediated synaptic transmission and long term potentiation in rat hippocampal slices. *Neurosci. Lett.*, *80*, 111-114.

Collingridge, G. L., Kehl, S. J. & McLennan, H. (1893). Excitatory amino acids in synaptic transmission in the schaffer collateral-commissural pathway of the rat hippocampus. *J. Physiol.*, *334*, 33-46.

Daniel, J. M., Fader, A. J., Spencer, A. L. & Dohanich, G. P. (1997). Estrogen enhances performance of female rats during acquisition of a radial arm maze. *Hormones and Behavior*, *32*(3), 217-225.

Daniel, J. M., Hulst, J. L. & Berbling, J. L. (2006). Estradiol replacement enhances working memory in middle-aged rats when initiated immediately after ovariectomy but not after a long-term period of ovarian hormone deprivation. *Endocrinology*, *147*(1), 607-614.

Daniel, J. M. & Lee, C. D. (2004). Estrogen replacement in ovariectomized rats affects strategy selection in the Morris water maze. *Neurobiology of Learning and Memory*, *82*, 142-149.

Davidge, S. T., Zhang, Y. & Stewart, K. G. (2001). A comparison of ovariectomy models for estrogen studies. *Am J Physiol Regul Integr Comp Physiol*, *280*, R904-R907.

Diz-Chaves, Y., Kwiatkowska, A., Von Hulst, H., Pernia, O., Carrero, P. & Garcia-Segura, L. M. (2012). Behavioral effects of estradiol therapy in ovariectomized rats depend on the age when the treatment is initiated. *Experimental Gerontology*, *47*, 93-99.

Espeland, M. A., Rapp, S. R., Shumaker, S. A., Brunner, R., Manson, J. E., Sherwin, B. B., Hsia, J., Margolis, K. L., Hogan, P. E., Wallace, R., Dailey, M., Freeman, R. & Hays, J. (2004). Conjugated equine estrogens and global cognitive function in postmenopausal women: Women's Health Initiative Memory Study. *JAMA*, *291*, 2959–2968.

Fan, L., Zhao, Z., Orr, P. T., Chambers, C. H., Lewis, M. C. & Frick, K. M. (2010). Estradiol-induced object memory consolidation in middle-ages female mice requires dorsal hippocampal extracellualar signal-regulated kinase and phosphatidylinositol 3-kinase activation. *J. Neurosci.*, *30*, 4390-4400.

Farris, S. M., Robinson, G. E. & Fahrbach, S. E. (2001). Experience- and agerelated outgrowth of intrinsic neurons in the mushroom bodies of the adult worker honeybee. *J. Neurosci.*, *21*, 6395–6404.

Fernandez, S. M., Lewis, M. C., Pechenino, A. S., Harburger, L. L., Orr, P. T., Gresack, J. E., Schafe, G. E. & Frick, K. M. (2008). Estradiol-induced enhancement of object memory consolidation involves hippocampal extracellular signal-regulated kinase activation and membrane-bound estrogen receptors. *J. Neurosci.*, *28*, 8660-8667.

Foster, T. C., Sharrow, K. M., Kumar, A. & Masse, J. (2003). Interaction of age and chronic estradiol replacement on memory and markers of brain aging. *Neurobiology of Aging*, *24*, 839-852.

Frankfurt, M., Gould, E., Woolley, C. C. & McEwen, B. S. (1990). Gonadal steroids modify spine density in ventromedial hypothalamic neurons: a Golgi study in the adult rat. *Neuroendocrinology*, *51*, 530-535.

Frankfurt, M., Gould, E., Woolley, C. S. & McEwen, B. S. (1990). Gonadal steroids modify dendritic spine density in ventromedial hypothalamic neurons: A golgi study in the adult rat. *Neuroendocrinology*, *51*, 530-535.

Frick, K. M., Fernandez, S. M., Bennett, J. C., Prange-Kiel, J., MacLusky, N. J. & Leranth, C. (2004). Behavioral training interferes with the ability of gonadal hormones to increase CA1 spine synapse density in ovariectomized female rats. *Eur J Neurosci.*, *19*, 3026-3032.

Frye, C. A. & Rhodes, M. E. (2002). Enhancing effects of estrogen on inhibitory avoidance performance may be in part independent of intracellular estrogen receptors in the hippocampus. *Brain Research*, *956*(2), 285-293.

Galea, L. A., Wide, J. K., Paine, T. A., Holmes, M. M., Ormerod, B. K. & Floresco, S. B. (2001). High levels of estradiol disrupt conditioned place preference learning, stimulus response learning and reference memory but have limited effects on working memory. *Behavioural Brain Research*, *126*(1-2), 115-126.

Ganeshina, O., Berry, R. W., Petralia, R. S., Nicholson, D. A. & Geinisman, Y. (2004). Synapses with a segmented, completely partitioned postsynaptic density express more AMPA receptors than other axospinous synaptic junctions. *Neuroscience*, *125*, 615-623.

Gibbs, R. B. (2000). Long-term treatment with estrogen and progesterone enhances acquisition of a spatial memory task by ovariectomized aged rats. *Neurobiology of Aging*, *21*, 107-116.

Gould, E., Woolley, C. S., Frankfurt, M. & McEwen, B. S. (1990). Gonadal steroids regulate dendritic spine density in hippocampal pyramidal cells in adulthood. *Journal of Neuroscience*, *10*, 1286-1291.

Harris, K. M., Jensen, F. E. & Tsao, B. (1992). Three-dimensional structure of dendritic spines and synapses in rat hippocampus (CA1) at postnatal day 15 and adult ages: implications for the maturation of synaptic physiology and long-term potentiation. *J. Neurosci.*, *12*, 2685–705.

Harris, K. M., Jensen, F. E. & Tsao, B. (1992). Three-dimensional structure of dendritic spines and synapses in rat hippocampus (CA1) at postnatal day 15 and adult ages: implications for the maturation of synaptic physiology and long-term potentiation. *J. Neurosci.*, *12*, 2685–705.

Hogervorst, E., Williams, J., Budge, M., Riedel, W. & Jolles, J. (2000). The nature of the effect of female gonadal hormone replacement therapy on cognitive function in postmenopausalwomen: a meta-analysis. *Neuroscience*, *101*, 485–512.

Hojo, Y., Murakami, G., Mukai, H., Higo, S., Hatanaka, Y., Ogiue-Ikeda, M., Ishii, H., Kimoto, T. & Kawato, S. (2008). Estrogen synthesis in the brain- Role in synaptic plasticity and memory. *Molecular and Cellular Endocrinology*, *290*, 31-43.

Holmes, M. M., Wide, J. K. & Galea, L. A. (2002). Low levels of estradiol facilitate, whereas high levels of estradiol impair, working memory performance on the radial arm maze. *Behavioral Neuroscience*, *116*(5), 928-934.

Hubener, M. & Bonhoeffer, T. (2010). Searching for engrams. *Neuron*, *67*, 363-371.

Inagaki, T., Gautreaux, C. & Luine, V. (2010). Acute estrogen treatment facilitates recognition memory consolidation and alters monoamine levels in memory-related brain areas. *Hormones and Behavior*, *58*, 415-426.

Kiss, A., Delattre, A. M., Pereira, S. I. R., Carolino, R. G., Szawka, R. E., Anselmo-Franci, J. A., Zanata, S. & Ferraz, A. C. (2013). Estradiol replacement in young, adult and middle-aged female ovariectomized rats promotes improvement pf spatial reference memory and an antidepressant effect and alters monoamines and BDNF levels in memory- and depression-related brain areas. *Behavioral Brain Research*, *227*, 100-108.

Knafo, S., Ariav, G., Barkai, E. & Libersat, F. (2004). Olfactory learning-induced increase in spine density along the apical dendrites of CA1 hippocampal neurons. *Hippocampus*, *14*, 819–825.

Konkle, A. T. M. & McCarthy, M. M. (2011). Developmental time course of estradiol, testosterone, and dihydrotestosterone levels in discrete regions of male and female rat brain. *Neuroendocrinology*, *152*, 223-235.

Korol, D. L. (2004). Role of estrogen in balancing contributions from multiple memory systems. *Neurobiology of Learning and Memory*, *82*(3), 309-323.

Korol, D. L. & Kolo, L. L. (2002). Estrogen-induced changes in place and response learning in young adult female rats. *Behavioral Neuroscience*, *116*(3), 411-420.

Korol, D. L., Malin, E. L., Borden, K. A., Busby, R. A. & Couper-Leo, J. (2004). Shifts in preferred learning strategy across the estrous cycle in female rats. *Hormones and Behavior*, *45*(5), 330-338.

Launer, L. J., Andersen, K., Dewey, M. E., Letenneur, L., Ott, A., Amaducci, L. A., Brayne, C.,Copeland, J. R. M., Dartigues, J. -F., Kragh-Sorensen, P., Lobo, A., Martinez-Lage, J. M., Stijnen, T. & Hofman, A. (1999). Rates and risk factors for dementia and Alzheimer's disease. *Neurology*, *52*, 78–84.

LeBlanc, E. S., Janowsky, J., Chan, B. K. S. & Nelson, H. D. (2001). Hormone replacement therapy and cognition: Systematic review and meta-analysis. *JAMA*, *285*, 1489–1499.

Leranth, C., Shanabrough, M. & Redmond, D. E. (2002). Gonadal hormones are responsible for maintaining the integrity of spine synapses in the CA1 hippocampal subfield of female nonhuman primates. *Journal Comp Neuro.*, *447*, 34-42.

Leuner, B. & Shors, T. J. (2004). New spines, new memories. *Molecular Neurobiology*, *29*, 117-130.

Leuner, B., Falduto, J. & Shors, T. J. (2003). Associative memory formation increases the observation of dendritic spines in the hippocampus. *J., Neurosci.*, *23*, 659-665.

Li, C., Brake, W. G., Romeo, R. D., Dunlop, J. C., Gordon, M., Buzescu, R., Magarinos, A. M., Allen, P. B., Greengard, P., Luine, V. & McEwen, B. S. Estrogen alters hippocampal dendritic spine shape and enhances synaptic protein immunoreactivity and spatial memory in female mice. *PNAS*, *101*, 2185-2190.

Lipatova, O. & Toufexis, D. J. (2013). Estrogen enahnces the retention of spatial reference memory in the open field tower task, but disrupts the expression of spatial memory following a novel start position. *Neurobiology of learning and memory*, *99*, 50-58.

Luine, V., Jacome, L. F. & Maclusky, N. J. (2003). Rapid enhancements of visual and place memory by estrogens in rats. *Endocrinology*, *144*, 2836-2844.

Maclusky, N. J., Luine, V. N., Hajszan, T. & Leranth, C. (2005). The 17α and 17β isomers of estradiol both induce rapid spine synapse formation in the CA1 hippocampal subfield of ovariectomized female rats. *Endocrinology*, *146*, 287-293.

Matsuzaki, M., Ellis-Davies, G. C., Nemoto, T., Miyashita, Y., Iino, M. & Kasai, H. (2001). Dendritic spine geometry is critical for AMPA receptor expression in hippocampal CA1 pyramidal neurons. *Nat. Neurosci.*, *4*, 1086–1092.

Matsuzaki, M., Honkura, N., Ellis-Davies, G. C. R. & Kasai, H. (2004). Structural basis of long-term potentiation in single dendritic spines. *Nature*, *429*, 761-766.

McEwen, B., Akama, K., Alves, S., Brake, W. G., Bulloch, K., Lee, S., Li, C., Yuen, G. & Milner, T. A. (2001). Tracking the estrogen receptor in neurons: Implications for estrogen-induced synapse formation. *PNAS*, *98*, 7093-7100.

McEwen, B. S. & Alves, S. E. (1999). Estrogen actions in the central nervous system. *Endocrine Reviews*, *20*, 279-307.

McGaugh, J. L. (1989). Dissociating learning and performance: drug and hormone enhancement of memory storage. *Brain Res. Bull.*, *23*, 339–345.

McGaugh, J. L. (2000). Memory-A century of consolidation. *Science*, *287*, 248-251.

McLaughlin, K. J., Bimonte-Nelson, H., Neisewander, J. L. & Conrad, C. D. (2008). Assessment of estradiol influence on spatial tasks and hippocampal CA1 spines: Evidence that the duration of hormone deprivation after ovariectomy compromises 17β-estradiol effectiveness in altering CA1 spines. *Hormones and Behavior*, *54*, 386-395.

Meyer, K. & Korz, V. (2013). Age dependent differences in the regulation of hippocampal steroid hormones and receptor genes: Relations to motivation and cognition in male rats. *Hormones and Behavior*, *63*, 376-384.

Milner, T., McEwen, B. S., Hayashi, S., Li, C. J., Reagan, L. P. & Alves, S. E. (2001). Ultrastructural evidence that hippocampal alpha estrogen receptors are located at extranuclear sites. *J Comp Neur.*, *429*, 355-371.

Milner, T. A., Ayoola, K., Drake, C. T., Herrick, S. P., Tabori, N. E., McEwen, B. S., Warrier, S. & Alves, S. E. (2005). Ultrastructural localization of estrogen receptor β immunoreactivity in the rat hippocampal formation. *J Comp Neur.*, *491*, 81-95.

Morris, R. G. (1989). Synaptic plasticity and learning: Selective impairment of learning in rats and blockade of long-term potentiation in vivo by the *N*- Methyl-D-Aspartate Receptor Antagonist AP5. *J. Neurosci.*, *9*, 3040-3057.

Morris, R. G., Hagan, J. J. & Rawlins, J. N. (1986). Allocentric spatial learning by hippocampectomised rats: a further test of the "spatial mapping" and "working memory" theories of hippocampal function. *Q. J. Exp. Psychol. B.*, *38*, 365-395.

Okamoto, K. -I., Nagai, T., Miyawaki, A. & Hayashi, Y. (2004). Rapid and persistent modulation of actin dynamics regulates postsynaptic reorganization underlying bidirectional plasticity. *Nat. Neurosci.*, *7*, 1104-1112.

Osterlund, M. K., Keller, E. & Hurd, Y. L. (2000). The human forebrain has discrete estrogen receptor alpha messenger RNA expression: high levels in the amygdaloid complex. *Neuroscience*, *95*, 333–342.

Packard, M. G. & Teather, L. A. (1997). Posttraining estradiol injections enhance memory in ovariectomized rats: Cholinergic blockade and synergism. *Neurobiology of Learning and emory*, *68*, 172-188.

Packard, M. G. (1998). Posttraining estrogen and memoryodulation. *Hormones and Behavior*, *34*, 126-139.

Perez, S. E., Chen, E. -Y. & Mufson, E. J. (2003). Distribution of estrogen receptor alpha and beta immunoreactive profiles in the postnatal rat brain. *Dev Brain Res.*, *145*, 117-139.

Pleil, K. E. & Williams, C. L. (2010). The development and stability of estrogen-modulated spatial navigation strategies in female rats. *Hormones and Behavior*, *57*, 360-367.

Rapp, S. R., Espeland, M. A., Shumaker, S. A., Henderson, V. W., Brunner, R. L., Manson, J. E., Gass, M. L. S., Stefanick, M. L., Lane, D. S., Hays, J., Johnson, K. C., Coker, L. H., Dailey, M. & Bowen, D. (2003). Effect of estrogen plus progestin on global cognitive function in postmenopausal women. The Women's Health Initiative Memory Study: a randomized controlled trial. *JAMA*, *289*, 2663–2672.

Restivo, L., Roman, F. S., Ammassari-Teule, M. & Marchetti, E. (2006). Simultaneous olfactory discrimination elicits a strain-specific increase in dendritic spines in the hippocampus of inbred mice. *Hippocampus*, *16*, 472–479.

Restivo, L., Vetere, G., Bontempi, B. & Ammassari-Teule, M. (2009). The formation of recent and remote memory is associated with time-dependent formation of dendritic spines in the hippocampus and anterior cingulate cortex. *J. Neurosci.*, *29*, 8206-8214.

Rodgers, S. P., Bohacek, J. & Daniel, J. M. (2010). Transient estradiol exposure during middle age in ovariectomized rats exerts lasting effects on cognitive function and the hippocampus. *Neuroendocrinology*, *151*, 1194-1203.

Sandstrom, N. J. & Williams, C. L. (2001). Memory retention is modulated by acute estradiol and progesterone replacement. *Behavioral Neuroscience*, *115*(2), 384-393.

Scharfman, H. E., Hintz, T. M., Gomez, J., Stormes, K. A., Barouk, S. & Malthankar-Phatak, G. H. et al. (2007). Changes in hippocampal function of ovariectomized rats after sequential low doses of estradiol to simulate the preovulatory estrogen surge. *European Journal of Neuroscience*, *26*(9), 2595-2612.

Sherwin, B. B. (1999). Can estrogen keep you smart? Evidence from clinical studies. *J. Psychiatry Neurosci.*, *24*, 315–321.

Sherwin, B. B. (2006). Estrogen and cognitive aging in women. *Neuroscience*, *138*, 1021–1026.

Sherwin, B. B. & Henry, J. F. (2008). Brain aging modulates the neuroprotective effects of estrogen on selective aspects of cognition in women: a critical review. *Front Neuroendocr.*, *29*, 88–113.

Shughrue, P., Scrimo, P., Lane, M., Askew, R. & Merchenthaler, I. (1997a). The distribution of estrogen receptor-β mRNA in forebrain regions of the estrogen receptor-α knockout mouse. *Endocrinology*, *138*, 5649–5652.

Shughrue, P. J. & Merchenthaler, I. (2000). Evidence for novel estrogen binding sites in the rat hippocampus. *Neuroscience*, *99*, 605-612.

Shughrue, P. J., Lane, M. V. & Merchenthaler, I. (1997b). Comparative distribution of estrogen receptor-α and -β mRNA in the rat central nervous system. *J. Comp. Neurol.*, *388*, 507–525.

Shumaker, S. A., Legault, C., Thal, L., Wallace, R. B., Ockene, J. K., Hendrix, S. L., Jones III, B. N., Assaf, A. R., Jackson, R. D., Kotchen, J. M., Wassertheil-Smoller, S. & Wactawski-Wende, J. (2003). Estrogen plus progestin and the incidence of dementia and mild cognitive impairment in postmenopausal women. The Women's Health Initiative Memory Study: a randomized controlled trial. *JAMA*, *289*, 2651–2662.

Shumaker, S. A., Legault, C., Kuller, L., Rapp, S. R., Thal, L., Lane, D. S., Fillit, H., Stefanick, M. L., Hendrix, S. L., Lewis, C. E., Masaki, K. & Coker, L. H. (2004). Conjugated equine estrogens and incidence of probable dementia and mild cognitive impairment in postmenopausal women: Women's Health Initiative Memory Study. *JAMA*, *291*, 2947–2958.

Solum, D. T. & Handa, R. J. (2001). Localization of estrogen receptor alpha (ER alpha) in pyramidal neurons of the developing rat hippocampus. *Brain Research. Developmental Brain Research*, *128*(2), 165-175.

Spencer, J. L., Waters, E. M., Romeo, R. D., Wood, G. E., Milner, T. A. & McEwen, B. S. (2008). Uncovering the mechanisms of estrogen effects on hippocampal function. *Frontiers in Neuroendocrinology*, *29*(2), 219-237.

Srivastava, D. P. & Penzes, P. (2011). Rapid estradiol modulation of neuronal connectivity and its implications for disease. *Frontiers in Endocrinology*, *2*, 1-17.

Srivastava, D. P., Woolfrey, K. M., Jones, K. A., Shum, C. Y., Lash, L. L., Swanson, G. T. & Penzes, P. (2008). Rapid enhancement of two-step wiring plasticity by estrogen and NMDA receptor activity. *PNAS*, *105*, 14650-14655.

Stackman, R. W., Blasberg, M. E., Langan, C. J. & Clark, A. S. (1997). Stability of spatial working memory across the estrous cycle of Long-Evans rats. *Neurobiology of Learning and Memory*, *67*(2), 167-171.

Talboom, J. S., Williams, B. J., Baxley, E. R., West, S. G. & Bimonte-Nelson, H. A. (2008). Higher levels of estradiol replacement correlate with better spatial memory in surgically menopausal young and middle-aged rats. *Neurobiology of Learning and Memory*, *90*, 155-163.

Tang,Y., Janssen, W. G. M., Hao, J., Roberts, J. A., McKay, H., Lasley, B., Allen, P. B., Greengard, P., Rapp, P. R., Kordower, J. H., Hof, P. & Morrison, J. H. (2004). Estrogen replacement increases spinopholon-immunoreactive spine number in the prefrontal cortex of female rhesus monkeys. *Cerebral Cortex*, *14*, 215-223.

Walf, A. A., Rhodes, M. E. & Frye, C. A. (2006). Ovarian steroids enhance object recognition in naturally cycling and ovariectomized, hormone-primed rats. *Neurobiology of Learning and Memory*, *86*, 35-46.

Wallace, M., Luine, V., Arellanos, A. & Frankfurt, M. (2006). Ovariectomized rats show decreased recognition memory and spine density in the hippocampus and prefrontal cortex. *Brain Research*, *1126*, 176-182.

Wang, V. C., Neese, S. L., Korol, D. & Schantz, S. L. (2009). Chronic estradiol replacement impairs performance on an operant delayed spatial alternation task in young, middle-aged, and old rats. *Hormones and Behavior*, *56*, 382-390.

Wang, V. C., Neese, S. L., Korol, D. & Schantz, S. L. (2011). Estradiol impairs response inhibition in young and middle-aged, but not old rats. *Neurotoxicology and Teratology*, *33*, 405-414.

Watman, B. C., Keeley, R. J. & Holahan, M. R. (2012). Estradiol treatment in preadolescent females enhances adolescent spatial memory and differentially modulates hippocampal region-specific phosphorylated ERK labeling. *Neuroscience Letters*, *528*, 114-119.

Wide, J. K., Hanratty, K., Ting, J. & Galea, L. A. (2004). High level estradiol impairs and low level estradiol facilitates non-spatial working memory. *Behavioural Brain Research*, *155*(1), 45-53.

Wolf, O. T. & Kirschbaum, C. (2002). Endogenous estradiol and testosterone levels are associated with cognitive performance in older women and men. *Horm. Behav.*, *41*, 259–266.

Woolley, C. S. & McEwen, B. S. (1992). Estradiol mediates fluctuation in hippocampal synapse density during the estrous cycle in the adult rat. *Journal Neurosci.* *12*, 2549-2554.

Woolley, C. S. & McEwen, B. S. (1994). Estradiol regulates hippocampal dendritic spine density via an *N*-methyl-D-Aspartate receptor-dependent mechanism. *J Neurosci.*, *14*, 7680-7687.

Woolley, C. S., Gould, E., Frankfurt, M. & McEwen, B. S. (1990). Naturally occurring fluctuation in dendritic spine density on adult hippocampal pyramidal neurons. *Journal of Neuroscience*, *10*, 4035-4039.

Woolley, C. S., Weiland, N. G., McEwen, B. S. & Schwartzkronin, P. A. (1997). Estradiol increases the sensitivity of hippocampal CA1 pyramidal cells to NMDA receptor-mediated synaptic input: Correlation with dendritic spine density. *J Neurosci.*, *17*, 1848-1859.

Yaffe, K., Sawaya, G., Lieberburg, I. & Grady, D. (1998). Estrogen therapy in postmenopausal women: effects on cognitive function and dementia. *JAMA*, *279*, 688–695.

Zandi, P. P., Carlson, M. C., Plassman, B. L., Welsh-Bohmer, K. A., Mayer, L. S., Steffens, D. C. & Breitner, J. C. S. (2002). Hormone replacement therapy and incidence of Alzheimer disease in older women. *JAMA*, *288*, 2123–2129.

Zhou, Q., Homma, K. J. & Poo, M. M. (2004). Shrinkage of dendritic spines associated with long-term depression of hippocampal synapses. *Neuron*, *44*, 749–757.

Zurkovsky, L., Brown, S. L. & Korol, D. L. (2006). Estrogen modulates place learning through estrogen receptors in the hippocampus. *Neurobiology of Learning and Memory*, *86*(3), 336-343.

Zurkovsky, L., Brown, S. L., Boyd, S. E., Fell, J. A. & Korol, D. L. (2007). Estrogen modulates learning in female rats by acting directly at distinct memory systems. *Neuroscience*, *144*(1), 26-37.

In: Estradiol: Synthesis, Health Effects and Drug Interactions ISBN: 978-1-62808-962-2
Editors: Ricco Palmeri and Sal Grimaudo

Chapter 8

Estradiol in the Environment: Analysis and Occurrence

J. C. Bravo Yagüe, R. M. Garcinuño Martínez, A. Gallego Picó, D. González Gómez, P. Fernández Hernando and J. S. Durand Alegría*

GTyMAQ Research Group, Department of Analytical Sciences, Faculty of Sciences, UNED, Madrid, Spain

Abstract

In last decades, increases in the occurrence of certain abnormalities in development of wildlife species brought world-wide attention to scientific community about environmental contaminants. Estradiol is a steroidal natural hormone produced by humans and animals that is excreted in urine and feces, reaching the natural environment mainly through discharge from wastewater treatment plants (WWTP). The environmental occurrence of estradiol leads to increase the frequency of appearance of reproductive disorders and cancer in wildlife and probably in humans, being nanogram-per-liter levels of this compound able to produce endocrine disruption in living organisms. Reported concentrations of estradiol in environmental matrices are usually very low and the analytical difficulties associated with the determination of this estrogen in environment have been overcome by using preconcentration and clean up steps followed by highly sensitive analytical methods and the number of analytical methods currently available for the determination of estradiol in environmental matrices is still limited.

The purpose of this chapter is to provide a general overview on estradiol occurrence and analysis in environmental matrices.

Keywords: Estrogens, Estradiol, Endocrine Disruptors, EDCs, Environmental analysis

* Corresponding Author address: Email: rmgarcinuno@ccia.uned.es.

Introduction

For over half a century, evidences have appeared on the hormone-like effects of environmental chemicals in fish, wildlife and humans (Colborn et al., 1993). These effects were discovered long after these chemicals were released into the environment. Compounds with potential to alter the normal endocrine function of animals and humans, such as environmental estrogens have been referred to as endocrine disrupting chemicals (EDCs). With the publication of the book "Our stolen future" (Colborn et al., 1996), where evidences of the effects of endocrine disrupting chemicals (EDCs) on the wildlife populations were revealed, endocrine disruption became a public, political, and scientific issue. Since then, the list of suspected endocrine disrupting chemicals has been steadily growing, and the research in this field has made substantial progress (Hotchkiss et al., 2008).

Several definitions have been proposed to define Endocrine Disruptor by Recognized Organizations: According to United States Environmental Protection Agency, USEPA, an endocrine disruptor is an exogenous agent that interferes with the synthesis, secretion, transport, binding, action, or elimination of natural hormones in the body which are responsible for the maintenance or homeostasis, reproduction, development and or behavior (Kavlock et al., 1996). European Union, EU, defines an endocrine disruptor as an exogenous substance that causes adverse health effects in an intact organism, or its progeny, secondary to changes in endocrine function. A potential endocrine disruptor is a substance that possesses properties that might be expected to lead to endocrine disruption in an intact organism (European Commission, 1996). World Health Organization, WHO, defines an endocrine disruptor as an exogenous substance or mixture that alters functions of the endocrine system and consequently causes adverse effects in an intact organism, or its progeny, or (sub) populations (Damstra et al., 2002). EU and WHO definitions consider both the mode of action (i.e. the ability to interfere with hormone action) and the ability to produce adverse effects (cause harm). USEPA definition does not imply that all chemicals that interfere with any aspect of hormone action are a significant risk. Risk will depend on the exposure and the potency of the chemical.

Estrogens are hormones that are responsible for the development and maintenance of female secondary sex characteristics, reproductive function, regulation of the menstrual cycle, and maintenance of pregnancy. It is important to note that hormones are effective at very low concentrations, meaning that any disturbance or alteration of their normal regulatory processes could have dramatic effects on organ activity and subsequently on the development and overall functioning of the organism. Endogenous estrogens are excreted in the urine, bile or feces and, once eliminated by the body, are considered as exogenous estrogens. Among the naturally occurring estrogens, 17 β-estradiol (E2) and estrone (E1) are of major concern, because they exert their endocrine disrupting effect at lower concentrations than most other steroids and xeno-estrogens. The other free estrogens excreted by animals and humans, included 17 α-estradiol are considered weak estrogens. Therefore, unless otherwise stated, estradiol in this Chapter is used to mean free 17 β-estradiol. Due to its potential health effects and occurrence, E2 was included in 2009 in the USEPA Third Drinking Water Contaminant Candidate List (CCL 3) (USEPA, 2009a) that is a list of contaminants that are currently not subject to any proposed or promulgated national primary drinking water regulations, that are known or anticipated to occur in public water systems, and which may require regulation under the Safe Drinking Water Act (SDWA). Additionally, 17 β-estradiol has been included in the Proposal for a Directive of the European Parliament and of the Council amending Directives 2000/60/EC (Water Framework Directive) which contains the list of priority substances in the field of water policy.

Estradiol is released into environment mainly via excretion, mostly through urban wastewater, since population in the world is increasing rapidly, especially in urban areas. E2 is not sufficiently eliminated during treatment of the wastewater and a fraction of it is finally released into surface waters and can cause adverse biological responses in fish or other wildlife. It can also enter the environment due to runoffs and soil leaching after the agricultural application of biosolids and manure contributing to the release of estradiol in the environment. The presence of estradiol in environmental samples has been associated to a number of biological responses over different species of fish, amphibians and reptiles. Many studies on the effects of E2 in fish have been carried out. It was reported by Routledge et al. (1998) that feminization of fish occurs at concentrations as low as 14 ng L^{-1} of 17β-estradiol. Tyler and Routledge (1998) observed an induction of vitellogenin in male rainbow trout exposed at 1 to 10 ng L^{-1} over a 3-week period. Nakamura et al. (1984) reported feminization of 84 to 100% of salmon for an estradiol concentration of 2000 ng L^{-1}. Studies relevant to the assessment of potential endocrine disrupting effects of estradiol in wildlife were carried out by WRc-NSF Company in the context of endocrine disrupter priority list of actions, within the European Commission Strategy for Endocrine Disrupters (Johnson and Harvey, 2002). Based on available data, the U.K. Environment Agency has derived a predicted-no-effect-concentration (PNEC) for 17β-estradiol of 1 ng L^{-1} (U. K. Environment Agency, 2000). Although cause-effect relationships between environmental E2 exposure and adverse effects in humans are difficult to establish, evidence suggests E2 exposure induces breast cancer.

Sources

Estradiol enter the environment by many sources and pathways, including direct discharge from municipal wastewater treatment plants that causes a contamination from discrete locations and diffuse sources such as agricultural runoff from animal wastes and land application of biosolids and manure fertilizers.

Estradiol from Human Excretion

Human excretion is one of the major sources of contamination by estrogens, particularly wastewater receiving these compounds. The total daily excretion rate of E2 varies greatly depending on stage of the menstrual cycle and on age, being greater from pregnant women. Based on the survey and previous measurements of human estrogen excretion, Johnson et al. (2000) estimated the daily excretion of estradiol from males were 1.6 μg/day and menstruating females were excreting 3.5 μg/day of E2, in their urine, whereas menopausal women were excreting 2.3 μg/day of E2. Pregnant women were excreting 259 μg/day of E2. Excretion of 14 μg/day of conjugated E2 from female inhabitants of a Roman condominium were reported by D' Ascenzo et al. (2003). According to Adlercreutz et al. (1986) women can excrete with urine 2.4 μg E2 per day, being eliminated by feces approximately 0.4 μg/day (Adlercreutz et al., 1994).

Estradiol is not only produced naturally in the body but also introduced synthetically. Estradiol used in estrogen replacement therapy and in oral contraceptives is a clearly identifiable source of estrogen. Most combined oral contraceptive pills contain ethynilestradiol (EE2) with progestins; however, in last years new contraceptive pills containing 17β-estradiol have been launched (Christin-Maitre et al., 2013). The amount of E2 used for pharmaceutical purposes contributes less than 5% compared with the natural E2 excretion (Christensen, 1998). Since population grows continuously and more people live in large cities, excreted E2 enter the environment mainly via the effluents of the Wastewater Treatment Plants.

Application of biosolids resulting from treatment of sewage sludge as fertilizers and soil amendments could result as a possible source of hormones to the environment. In the United States, it is estimated that the average WWTP produces 240 kg dry weigh of solids per million liters of wastewater treated, resulting in approximately 8 million tons of biosolids produced per year, of which about 50% is land applied (Kinney et al., 2006). A survey conducted by USEPA has reported the presence of estrogen hormones in biosolid ranging from 22 to 355 ng g^{-1} (USEPA 2009b). Andaluri et al. (2012) detected 230 ng g^{-1} dry weigh of E2 in biosolids from an activated-sludge municipal WWTP in the U.S.

Estradiol from Animal Excretion

The other major source of estradiol is livestock, that excrete the same natural estrogens as humans, which end up in the environment throw animal waste disposal, being of great concern the possibly runoff from farm and agricultural lands. Although the use of 17β-estradiol as growth promoter is banned in many regions (e.g., European Union), the possibility of widespread abuse of hormonal substances by unscrupulous farmers and veterinary professionals still exist, mainly due to the economic benefits that these substances provide in animal husbandry and the existence of authorized drugs in some countries, since the use of hormones as growth promoters is still a legal practice in some parts of the world (Stephany, 2001). Estradiol excretion rates and routes differ by species. Cattle excrete much more 17α-estradiol than 17β-estradiol, and mostly en feces, whereas swine and poultry excrete estrogens mostly in urine and 17α-estradiol rarely occurs (Hanselman et al., 2003). Since urine and feces are not used separately in commercial animal production systems, the route of excretion would not appear to be an important environmental consideration (Knight, 1980). The contribution of livestock to the annual estradiol excretion could be considered the major source of estradiol reaching the environment. It is estimated that the United States dairy cow population excretes 80 tons of E2 per year, while the pig population excretes 8 tons E2 per year (Johnson et al., 2006). Liu et al. (2012a) studied the occurrence of 28 steroids in three swine farms and three dairy cattle farms in Chine, one of the largest animal farming countries in the world, and estimated that total contribution of E2 to the environment in China were 2520 and 3580 kg/year from swine and dairy cattle, respectively.

Recent studies suggest that land application of animal manure could be an important source of steroidal hormones for agricultural runoff (Jenkins et al., 2008; Jenkins et al., 2009). In poultry waste, a concentration ranging from 14 to 533 ng g^{-1} dry weight with an average of

44 ng g^{-1} for E2 was reported by Shore et al. (1995). E2 was detected at concentrations of 150 and 17 ng g^{-1} dry weigh in poultry manure and cattle manure from concentrated animal feeding operations (CAFOs) in the U. S. (Andaluriet al., 2012). Concentrations of 4.95 ng g^{-1} of E2 in raw poultry manure was reported by Dutta et al. (2012). In addition to manure application for fertilizer, livestock waste can enter the environment when rain causes overflow, or from runoff and leaching into the soil near manure storage facilities. Contribution of wild animals and domestic pets to the amount of estradiol released to the environment is practically unknown.

Occurrence

Estradiol in Environmental Waters

In present-day cities human waste is released to the sewer system which leads it to the municipal WWTP where the E2 can be removed. An incomplete removal of this compound can cause its occurrence in receiving waters. Liu et al. (2012b) studied the occurrence of 28 steroids in wastewater of two WWTPs in Guangdong, China, that apply different treatment technologies: activated sludge treatment technology following by chlorination and oxidation ditch following by chlorination. Concentrations of E2 in influent of WWTPs ranged from 12 to 23.9 ng L^{-1}. Although the treatment used in the WWTPs were very effective to eliminate estradiol, it still was detected in the final effluents an concentrations up to 4,8 ng L^{-1} . Values of E2 detected in the largest wastewater treatment plant in Beijing, China, ranged from 3,7 to 140 ng L^{-1} in influents and 3.9 ng L-1 in effluent (Zhou et al., 2012). Ying et al. (2002) provided an overview of E2 concentrations in effluents of sewage treatment plants in different countries, ranging up to 64 ng L^{-1}. Jiang et al. (2005) carried out a study of the concentration of selected EDCs in two WWTPs in UK, where concentrations of E2 in influents from 132 to 224 ng L^{-1} were found. A recent review by Combalbert and Hernandez-Raquet, (2010) contains more data on various levels of hormones in human waste and reported that E2 concentrations varies between 0.5 and 125 ng L^{-1} in human raw sewage effluents.

Several studies have shown that disposal of biosolids and animal manure to agricultural land could lead to movement of estrogens into surface and ground water (Barber et al., 2009). E2 concentrations ranging from 19 to 389 ng L^{-1} were observed in runoff following poultry litter application depending on tillage conditions (Nichols et al., 1997). Finlay-Moore et al. (2000) measured 20-2530 ng L^{-1} of 17β-estradiol in runoff water from poultry (broiler) litter-ammended grasslands. Pailler et al. (2009) measured the runoff water in a small mixed-land use, rural catchment, in Luxemburg and found E2 at concentration of 6 ng L^{-1}. Jenkins et al. (2009) observed a concentration range of 8 to 79 ng L^{-1} for E2 in surface runoff from agricultural soils receiving poultry litter. Groundwater has been reported to be contaminated with E2 (Peterson et al., 2001; Shore et al., 1995). Shore et al. (1995) believed that a constant E2 concentration of about 5 ng L^{-1} in spring water was caused by infiltration of E2 through the soil profile to the groundwater. Peterson et al. (2000) measured E2 concentrations ranging from 6 to 66 ng L^{-1} in mantled karst aquifers in northwest Arkansas where poultry litter and cattle manure were applied. U.S. aquifers under areas covered in animal manure were found to have an E2 concentration of 37.6 ng L^{-1} in a research carried out by Khanal et al. (2006).

The presence of estrogenic compounds in surface waters has been noted since the early 80s (Richardson and Bowron, 1985). The main sources of Estradiol in surface waters are domestic wastewater because of the incomplete elimination of E2 in sewage treatment plants and surface runoff. Many papers reported the presence of estradiol in surface waters. In a recent paper, Velico and Suri (2009) reported concentrations of E2 ranging from 0.09 to 5.04 ng L^{-1} detected in surface water samples collected from 21 locations in Pennsylvania. Miege et al. (2009) quantified 0.1 to 2.3 ng L^{-1} of E2 in an affluent of the Seine River (Paris). A mean concentration of 10 ng L^{-1} in river water was observed in Hamadan city, west of Iran (Jafari et al., 2009).

Although the probability of adverse effects on human health due to E2 occurrence in drinking water is very low, the possibly health risk to residents has lead to increasing attention on drinking water safety.

Estradiol was isolated in drinking water in Israel although concentrations were unlikely to possess a significant risk to human health (Shore et al., 1993). Kuch and Balsmitter (2001) detected concentrations of E2 up to 2,1 ng L^{-1} in tap water originating from drinking water plants in Germany. E2 was detected at concentration of 30 ng L^{-1} in municipal water supplies in Arkansas (Lange et al., 2002). Concentrations of 0.1 ng L^{-1} have been reported in municipal drinking water network located in the city of Hamadan in the west of Iran (Jafari et al., 2009).

Estradiol in Environmental Solid Matrices

Due to its hydrophobic properties, E2 in surface water tends to be adsorbed by sediment particles. Hashimoto et al. (2005) reported E2 concentrations from 0.1 to 4.8 ng g^{-1} in sediment at 57 study sites in the inner part of Tokyo Bay. Reported concentrations of E2 in 28 riverine sediments from the Pearl River Delta in China were from 0.9 to 2.6 ng g^{-1} dry weight (dw) (Gong et al., 2011).

Froehner et al. (2012) investigated the occurrence of estrogens in surface sediments of mangrove forest along the Brazilian coast, where E2 concentration ranged from 0.03 to 39.77 ng g^{-1}. Estradiol was found at 0.22-2.48 ng g-1 in deep ocean sediments in the proximity of a deep ocean sewage outfall near Sydney (Braga et al., 2005).

As in the case of groundwater, estradiol enters soil compartment mainly via land application of biosolids, manure and wastewater irrigation. Finlay-Moore et al. (2000) measured estradiol concentrations in soil from large grazed and ungrazed grasslands ammended with broiler litter.

Estradiol bound to the soil with a reported concentration of about 650 ng kg^{-1} on manured soils as opposed to 150 ng kg^{-1} on control fields. Studies carried out in soils with long-term biosolids application and wastewater irrigation (Stumpe and Marschner, 2007) show that while estradiol can be transformed in agricultural settings, it likely persists long enough to potentially impact the quality of runoff water (Yang et al., 2012).

Thomson et al. (2009) carried out a study to determine the fate and transport of manure-borne E2 in soil.

A relationship was observed between E2 and dissolved organic carbon (DOC), which could potentially explain its greater than expected mobility and persistence.

Analysis

Sample Preparation

Traditionally, routine methods involve several sample preparation steps before instrumental analysis. This preparation starts with sampling and sample storage. Storage and handling in the laboratory must be such estradiol within the sample does not suffer sorption or transformation processes that lead to an inadequate measurement of its concentration. Due to possible photodegradation of E2, amber glass containers pre-cleaned with an organic solvent and rinsed with ultrapure water are the optimum storage for water samples collection. The volume of sample required depends on the later extraction step and the sensitivity of the analytical technique and can vary from 50 mL to 5 L. Salvador et al. (2007) developed an on-line method capable of E2 quantification in wastewater with less than 1 mL of water sample. Within recent years, a new approach for sample collection has been presented. It involves the extraction of estrogenic compounds directly on an adsorption medium, which is a permeable membrane. The device used is the passive-sampler. The main passive sampling tool is known as Polar Organic Chemical Integrative Sampler (POCIS). This device is left in the water for a period time (1 to 10 weeks), and the estrogenic compounds are extracted directly on the membrane (Zhang et al., 2008). Storage of water samples at 4ºC without preservation is possible if analysis is carried out in the subsequent 24-48 hours. The addition of preservative chemicals such as hydrochloric or sulphuric acid to a pH of 2-3, the preservative technique more used, or 1% formaldehyde to water samples in bottles allows no significant losses of E2 after 24 days of storage. For river water samples Estradiol degradation can be avoided for 60 days by passing the sample though the extraction cartridge (Carbograph-4), washing the cartridge with methanol, and storing it at -18 ºC (Baronti et al., 2000). In the case of solid samples frozen is the preferred method to prevent further microbial action.

It has been estimated that over 99% of the estrogenic activity in environmental water may be attributable to the presence of free steroid estrogens (Snyder et al., 2000). When determination of E2 in water samples is performed, a first step of filtration is usually carried out to eliminate high loads of organic material and suspended particles and is particularly necessary when subsequent extraction of the sample is based on the use of solid-phase extraction (SPE), because suspended solids could easily clog the adsorbent bed. Filtration is also recommended when the analysis is performed by immunochemical assay, to avoid undesired adsorption onto antibodies. The retention of E2 on the filter material is normally not a problem. Huang el al, 2001 reported E2 recoveries of 99% in 0.22 μm polypropylene filters used for wastewater effluent preparation. A similar effect eliminating suspended particles could be obtained by centrifuging the sample.

Extraction is the most critical step in sample preparation. As already mentioned, due to low concentrations estradiol occurs in the environment available analytical methods are often insufficiently sensitive and a preconcentration step must be performed, thus prior to separation and detection of E2 via instrumental techniques, samples are commonly subjected to an extraction procedure, used to concentrate and isolate the analyte. Extraction of estradiol from water samples is usually performed by solid-phase extraction (SPE), which involves passing the sample through a solid material selected to bind the estrogen of interest, using disks, columns or most frequently cartridges. Disks are not clogged as easily as cartridges by the suspended matter present in the samples and had a larger surface area for adsorbent-matrix contact, which result in higher extraction rates, however longer time of filtration is required. Important advantages of cartridges are lower consumption of elution solvents, shorter processing time and possibility of coupling with automated filtration systems. More advantages of SPE over other extraction techniques such as liquid-liquid extraction are availability of many different types of sorbents and experimental simplicity.

A wide variety of sorbents such as silica based (C18, C8), hydrophilic lipophilic balanced (HLB), mixed cation exchange (MCX), and mixed anionic exchange (MAX) have been applied to the extraction of E2 from environmental matrices although the majority of published methods use C18 (Koha et al., 2007; Stavrakakis et al., 2008) and Oasis HLB (polystyrenedivinylbenzene-N-vinylpyrolidone terpolymer) cartridges (Reddy et al., 2005; Beck et al., 2006). The main drawback of the use of these sorbents is their lack of selectivity that can be solved by the utilization of selective materials such as immunosorbents, which can retain selectively E2 in wastewater with recoveries higher than 80% (Ferguson et al., 2001), or molecularly imprinted polymers (Watabe et al., 2006; Jing et al., 2012) that allow selective extraction of E2 from contaminated waters with a more mechanical and chemical stability than immunosorbents. A comparison of various types of SPE commercial sorbents (LiChrolut EN, LiChrolut RP-18, Isolut ENV, Hysphere-Resin-GP, Oasis HLB) used for the extraction of E2 and several more estrogens in environmental matrices, included water and river sediments, have been made by Lopez de Alda and Barcelo (2001). In a similar way, Liu et al. (2004) carried out a comparative study of several cartridges (Strata, DSC, Isolute and Oasis HLB) for the extraction of E1, E2 and EE2 from river waters and obtained the better recoveries with the Oasis HLB cartridges. The main drawback of SPE is the time consumption and the large amount of organic solvents required. In recent years, miniaturized techniques such as solid-phase microextraction (SPME), Stir-Bar Sorptive Extraction (SBSE) and liquid-phase microextraction (LPME) have been reported as alternatives to SPE. Almeida et al. (2006) reported extraction of estradiol and other esteroidal hormones in water and urine matrices by SBSE coated with PDMS. Li et al. (2011) performed a clean-up procedure for the determination of estradiol in surface water based on Hollow-Fiber Liquid Phase Microextraction (HF-LPME) that provided an enrichment of 300.

Off-line SPE is the most frequently used method of extraction. However, in last years new on-line extraction methods have been developed (Rodriguez-Mozaz et al., 2007). As compared with off-line SPE, on-line SPE techniques have made it possible to develop a faster method reducing the sample preparation time and, thus, increasing the sample throuhput. Conditioning, washing, and elution steps can be performed automatically (Alvarez et al., 2008). The risk of sample contamination can be reduced and the method eliminates the analyte loss by evaporation, improves the accuracy and reduces the risk for the operator (Watabe et al., 2006).

The extraction of E2 from solid samples (soils, sediments and sludges) involves the use of organic solvents that induce co-extraction of many interferents and result in heterogeneous extracts being useful a centrifugation step to remove suspended particles before purification. This extraction is usually carried out by shaking, sonication or microwave-assisted extraction. Typically, estrogens are extracted from solid samples by use of polar or medium polarity organic solvents (e.g., methanol, acetone, hexane-acetone, diethylether-hexane). In the next step, SPE is commonly applied for the purification of the crude extract.

Purification of the extracts of water samples is not always necessary. However, a clean-up step is generally required for analysis of E2 of wastewater influents and heavily contaminated waters characterized by much higher organic matter content than wastewater effluent or surface waters. Purification is carried out to reduce non-targeted compounds coincidently eluted with E2 from the SPE sorbent. Purification is mainly performed on silica-gel cartridges and elution is done with a mixture of hexane or cyclohexane/acetone 65/35 (Zuehlke et al., 2005). Purification is essential for the analysis of E2 in solid samples and usually is performed by gel permeation chromatography followed by SPE clean-up with silica gel or C18 (Ternes et al., 2002).

Analytical Techniques

For many years, the environmental determination of steroid sex hormones has been dominated by the use of gas chromatography-mass spectrometry (GC-MS), although biological assays have also been used. However, in the last 10-15 years liquid chromatography (LC) techniques have replaced GC as they present advantages such as reduced sample pretreatment and their capacity to determine polar or thermally stable compounds. Combination of LC and MS has experienced rapid growth, due to instrumental developments. Biological techniques, e.g., immunoassay, are among the most sensitive analytical methods, but are limited by the availability of the specific antisera and are subject to cross-reactivity. GC–MS is an appropriate method for the separation of the noncomplex samples of estrogenic compounds. Finally, LC–MS is not limited by such factors as non-volatility and high molecular weight, and enables the determination estrogens without the need for derivatization. An advantage of GC-MS compared to LC-MS is the availability of the data library of mass espectra, which is useful for the identification of unknown peaks.

Immunochemical techniques are essential for rapid screening of steroid compounds in environmental samples. They are characterized by high output, relative low cost and the possibility of analyzing large amount of samples even in the field. Immunochemical methods are very useful; however, they present certain limitations. Their sensitivity is sometimes insufficient for trace analysis and the structural similarity of estrogens may occasionally cause incorrect positive results of determination, due to non-specific binding to the antibody.

Comparison between Enzyme-Linked Immunosorbent Assay (ELISA) and LC-MS-MS used in the measurement concentrations of E2 in environmental matrices shows a slight tendency for ELISA values to be higher than values of LC-MS-MS (Dutta et al., 2010). A microplate magnetic chemiluminescence enzyme immunoassay for screening of E2 in water samples was performed by Zhao and Lin (2005). The method specifically recognized E2, without crossreactions for three other major estrogenic compounds, with a detection limit of 5.4 ng L^{-1}.

GC is often used for analysis of E2 in experimental samples (Mouatassim-Soualli et al., 2003; Morteani et al., 2006; Muller et al., 2008). The advantages of GC involve high separation efficiency, a high speed of analysis, trace availability of highly sensitive detectors and environmental friendliness owing to the fact that the mobile phases are inert gases. At present, the most frequently used detection techniques are based on mass spectrometry (MS). To improve the stability of the estradiol and the sensitivity and precision of subsequent GC analysis the sample extract is usually derivatized. The most common derivatization technique is silylation, which is suitable for analytes containing an active hydrogen. To silylate estradiol, various derivatization reagents have been employed, e.g., N-methy-N-(trimethylsilyl) trifluoroacetamide (MSTFA) (Labadie and Budzinski, 2005; Peng et al., 2008), (N-O-Bis-(trimethylsilyl) trifluoroacetamide) (BSTFA) (Jeannot, et al., 2002; Hanselman et al., 2006), N-Methyl-N-tert-butyldimethylsilyltrifluoroacetamide (MTBSTFA) (Kelly, 2000). Acylation has also been used, in addition to silylation (Nakamura et al., 2001). A dual derivatization method has been developed for trace analysis of estradiol in river water, involving a SBDE step with in situ acylation (first derivatization), and quartz-wool assisted in-tube silylation (second derivatization), followed by GC-MS. The LOD for E2 in the river water was 0.5 ng L^{-1} (Kawaguchi et al., 2006). In occasions derivatization can be processed during SPE or SPME by modifying sorbent with a derivatization agent. Such a method was developed by Salvador et al. (2007), which used dansyl chloride for derivatization. Estradiol can be analyzed by GC directly, without derivatization; however, its conversion into more volatile derivative provides better results, improving E2 stability and sensitivity and precision of analysis by GC-MS or GC-MS/MS. Hajkova et al. (2007) carried out a multiresidue analysis of underivatized estrogens (estrone, 17 β-estradiol, 17 α-ethinylestradiol, dienestrol and diethylestilbestrol) in river sediments with several alternative GC-based approaches. Estradiol detection limits achieved by the use of GC-Q-MS, LP-GC-MS, GC-TOF-MS and GcxGC-TOF-MS were 5, 5, 12 and 2,5 ng g^{-1} dry weigh. To enhance spectral resolution and thus improve the detection selectivity, tandem GC-MS/MS can be used for determination of E2 in complex matrices. Although various ionization methods are available, electron ionization (EI) (Petrovic et al., 2001; Carpinteiro et al., 2004; Noppe et al., 2005; Noppe et al., 2007) and chemical ionization (CI) (Nakamura et al., 2000; Xiao et al., 2001; Fine et al., 2003) are the most common for the analysis of E2 with GC-MS. Analysis of estradiol in environmental solid matrices is more usually performed by GC-MS (Ternes et al., 2002; Isobe et al., 2006; Hajkova et al., 2007; Noppe et al., 2007) than LC-MS.

LC is one of the most used methods of analysis for environmental estradiol, especially in water samples. LC has some important advantages over GC, namely, estradiol samples can be analyzed directly, without derivatization, and aqueous samples do not require drying which is necessary in GC analysis. On the other hand, drawback of classical LC lies in a high consumption of solvents and, high cost of the instrumentation in case of LC-MS. As in the case of GC, the analysis itself is usually preceded by a SPE or SPME preconcentration step. For complex samples containing many compounds, LC is not enough for the unequivocal confirmation of estradiol, thus LC-MS/MS tandem can help eliminating the false identification and quantification of co-eluting compounds that can occur with single ion monitoring and improving the detection and quantification limits. There is a great variety in the instrumentation of mass spectrometric techniques, the ionization techniques (electrospray ionization, ESI, and atmospheric pressure chemical ionization, APCI), the ionization modes (negative ion, NI, and positive ion, PI) and in the monitoring modes (selected ion monitoring, SIM, and selected reaction monitoring, SRM). Nowadays, the interfaces more used for the analysis of E2 in the aquatic environment are ESI in negative ion mode (Isobe et al., 2003; Lagana et al., 2004; Benijts et al., 2004; Beck et al., 2005; Zuehlke et al., 2005). Alternatively, some studies reported use of ESI (Salvador et al., 2007; Vulliet et al., 2007) and APCI (Vanderford et al., 2003) in positive ion mode, being mostly LC methods applied in the SIM mode. The miniaturization is an important issue considered in all fields of analytical instrumentation including both parts of LC-MS coupling. The most widespread and well-established approach is ultrahigh performance liquid chromatography, UHPLC (Farre et al., 2007; Guillarme and Veauthey, 2012), which is based on the use of small particle size (sub-2 μm particles) in the stationary phase and short columns, at ultrahigh pressures (up to 1300 bars) yielding fast analyses and narrow chromatographic peaks. Moreover, UHPLC dramatically shortens analysis times, often to 10 min or less (Ibañez et al., 2008; Guillarme et al., 2010). Guedes-Alonso et al. (2013) performed a UHPLC-MS/MS method for the simultaneous determination of hormones in wastewater and a detection limit of 2.53 ng L^{-1} for E2 was achieved. LC is less used than GC for the analysis of estradiol in environmental solid matrices; however, in last years a number of methods have been developed to analyze E2 in this type of matrices by LC-MS/MS (Nieto et al., 2008; Gineys et al., 2010; Vega et al., 2011; Liu et al., 2011). The major drawback of LC-MS methods is the possibility of matrix effect due to the presence of co-eluting residual matrix impurities. This effect can affect ionization efficiency, resulting usually in signal suppression. Extensive cleaning of the samples can reduce ion suppression. Use of isotopically labeled internal standards is generally an efficient way to control matrix effect (Sojo et al., 2003).

References

A dlercreutz H, Fotsis T, Bannwart C, Hamalainen E, Bloigu S, Ollus A. Urinary estrogen profile determination in young finnish vegetarian and omnivorous women. *Journal of Steroid Biochemistry and Molecular Biology*. 1986;24(1):289-96.

Adlercreutz H, Gorbach SL, Goldin BR, Woods MN, Dwyer JT, Hamalainen E. Estrogen metabolism and excretion in oriental and caucasian women. *Journal of the National Cancer Institute*. 1994;86(14):1076-82.

Almeida C, Nogueira JMF. Determination of steroid sex hormones in water and urine matrices by stir bar sorptive extraction and liquid chromatography with diode array detection. *Journal of Pharmaceutical and Biomedical Analysis*. 2006;41(4):1303-11.

Alvarez Sanchez B, Priego Capote F, Ruiz Jimenez J, Luque de Castro MD. Automated solid-phase extraction for concentration and clean-up of female steroid hormones prior to liquid chromatography-electrospray ionization-tandem mass spectrometry: An approach to lipidomics. *Journal of Chromatography A*. 2008;1207(1-2):46-54.

Andaluri G, Suri RPS, Kumar K. Occurrence of estrogen hormones in biosolids, animal manure and mushroom compost. *Environmental Monitoring and Assessment*. 2012;184(2):1197-205.

Barber LB, Keefe SH, Leblanc DR, Bradley PM, Chapelle FH, Meyer MT, et al. Fate of Sulfamethoxazole, 4-Nonylphenol, and 17 beta-Estradiol in Groundwater Contaminated by Wastewater Treatment Plant Effluent. *Environmental Science & Technology*. 2009;43(13):4843-50.

Baronti C, Curini R, D'Ascenzo G, Di Corcia A, Gentili A, Samperi R. Monitoring natural and synthetic estrogens at activated sludge sewage treatment plants and in a receiving river water. *Environmental Science & Technology*. 2000;34(24):5059-66.

Beck IC, Bruhn R, Gandrass J, Ruck W. Liquid chromatography-tandem mass spectrometry analysis of estrogenic compounds in coastal surface water of the Baltic Sea. *Journal of Chromatography A*. 2005;1090(1-2):98-106.

Benijts T, Lambert W, De Leenheer A. Analysis of multiple endocrine disruptors in environmental waters via wide-spectrum solid-phase extraction and dual-polarity ionization LC-ion trap-MS/MS. *Analytical Chemistry*. 2004;76(3):704-11.

Braga O, Smythe GA, Schafer AI, Feitz AJ. Steroid estrogens in ocean sediments. *Chemosphere*. 2005;61(6):827-33.

Carpinteiro J, Quintana JB, Rodriguez I, Carro AM, Lorenzo RA, Cela R. Applicability of solid-phase microextraction followed by on-fiber silylation for the determination of estrogens in water samples by gas chromatography-tandem mass spectrometry. *Journal of Chromatography A*. 2004;1056(1-2):179-85.

Christensen FM. Pharmaceuticals in the environment - A human risk? *Regulatory Toxicology and Pharmacology*. 1998;28(3):212-21.

Christin-Maitre S, Laroche E, Bricaire L. A new contraceptive pill containing 17beta-estradiol and nomegestrol acetate. Women's health (London, England). 2013;9(1):13-23.

Colborn T, Saal FSV, Soto AM. Developmental effects of endocrine-disrupting chemicals in wildlife and humans. *Environmental Health Perspectives*. 1993;101(5):378-84.

Colborn T, Dumanoski D, Myers JP. Our stolen future: are we threatening our fertility, intelligence and, survival? A scientific detective story. Dutton, New York. 1996.

Combalbert S, Hernandez-Raquet G. Occurrence, fate, and biodegradation of estrogens in sewage and manure. *Applied Microbiology and Biotechnology*. 2010;86(6):1671-92.

Damstra T, Barlow S, Bergman A, Kavlock RJ, van der KraakGeds. Global assessment of the state-of-the-science of endocrine disruptors. Geneva: *World Health Organization*. WHO/PCS/EDC/02.2. 2002

D'Ascenzo G, Di Corcia A, Gentili A, Mancini R, Mastropasqua R, Nazzari M, et al. Fate of natural estrogen conjugates in municipal sewage transport and treatment facilities. *Science of the Total Environment*. 2003;302(1-3):199-209.

Dutta SK, Inamdar SP, Tso J, Aga DS. Concentrations of Free and Conjugated Estrogens at Different Landscape Positions in an Agricultural Watershed Receiving Poultry Litter. *Water Air and Soil Pollution*. 2012;223(5):2821-36.

Dutta S, Inamdar S, Tso J, Aga DS, Sims JT. Free and Conjugated Estrogen Exports in Surface-Runoff from Poultry Litter-Amended Soil. *Journal of Environmental Quality*. 2010;39(5):1688-98.

European Commission. European workshop on the impact of endocrine disruptors on human health and wildlife. In: Environment and climate research programme DX. Brussels. 1996.

Farre M, Kuster M, Brix R, Rubio F, de Alda M-JL, Barcelo D. Comparative study of an estradiol enzyme-linked immunosorbent assay kit, liquid chromatography-tandem mass spectrometry, and ultra performance liquid chromatography-quadrupole time of flight mass spectrometry for part-per-trillion analysis of estrogens in water samples. *Journal of Chromatography A*. 2007;1160(1-2):166-75.

Ferguson PL, Iden CR, McElroy AE, Brownawell BJ. Determination of steroid estrogens in wastewater by immunoaffinity extraction coupled with *HPLC-Electrospray-MS. Analytical Chemistry*. 2001;73(16):3890-5.

Fine DD, Breidenbach GP, Price TL, Hutchins SR. Quantitation of estrogens in ground water and swine lagoon samples using solid-phase extraction, pentafluorobenzyl/trimethylsilyl derivatizations and gas chromatography-negative ion chemical ionization tandem mass spectrometry. *Journal of Chromatography A*. 2003;1017(1-2):167-85.

Finlay-Moore O, Hartel PG, Cabrera ML. 17 beta-estradiol and testosterone in soil and runoff from grasslands amended with broiler litter. *Journal of Environmental Quality*. 2000;29(5):1604-11.

Froehner S, Machado KS, Stefan E, Bleninger T, da Rosa EC, Martins CdC. Occurrence of selected estrogens in mangrove sediments. *Marine Pollution Bulletin*. 2012;64(1):75-9.

Gineys N, Giroud B, Vulliet E. Analytical method for the determination of trace levels of steroid hormones and corticosteroids in soil, based on PLE/SPE/LC-MS/MS. *Analytical and Bioanalytical Chemistry*. 2010;397(6):2295-302.

Gong J, Ran Y, Chen D-Y, Yang Y. Occurrence of endocrine-disrupting chemicals in riverine sediments from the Pearl River Delta, China. *Marine Pollution Bulletin*. 2011;63(5-12):556-63.

Guedes-Alonso R, Sosa-Ferrera Z, Juan Santana-Rodriguez J. Simultaneous Determination of Hormonal Residues in Treated Waters Using Ultrahigh Performance Liquid Chromatography-Tandem Mass Spectrometry. *Journal of Analytical Methods in Chemistry*. 2013.

Guillarme D, Schappler J, Rudaz S, Veuthey J-L. Coupling ultra-high-pressure liquid chromatography with mass spectrometry. *Trac-Trends in Analytical Chemistry*. 2010;29(1):15-27.

Guillarme, D; Veuthey, JL, editors. UHPLC in Life Sciences. *Royal Society of Chemistry*. 2012.

Hajkova K, Pulkrabova J, Schurek J, Hajslova J, Poustka J, Napravnikova M, et al. Novel approaches to the analysis of steroid estrogens in river sediments. *Analytical and Bioanalytical Chemistry*. 2007;387(4):1351-63.

Hanselman TA, Graetz DA, Wilkie AC. Manure-borne estrogens as potential environmental contaminants: A review. *Environmental Science & Technology*. 2003;37(24):5471-8.

Hanselman TA, Graetz DA, Wilkie AC, Szabo NJ, Diaz CS. Determination of steroidal estrogens in flushed dairy manure wastewater by gas chromatography-mass spectrometry. *Journal of Environmental Quality*. 2006;35(3):695-700.

Hashimoto S, Horiuchi A, Yoshimoto T, Nakao M, Omura H, Kato Y, et al. Horizontal and vertical distribution of estrogenic activities in sediments and waters from Tokyo Bay, Japan. *Archives of Environmental Contamination and Toxicology*. 2005;48(2):209-16.

Hotchkiss AK, Rider CV, Blystone CR, Wilson VS, Hartig PC, Ankley GT, et al. Fifteen years after "Wingspread" - Environmental endocrine disrupters and human and wildlife health: Where we are today and where we need to go. *Toxicological Sciences*. 2008;105(2):235-59.

Huang CH, Sedlak DL. Analysis of estrogenic hormones in municipal wastewater effluent and surface water using enzyme-linked immunosorbent assay and gas chromatography/tandem mass spectrometry. *Environmental Toxicology and Chemistry*. 2001;20(1):133-9.

Ibanez M, Sancho JV, McMillan D, Rao R, Hernandez F. Rapid non-target screening of organic pollutants in water by ultraperformance liquid chromatography coupled to time-of-light mass spectrometry. *Trac-Trends in Analytical Chemistry*. 2008;27(5):481-9.

Isobe T, Shiraishi H, Yasuda M, Shinoda A, Suzuki H, Morita M. Determination of estrogens and their conjugates in water using solid-phase extraction followed by liquid chromatography-tandem mass spectrometry. *Journal of Chromatography A*. 2003;984(2):195-202.

Isobe T, Serizawa S, Horiguchi T, Shibata Y, Managaki S, Takada H, et al. Horizontal distribution of steroid estrogens in surface sediments in Tokyo Bay. *Environmental Pollution.* 2006;144(2):632-8.

Jafari AJ, Abasabad RP, Salehzadeh A. Endocrine disrupting contaminants in water resources and sewage in hamadan city of iran. *Iranian Journal of Environmental Health Science & Engineering.* 2009;6(2):89-96.

Jeannot R, Sabik H, Sauvard E, Dagnac T, Dohrendorf K. Determination of endocrine-disrupting compounds in environmental samples using gas and liquid chromatography with mass spectrometry. *Journal of Chromatography A.* 2002;974(1-2):143-59.

Jenkins MB, Endale DM, Schomberg HH, Hartel PG, Cabrera ML. 17 beta-Estradiol and testosterone in drainage and runoff from poultry litter applications to tilled and no-till crop land under irrigation. *Journal of Environmental Management.* 2009;90(8):2659-64.

Jenkins MB, Truman CC, Siragusa G, Line E, Bailey JS, Frye J, et al. Rainfall and tillage effects on transport of fecal bacteria and sex hormones 17 beta-estradiol and testosterone from broiler litter applications to a Georgia Piedmont Ultisol. *Science of the Total Environment.* 2008;403(1-3):154-63.

Jiang JQ, Yin Q, Zhou JL, Pearce P. Occurrence and treatment trials of endocrine disrupting chemicals (EDCs) in wastewaters. *Chemosphere.* 2005;61(4):544-50.

Jing Z, Chao XL, Li C, Xiang XZ, Guang QX, Ming SJ. Separation and determination of trace environmental estrogen through molecularly imprinted solid phase extraction coupled to high performance liquid chromatography. *Journal of Environmental Science and Health Part a-Toxic/Hazardous Substances & Environmental Engineering.* 2012;47(12):1889-96.

Johnson I, Harvey P.Study on the scientific evaluation of 12 substances in the context of endocrine disrupter priority list of actions. WRc-NSF. Report No.: UC 6052, 2002.

Johnson AC, Belfroid A, Di Corcia A. Estimating steroid oestrogen inputs into activated sludge treatment works and observations on their removal from the effluent. *Science of the Total Environment.* 2000;256(2-3):163-73.

Johnson AC, Williams RJ, Matthiessen P. The potential steroid hormone contribution of farm animals to freshwaters, the United Kingdom as a case study. *Science of the Total Environment.* 2006;362(1-3):166-78.

Kavlock RJ, Daston GP, DeRosa C, FennerCrisp P, Gray LE, Kaattari S, et al. Research needs for the risk assessment of health and environmental effects of endocrine disruptors: A report of the US EPA-sponsored workshop. *Environmental Health Perspectives.* 1996;104:715-40.

Kawaguchi M, Ito R, Sakui N, Okanouchi N, Saito K, Nakazawa H. Dual derivatization-stir bar sorptive extraction-thermal desorption-gas chromatography-mass spectrometry for determination of 17 beta-estradiol in water sample. *Journal of Chromatography A.* 2006;1105(1-2):140-7.

Kelly C. Analysis of steroids in environmental water samples using solid-phase extraction and ion-trap gas chromatography-mass spectrometry and gas chromatography-tandem mass spectrometry. *Journal of Chromatography A.* 2000;872(1-2):309-14.

Khanal SK, Xie B, Thompson ML, Sung S, Ong S-K, Van Leeuwen J. Fate, transport, and biodegradation of natural estrogens in the environment and engineered systems. *Environmental Science & Technology.* 2006;40(21):6537-46.

Kinney CA, Furlong ET, Zaugg SD, Burkhardt MR, Werner SL, Cahill JD, et al. Survey of organic wastewater contaminants in biosolids destined for land application. *Environmental Science & Technology.* 2006;40(23):7207-15.

Knight WM. In: Strogens in the Environment Dev. Toxicol. Environ. Sci. 5, McLachlan JA, Ed.; Elsevier/North-Holland: New York, 1980; pp 391-401.

Koha YKK, Chiu TY, Boobis A, Cartmell E, Lester JN, Scrimshaw MD. Determination of steroid estrogens in wastewater by high performance liquid chromatography - tandem mass spectrometry. *Journal of Chromatography A.* 2007;1173(1-2):81-7.

Kuch HM, Ballschmiter K. Determination of endocrine-disrupting phenolic compounds and estrogens in surface and drinking water by HRGC-(NCI)-MS in the picogram per liter range. *Environmental Science & Technology.* 2001;35(15):3201-6.

Labadie P, Budzinski H. Determination of steroidal hormone profiles along the Jalle d'Eysines River (near Bordeaux, France). *Environmental Science & Technology.* 2005;39(14):5113-20.

Lagana A, Bacaloni A, De Leva I, Faberi A, Fago G, Marino A. Analytical methodologies for determining the occurrence of endocrine disrupting chemicals in sewage treatment plants and natural waters. *Analytica Chimica Acta.* 2004;501(1):79-88.

Lange IG, Daxenberger A, Schiffer B, Witters H, Ibarreta D, Meyer HHD. Sex hormones originating from different livestock production systems: fate and potential disrupting activity in the environment. *Analytica Chimica Acta.* 2002;473(1-2):27-37.

Li H, Jiang Y, Liu Y. Enrichment and Determination of Trace Estradiol in Environmental Water Samples by Hollow-Fiber Liquid-Phase Microextraction Prior to HPLC. *Journal of Chromatographic Science.* 2011;49(9):676-82.

Liu R, Zhou JL, Wilding A. Simultaneous determination of endocrine disrupting phenolic compounds and steroids in water by solid-phase extraction-gas chromatography-mass spectrometry. *Journal of Chromatography* A. 2004;1022(1-2):179-89.

Liu S, Ying G-G, Zhang R-Q, Zhou L-J, Lai H-J, Chen Z-F. Fate and occurrence of steroids in swine and dairy cattle farms with different farming scales and wastes disposal systems. *Environmental Pollution.* 2012;170:190-201.

Liu S, Ying G-G, Zhao J-L, Chen F, Yang B, Zhou L-J, et al. Trace analysis of 28 steroids in surface water, wastewater and sludge samples by rapid resolution liquid chromatography-electrospray ionization tandem mass spectrometry. *Journal of Chromatography A.* 2011;1218(10):1367-78.

Liu S, Ying G-G, Zhao J-L, Zhou L-J, Yang B, Chen Z-F, et al. Occurrence and fate of androgens, estrogens, glucocorticoids and progestagens in two different types of municipal wastewater treatment plants. *Journal of Environmental Monitoring.* 2012;14(2):482-91.

Lopez de Alda MJ, Barcelo D. Use of solid-phase extraction in various of its modalities for sample preparation in the determination of estrogens and progestogens in sediment and water. *Journal of chromatography A.* 2001;938(1-2):145-53.

Miege C, Karolak S, Gabet V, Jugan ML, Oziol L, Chevreuil M, et al. Evaluation of estrogenic disrupting potency in aquatic environments and urban wastewaters by combining chemical and biological analysis. *Trac-Trends in Analytical Chemistry.* 2009;28(2):186-95.

Morteani G, Moeller P, Fuganti A, Paces T. Input and fate of anthropogenic estrogens and gadolinium in surface water and sewage plants in the hydrological basin of Prague (Czech Republic). *Environmental Geochemistry and Health*. 2006;28(3):257-64.

Mouatassim-Souali A, Tamisier-Karolak SL, Perdiz D, Cargouet M, Levi Y. Validation of a quantitative assay using GC/MS for trace determination of free and conjugated estrogens in environmental water samples. *Journal of Separation Science*. 2003;26(1-2):105-11.

Muller M, Rabenoelina F, Balaguer P, Patureau D, Lemenach K, Budzinski H, et al. Chemical and biological analysis of endocrine-disrupting hormones and estrogenic activity in an advanced sewage treatment plant. *Environmental Toxicology and Chemistry*. 2008;27(8):1649-58.

Nakamura M. Effects of estradiol-17-beta on gonadal sex-differentiation in 2 species of salmonids, the masu salmon, oncorhynchus-masou, and the chum salmon, o-keta. *Aquaculture*. 1984;43(1-3):83-90.

Nakamura S, Sian TH, Daishima S. Determination of estrogens in river water by gas chromatography-negative-ion chemical-ionization mass spectrometry. *Journal of Chromatography A*. 2001;919(2):275-82.

Nakamura S, Takino M, Daishima S. Determination of chlorophenols, bisphenol A and 17 beta-estradiol by gas chromatography/negative-ion chemical-ionization mass spectrometry. *Bunseki Kagaku*. 2000;49(3):181-7.

Nichols DJ, Daniel TC, Moore PA, Edwards DR, Pote DH. Runoff of estrogen hormone 17 beta-estradiol from poultry litter applied to pasture. *Journal of Environmental Quality*. 1997;26(4):1002-6.

Nieto A, Borrull F, Pocurull E, Marce RM. Determination of natural and synthetic estrogens and their conjugates in sewage sludge by pressurized liquid extraction and liquid chromatography-tandem mass spectrometry. *Journal of Chromatography A*. 2008;1213(2):224-30.

Noppe H, De Wasch K, Poelmans S, Van Hoof N, Verslycke T, Janssen CR, et al. Development and validation of an analytical method for detection of estrogens in water. *Analytical and Bioanalytical Chemistry*. 2005;382(1):91-8.

Noppe H, Verslycke T, De Wulf E, Verheyden K, Monteyne E, Van Caeter P, et al. Occurrence of estrogens in the Scheldt estuary: A 2-year survey. E*cotoxicology and Environmental Safety*. 2007;66(1):1-8.

Pailler J-Y, Guignard C, Meyer B, Iffly J-F, Pfister L, Hoffmann L, et al. Behaviour and Fluxes of Dissolved Antibiotics, Analgesics and Hormones During Flood Events in a Small Heterogeneous Catchment in the Grand Duchy of Luxembourg. *Water Air and Soil Pollution*. 2009;203(1-4):79-98.

Peng X, Yu Y, Tang C, Tan J, Huang Q, Wang Z. Occurrence of steroid estrogens, endocrine-disrupting phenols, and acid pharmaceutical residues in urban riverine water of the Pearl River Delta, South China. *Science of the Total Environment*. 2008;397(1-3):158-66.

Peterson EW, Davis RK, Orndorff HA. 17 beta-estradiol as an indicator of animal waste contamination in mantled karst aquifers. *Journal of Environmental Quality*. 2000;29(3):826-34.

Petrovic M, Eljarrat E, de Alda MJL, Barcelo D. Analysis and environmental levels of endocrine-disrupting compounds in freshwater sediments. T*rac-Trends in Analytical Chemistry*. 2001;20(11):637-48.

Reddy S, Iden CR, Brownawell BJ. Analysis of steroid conjugates in sewage influent and effluent by liquid chromatography-tandem mass spectrometry. *Analytical Chemistry.* 2005;77(21):7032-8.

Richardson ML, Bowron JM. The fate of pharmaceutical chemicals in the aquatic environment. *Journal of Pharmacy and Pharmacology.* 1985;37(1):1-12.

Rodriguez-Mozaz S, Lopez de Alda MJ, Barcelo D. Advantages and limitations of on-line solid phase extraction coupled to liquid chromatography-mass spectrometry technologies versus biosensors for monitoring of emerging contaminants in water. *Journal of Chromatography A.* 2007;1152(1-2):97-115.

Routledge EJ, Sheahan D, Desbrow C, Brighty GC, Waldock M, Sumpter JP. Identification of estrogenic chemicals in STW effluent. 2. In vivo responses in trout and roach. *Environmental Science & Technology.* 1998;32(11):1559-65.

Salvador A, Moretton C, Piram A, Faure R. On-line solid-phase extraction with on-support derivatization for high-sensitivity liquid chromatography tandem mass spectrometry of estrogens in influent/effluent of wastewater treatment plants. *Journal of Chromatography* A. 2007;1145(1-2):102-9.

Shore LS, Correll DL, Chakraborty PK. Relationship of fertilization with chick manure and concentrations of estrogens in small streams. In: Steele K, editor. Animal waste and the land –water interface. Boca Raton, FL: *CRC Press*; 1995. p. 155– 62.

Snyder EM, Snyder SA, Giesy JP, Blonde SA, Hurlburt GK, Summer CL, et al. SCRAM: A scoring and ranking system for persistent, bioaccumulative, and toxic substances for the North American Great Lakes - Part II. Bioaccumulation potential and persistence. *Environmental Science and Pollution Research.* 2000;7(2):116-21.

Sojo LE, Lum G, Chee P. Internal standard signal suppression by co-eluting analyte in isotope dilution LC-ESI-MS. *Analyst.* 2003;128(1):51-4.

Stavrakakis C, Colin R, Hequet V, Faur C, Le Cloirec P. Development and statistical validation of a quantitative method for the determination of steroid hormones in environmental water by column liquid chromatography/tandem mass spectrometry. *Journal of Aoac International.* 2008;91(1):237-46.

Stephany RW. Hormones in meat: different approaches in the EU and in the USA. Apmis. 2001;109:S357-S63.

Stumpe B, Marschner B. Long-term sewage sludge application and wastewater irrigation on the mineralization and sorption of 17 beta-estradiol and testosterone in soils. *Science of the Total Environment.* 2007;374(2-3):282-91.

Ternes TA, Andersen H, Gilberg D, Bonerz M. Determination of estrogens in sludge and sediments by liquid extraction and GC/MS/MS. *Analytical Chemistry.* 2002;74(14):3498-504.

Thompson ML, Casey FXM, Khan E, Hakk H, Larsen GL, DeSutter T. Occurrence and pathways of manure-borne 17 beta-estradiol in vadose zone water. *Chemosphere.* 2009;76(4):472-9.

Tyler CR, Routledge EJ. Oestrogenic effects in fish in English rivers with evidence of their causation. *Pure and Applied Chemistry.* 1998;70(9):1795-804.

U. K. Environment Agency. Endocrine Disrupting Substances in the Environment: *The Environment Agency's Strat*egy. 2000.

USEPA. Final Contaminant Candidate List 3. Chemicals: Identifying the Universe. *Office of Water. EPA* 815-R-09-006. 2009a.

USEPA. Targeted National Sewage sludge survay sampling and analysis technical report. *Office of Water. EPA*-822-R-08-016. 2009b.

Vanderford BJ, Pearson RA, Rexing DJ, Snyder SA. Analysis of endocrine disruptors, pharmaceuticals, and personal care products in water using liquid chromatography/tandem mass spectrometry. *Analytical Chemistry*. 2003;75(22):6265-74.

Vega-Morales T, Sosa-Ferrera Z, Santana-Rodriguez JJ. Determination of various estradiol mimicking-compounds in sewage sludge by the combination of microwave-assisted extraction and LC-MS/MS. *Talanta*. 2011;85(4):1825-34.

Velicu M, Suri R. Presence of steroid hormones and antibiotics in surface water of agricultural, suburban and mixed-use areas. *Environmental Monitoring and Assessment*. 2009;154(1-4):349-59.

Vulliet E, Baugros J-B, Flament-Waton M-M, Grenier-Loustalot M-F. Analytical methods for the determination of selected steroid sex hormones and corticosteriods in wastewater. *Analytical and Bioanalytical Chemistry*. 2007;387(6):2143-51.

Watabe Y, Kubo T, Nishikawa T, Fujita T, Kaya K, Hosoya K. Fully automated liquid chromatography-mass spectrometry determination of 17 beta-estradiol in river water. *Journal of Chromatography A*. 2006;1120(1-2):252-9.

Xiao XY, McCalley DV, McEvoy J. Analysis of estrogens in river water and effluents using solid-phase extraction and gas chromatography-negative chemical ionisation mass spectrometry of the pentafluorobenzoyl derivatives. *Journal of Chromatography A*. 2001;923(1-2):195-204.

Yang Y-Y, Gray JL, Furlong ET, Davis JG, ReVello RC, Borch T. Steroid Hormone Runoff from Agricultural Test Plots Applied with Municipal Biosolids. *Environmental Science & Technology*. 2012;46(5):2746-54.

Ying GG, Kookana RS, Ru YJ. Occurrence and fate of hormone steroids in the environment. *Environment International*. 2002;28(6):545-51.

Zhang Z, Hibberd A, Zhou JL. Analysis of emerging contaminants in sewage effluent and river water: Comparison between spot and passive sampling. *Analytica Chimica Acta*. 2008;607(1):37-44.

Zhao LX, Lin JM. Development of a micro-plate magnetic chemiluminescence enzyme immunoassay (MMCLEIA) for rapid- and high-throughput analysis of 17 beta-estradiol in water samples. *Journal of Biotechnology*. 2005;118(2):177-86.

Zhou Y, Zha J, Wang Z. Occurrence and fate of steroid estrogens in the largest wastewater treatment plant in Beijing, China. *Environmental Monitoring and Assessment*. 2012;184(11):6799-813.

Zuehlke S, Duennbier U, Heberer T. Determination of estrogenic steroids in surface water and wastewater by liquid chromatography-electrospray tandem mass spectrometry. *Journal of Separation Science*. 2005;28(1):52-8.

In: Estradiol: Synthesis, Health Effects and Drug Interactions ISBN: 978-1-62808-962-2
Editors: Ricco Palmeri and Sal Grimaudo

Chapter 9

Use of Combined Therapy of Estrogens with Antidepressants for Depressive Disorders: A Preclinical Review

Erika Estrada-Camarena,[1] Silvia Mejía-Mauries,[1] Nelly Maritza Vega-Rivera,[1,2] Alfredo Gallardo-Tenorio[1] and Alonso Fernández-Guasti[2,*]

[1]Laboratory of Neuropsychopharmacology, Direction of Neurosciences, National Institute of Psychiatry, México, D.F., Mexico

[2]Departament of Pharmacobiology, Center for Research and Advanced Studies (CINVESTAV), México, D.F., Mexico

Abstract

Depression is an important health problem, particularly in women around perimenopause. Controversial results exist in the efficacy of the combination of estrogens with antidepressants for depression treatment. Indeed, the use of estrogens as replacement therapy or as co-adjuvant with antidepressants has been subject of intense debate due to the possibility that estrogens may induce carcinogenic effects. However, recent reports indicate that the age of intervention -in relation with the menopause onset- is a crucial factor to explain the failure or success of the combined treatment with estrogens and antidepressants.

Other feature that contributes to the controversy is the type of compounds. Thus, the estrogenic compounds -with divergent neuropharmacological properties- differentially interact with the dissimilar kind of antidepressants: selective serotonin reuptake inhibitors, mixed reuptake inhibitors, tricyclics, atypical and monoamine-oxidase inhibitors.

The present review analyzes these two factors: age of treatment in relation to loss of ovarian function and type of estrogen/antidepressant. Thus, in the first part is presented a

* Corresponding author: Fernández-Guasti Alonso. Centro de Investigación y Estudios Avanzados, Departamento de Farmacobiología, Calzada de los Tenorios 235, Colonia Granjas Coapa,México 14330 D.F., Mexico. Tel.:+52 55 54 83 28 70; Fax:+52 55 54 83 28 63. E-mail address: jfernand@cinvestav.mx.

brief panorama of clinical and preclinical data of combining estrogenic compounds (17-β estradiol, E_2 and 17-α ethinyl-estradiol, EE_2) and antidepressants that we have used in basic research studies: two selective serotonin reuptake inhibitors (fluoxetine and citalopram), a mixed serotonin-noradrenaline reuptake inhibitor (venlafaxine) and a tricyclic compound preferentially with noradrenergic actions (desipramine).

Secondly, the antidepressant effects of the selective serotonin reuptake inhibitors are analyzed in relation to the subject's age and the time of loss of ovarian activity (menopause or ovariectomy) in clinical and preclinical studies. Finally, the participation of different monoaminergic and estrogen receptors as mediators of the synergism observed between estrogens and antidepressants is discussed.

Keywords: 17β estradiol, 17α ethynyl-estradiol, SSRIs, menopause, antidepressant-like effect, aging

Introduction

Menopause is defined as the permanent cessation of menstruation, resulting from loss of ovarian activity. This condition is recognized after 12 consecutive months of amenorrhea (Burger et al., 2008). The World Health Organization defines perimenopause as the period (2-8 years) preceding menopause and 1 year after final menses (Burger et al., 2008; Parry, 2008). During this period significant hormonal changes occur, for example there is an increase in follicle stimulating hormone (FSH) concentrations, variation in estrogen levels and frequent anovulatory cycles (Burger et al., 2008). After one year of amenorrhea (post-menopause) women present a well-defined hormonal profile with low levels of ovarian steroids and high gonadotrophin values (Soares and Cohen, 2001). This stage is characterized by vasomotor symptoms such as hot flashes, increased risk of osteoporosis, sexual dysfunction, psychosocial impairment and depressive symptoms (Soares et al., 2003; Soares and Cohen, 2001).

Interestingly, the incidence of major depression is three to five times higher in early perimenopause than in other periods of the reproductive life as compared with men (Riecher-Rossler and Geyter, 2007). Conversely, reduced risk for depression is reported in post-menopausal women (Payne et al., 2007; Riecher-Rossler and Geyter, 2007) when hormone levels appear stable. Thus, women without history of depression exhibited a stronger association between depressive symptoms and oscillations in estrogen levels and high levels of FSH and luteinizing hormone (LH) (Freeman et al., 2006), reinforcing the notion that perimenopause represents a period of particular vulnerability to this disease (Soares, 2010).

A treatment for depressive states associated to perimenopause is estrogen replacement therapy (ERT), because of its beneficial effects on other climacteric symptoms like osteoporosis and hot flashes (Rozenberg et al., 2013).

However, controversial results about its efficacy to reduce depression *versus* adverse actions restrict its utilization (Studd and Napi, 2012; Rozenberg et al., 2013). The use of a combined therapy of antidepressants with ERT to treat depression and climacteric symptoms may result advantageous: for example, ERT may shorten the onset of the therapeutic effect of antidepressants and may help to reduce vasomotor symptoms, to prevent osteoporosis and cardiovascular insults, and to promote neuroprotection (Estrada-Camarena et al., 2008; Studd, 2011).

Nevertheless, numerous controversies have related the use of ERT combined with antidepressants with the risk of cancer development, particularly in long-term users, in women with breast cancer history and on the time of intervention in relation to menopause onset (Soares, 2010; Chlebowski and Anderson, 2012).

In the first section of this chapter we present a brief panorama of clinical and preclinical data of combining estrogens and antidepressants, primarily selective serotonin reuptake inhibitors (SSRI´s), mixed reuptake inhibitors and tricyclics. Thereafter, a review of factors that underlies their action as well as the possible mechanisms involved in their antidepressant-like effects is presented.

1. Clinical and Preclinical Data of the Synergism between Estrogens and Antidepressants

1.1. Controversy in the Synergism between Estrogens and Antidepressants in Clinical Trials

In order to evaluate the role of the endocrine status in the response to antidepressants, it is conceivable to design studies where after assigning a woman to a pre or post-menopausal status, the antidepressant response is monitored. Few studies have been specifically designed with this purpose. For example a prospective open label study compared the response to several kinds of antidepressants, mainly SSRI's, in women with major depression -according to DSM-IV criteria- and selected as premenopausal or menopausal (Pae et al., 2009). Endocrine status was determined by the quantification of FSH, LH and estradiol levels; while depressive severity was evaluated by the Hamilton Depression Rating scale-17 (HamD-17), the Montgomery-Asberg Depression Rating Scale (MARDS) and the Clinical Global Impression Scale (CGI-S). Premenopausal women were younger (36±5 years) and showed lower FSH and LH levels, and high estradiol concentrations than post-menopausal women (61±6 years). Authors found a significant effect of the menopausal status, the age and the FSH levels on the depression severity, with pre-menopausal women being less depressed and more responsive to treatment than post-menopausal (Pae et al., 2009). Albeit this study is illustrative its main limitation is the low number of subjects and the lack of distinction between the different sorts of antidepressants.

The increase in the therapeutic effect of several antidepressants when combined with different estrogens, mainly conjugated equine estrogens (CEE) and 17β-estradiol (E_2), has been explored in clinical trials. Next we offer a series of controversial findings after combining various kinds of antidepressants: SSRI´s, fluoxetine, sertraline, citalopram and fluvoxamine; a mixed reuptake inhibitor, venlafaxine, or an atypical antidepressant, mirtazepine with different estrogen formulations alone or mixed with progestins (mainly medroxyprogesterone acetate, MPA), or androgens in perimenopausal and postmenopausal women varying in ages. Divergent results -positive, negative or no effect- have been reported in these trials. The nature of these discrepancies may rely on methodological differences.

For example, Schneider et al. (1997) analyzed the combination of ERT with fluoxetine (20 mg/kg) in a randomized trial in elderly women (60-70 years old) with unipolar major depression according to DSM-IIIR.

Seventy two women received ERT that consisted of CEE, estradiol, estropipate, transdermal estradiol, 17-α ethyinyl-estradiol (EE_2), estrogen mixed with methyl-testosterone or even non-specified esterified estrogens. Interestingly, the patients under treatment with ERT who received fluoxetine had a substantially greater mean Ham-D percentage improvement than patients on ERT who received placebo: 40% *vs.* 17%, respectively. Authors concluded that ERT augments fluoxetine response in elderly depressed patients (Schneider et al., 1997). Nonetheless, it must be mentioned that 68 of the 72 women receiving ERT and 32 of 286 that were not treated with ERT were hysterectomized without knowing if this factor influences the antidepressant effect of fluoxetine alone or in combination. Against these results, Amsterdam et al., (1999) failed to find an increased antidepressant effect of the same dose of fluoxetine (20 mg/kg) when combined with ERT in women aged around 45 years and with major depression. In this study patients were treated with ERT alone or estrogens mixed with MPA plus fluoxetine. The study was divided in two phases: a 12-week open-label with a fixed fluoxetine dose and a double blind one year relapse prevention phase. Authors did not find statistical differences in the mean Ham-D scores among groups during treatment or after it. Interestingly, the main difference between Schneider's and Amsterdam's works was the patient's age at intervention: 60-70 for the former *versus* around 45 for the latter.

In a follow-up study Schneider et al. in 2001 analyzed the possible synergism between ERT and sertraline, another SSRI. The sample also consisted of 60-70 years old women with major depression. The scales used to determine depression severity were the Ham-D and the CGI Scale. Thirty four subjects received estrogens (CEE, transdermal estradiol, esterified estrogens) plus sertraline and 93 got sertraline alone. Authors found a better response in the ERT-sertraline group than after the SSRI alone. Authors also analyzed the age factor and found that women in the range of 60-64 years old that took ERT plus sertraline responded better than the other age groups (65-69 or over 70 years old). This study concluded that ERT had a modest but significant improvement on the sertraline antidepressant effect (Schneider et al., 2001).

The introduction of other SSRI´s invited various authors to analyze their interaction with estrogens for the treatment of depression in women. Thus, Soares et al. (2003) examined the efficacy of citalopram alone or in combination with ERT for depression and menopause related symptoms treatment in premenopausal *versus* postmenopausal women with major depression. In this study authors explored the effect of citalopram (20-60 mg/day) as adjunctive treatment with ERT (transdermal estradiol) in non-responder women between 40-60 years old during 8-weeks. Menopausal status was corroborated by FSH determinations and interview. Remission of depression was defined according to MADRS scores. Authors reported that women under combined treatment showed MADRS score's improvement after 4 weeks, reaching a maximal median MADRS score at the end of the experiment. Similar findings were reported with CGI scores.

Also a significant reduction in anxiety and somatic, but not vasomotor, symptoms were observed after the combined treatment. Unfortunately, the study included a small sample (n=13) and did not discern if there were differences between pre- and post-menopausal women in the ERT plus citalopram response. By contrast, another trial failed to find an increased antidepressant effect of citalopram when combined with ERT (Kornstein et al., 2013). Premenopausal (n=896) and postmenopausal (n=544) women were treated with citalopram for 12-14 weeks.

Baseline demographic and clinical characteristics were used in adjusted analysis of the effect of menopausal status and use of hormonal contraceptives or menopausal hormonal replacement therapy (HRT) on outcomes. Remission was defined as a final HamD-17 value ≤ 7 or Quick Inventory of Depressive Symptomatology-Self-Report (QIDS-SR) score ≤ 5 and response as $\geq 50\%$ decrease from the baseline QIDS-SR score. Premenopausal women taking hormonal contraceptives had significantly greater unadjusted remission rates than women not taking contraception; however, these differences were lost when results were adjusted. In line, the response and remission rates did not differ between postmenopausal women taking *versus* not taking HRT. The authors concluded that citalopram treatment outcome was not affected by menopausal status or hormonal treatment (Kornstein et al., 2013).

Another aspect that should be taken into account in the analysis of such interaction is the relief of climacteric symptoms, which generally include depression. In this sense, several clinical reports indicate that particularly SSRI´s and venlafaxine are suitable alternatives to treat these symptoms. In this line, a single-blind, non-randomized trial evaluated the efficacy of citalopram alone or in combination with estrogens on climacteric symptoms (Kalay et al., 2007). The study included 100 natural or surgical menopausal women. The climacteric symptoms were evaluated using the Kupperman index and the Menopause Specific Quality of Life Questionnaire (MENQOL) that includes the analysis of hot flashes, sweating, insomnia, nervousness, depression, vertigo, fatigue, joint ache, headache, palpitation and vaginal dryness. All post-menopausal women had 2-8 years of menopause onset and were distributed in four groups (n=25 each): placebo, citalopram (20-40 mg/day), placebo plus HRT and citalporam plus HRT. In this study HRT consisted in CEE (0.625 mg/day) plus MPA (5 mg/day), E_2 (2 mg/day) and norethisterone acetate (1 mg/day) or CEE (0.625 mg/day) alone for hysterectomized women. Results showed that citolapram alone or in combination with HRT reduced the Kupperman scores and some parameters of the MENQOL index, including hot flashes, psychosocial and physical functioning, but had negative results on sexual dysfunction. The authors concluded that citalopram is effective for patients who do not want to take HRT for the alleviation of climacteric symptoms and an adjuvant treatment with HRT. It is important to note that few clinical studies have explored different estrogen doses (lower than 0.625 mg/day for CEE) and short-term treatments. One of them performed by Nagata and coworkers in 2005 reported that the combination of a low dose of CEE (0.325 mg/day) with the SSRI, fluvoxamine (50 mg/day) during 8-weeks in oophorectomized post-menopausal women (aged 41-55 years old) reduce the climacteric symptoms including depression, anxiety and hot flashes. Depression, anxiety and climacteric symptoms were measured using SDS, SRQ-D, state-trait anxiety test (STAI) and Kupperman scores, respectively. Interestingly, this study included women with cervical cancer. Authors concluded that a low-dose and short-term treatment with estrogen + SSRI is effective and safe for oophorectomized women in relieving the hot flashes and depression associated with climacteric symptoms (Nagata et al., 2005).

In basic research experiments (*vida infra*), in addition to SSRI´s, we have evaluated the antidepressant-like effect of noradrenergic (desipramine) and mixed noradrenergic-serotonergic reuptake inhibitors (venlafaxine) alone and in combination with estrogens. As far as we know there are no clinical trials that evaluate the combination of selective antidepressants acting at the catecholaminergic transmission (for example, bupropion or desipramine) and estrogens as a strategy to increase the antidepressant- or anticlimacteric-actions.

However, other drugs such as atypical antidepressants like mirtazapine or the mixed noradrenergic-serotonergic reuptake inhibitor, venlafaxine have been explored. Thus, Dias et al. (2006) evaluated the effect of venlafaxine in a 24 weeks study that included seventy-two menopausal, 50-60 years old women diagnosed with depression according to MADRS. Primary efficacy outcome was remission according to the MADRS, whereas secondary efficacy measures included the CGI. All women received venlafaxine alone or in combination with one of the following HRT combinations: CEE (0.625 mg) + MPA (2.5 mg) + methyltestosterone (2.5 mg); estrogen + MPA; methyltestosterone; and a group without HRT. The combination of methyl-testosterone plus venlafaxine induced a significant improvement on the MADRS scores compared with placebo, whereas estradiol+MPA+methyl-testosterone plus venlafaxine and estradiol+MPA plus venlafaxine had a significant improvement on CGI rates compared with placebo. Authors conclude that HRT increases the antidepressant efficacy of venlafaxine; however, it is difficult to elucidate which hormone played the main synergistic role (Dias et al., 2006). Regarding mirtazapine, Joffe et al. (2001) designed the following study: perimenopausal and postmenopausal women aged 40-61 unresponsive to ERT who met the criteria for major depression (according to DSM-IV) were treated with 30-45 mg/day mirtazapine for 8 weeks and assessed every 2 weeks with the HamD-17, Beck Depression Inventory (BDI), and CGI Scale. Remission was defined as a HamD-17 score ≤ 7 at week 8.

Authors described that remission was achieved by 14 of the 16 (87.5%) women treated with mirtazapine, regardless whether depression preceded or not ERT. Therapeutic response also appeared independent of menopausal status: perimenopausal *versus* postmenopausal, ERT preparation, and concomitant use of MPA. Authors concluded that mirtazapine is an effective treatment for major depression in perimenopausal and postmenopausal women whose depression precedes ERT use and does not respond to ERT or whose depression develops after ERT is initiated.

As aforementioned the analysis of the interaction between antidepressants and estrogens in clinical studies is highly controversial possibly due to: (1) the different antidepressants and HRT used, (2) their dosages and length of treatment, (3) the intervention time in relation with the cessation of menses, (4) the sample's age, endocrine condition and uterine surgery, and even (5) the scales and criteria used to determine depression, remission, response, climacteric symptoms and menopause. Due to the intricate control of these variables in clinics, preclinical work may help to analyze whether a specific combination effectively provokes an antidepressant-like response under controlled conditions. In addition, the use of animal models permits to experimentally explore the specific influence of some of these variables.

2. Basic Trials

2.1. Can Rodents Represent an Animal Model of Menopause?

In rats reproductive senescence is initiated by a period known as estropause, characterized by irregular cycles followed by constant estrous and finally by a persistent diestrous stage. In contrast with women, the rat ovary retains the capacity to secrete estrogens all along the life span (reviewed in Yin and Gore, 2006).

Thus, rats' estropause is not analogous to human menopause, and for this reason the ovaries extirpation (ovariectomy; OVX), preferably in aged subjects, is used as a strategy to induce an endocrine condition that resembles human menopause. Naturally, OVX produces a sharp decline in estrogen and progesterone levels accompanied by an increase in FSH and LH concentrations (Chakraborty and Gore, 2004), signs of osteoporosis (Gurkan et al., 1986; Kalu et al., 1998), increase in tail skin temperature (Kobayashi et al., 2000; Okada et al., 1997), and importantly, enhancement in experimental anxiety (Picazo et al., 2006) and depressive-like behaviors (Bekku et al., 2006; Estrada-Camarena et al., 2011). Regarding the latter, OVX in mice (Bekku et al., 2005) and rats (Estrada-Camarena et al., 2011; Vega-Rivera et al., 2013) temporarily increases the expression of passive behaviors in the forced swimming test (FST, an animal model of depression). These data are in agreement with clinical reports indicating that perimenopause may be associated with depression and has a critical expression period defined by ovarian endocrine oscillations (Parry, 2008; Soares and Zitek, 2008; Soares, 2010).

Most of the studies exploring the interaction between estrogens and antidepressants in basic research have used young adult ovariectomized animals and it is important to consider that aging is a determinant factor that contributes to depression development in concert with reproductive senescence (Chakraborty and Gore, 2004; de Chaves et al., 2009; Recamier-Carballo and Fernandez-Guasti, 2012).

2.2. An Animal Model for the Screening of Antidepressant-Like Effects

The depressive human disorder includes a set of signs and symptoms with complex etiology and therefore it is difficult to find a satisfactory animal model that mimics it. In psychopharmacology it is assumed that the animal models should fulfill various validity criteria (Willner, 1995).

In this way, the forced swimming test (FST) is an animal model of acute stress where rodents are forced to swim for 15 minutes in a cylinder with water at 23-25 ºC (Porsolt et al., 1977). During the first minutes rodents make vigorous movements in order to try to resolve the situation; however, after 5-10 minutes the animal adopts an immobility posture characterized by the minimal movements to keep the head above the water (Porsolt et al., 1977, López-Rubalcava et al., 2009; Recamier and Fernandez-Guasti, 2012). It is assumed that the immobility posture reflects a depressive-like behavior because the animals stop all attempts to escape the situation (Porsolt et al., 1977; Cryan et al., 2005). Interestingly, only drugs with antidepressant effects in clinics reduce the immobility behavior without altering general motor activity. Thus, this model meets the predictive and face validity criteria because immobility is a sign of despair, characteristic of depression (face validity) and is selective to antidepressants (predictive validity) (Cryan et al., 2005).

Besides, by using the modified version of the FST it is possible to infer the mechanism of action involved in the antidepressant-like action of a given drug (Detke et al., 1995). In this sense, all antidepressants decrease the immobility behavior by increasing the active behaviors: swimming and climbing. Interestingly, the SSRI´s, like fluoxetine, increase swimming behavior; while cathecolaminergic inhibitors, such as desipramine, bupropion and reboxetine, increase climbing behavior (Detke et al., 1995; Cryan et al., 2005; López-Rubalcava et al., 2012).

The FST is also sensitive to endocrine oscillations along the estrous cycle (Martinez-Mota et al., 1999; Estrada-Camarena et al., 2011), and to endocrine manipulations including OVX (Bekku et al., 2006; Estrada-Camarena et al., 2011; Vega-Rivera et al., 2013), progesterone withdrawal (Saavedra et al., 2006) and aging (de Chaves et al., 2009; Moretti et al., 2011; Recamier-Carballo and Fernandez-Guasti, 2012). As a result, the animal model is sensitive to the antidepressant-like effects of endogenous or exogenous estrogens and progestins (Martínez-Mota et al., 1999; Estrada-Camarena et al., 2003; Galea et al., 2001).

Therefore, using OVX animals and the FST, as the main model for the screening of antidepressant actions, in the next section we review some basic studies where the synergism between estrogens and antidepressants was explored.

2.3. Evidence of the Synergism between Estrogens and Antidepressants in Basic Research

The antidepressant-like action of some estrogens -17β-estradiol, 17α-ethynyl-estradiol, estradiol benzoate, estradiol valerate, diaryl-propinitrile, cumestrol, G1 and raloxifene- have been reported after an acute or chronic administration in OVX animals in the FST (for review see López-Rubalcava, 2012). Specifically, for E_2 and EE_2 a dose response curve showed that a single administration reduced the immobility behavior; however, E_2 enhanced swimming, whereas EE_2 increased swimming and climbing (Estrada-Camarena et al., 2003). According to the interpretation of the selective increase of active behaviors depending on the stimulation of the serotonergic or cathecolaminergic systems (*vide supra*), E_2 may be modulating the serotonergic activity, while EE_2 could be working on all three monoaminergic systems (López-Rubalcava et al., 2012). In addition, EE_2 was more potent than E_2 in inducing antidepressant-like effects (for review López-Rubalcava et al., 2012).

On the other hand, OVX rodents respond to most classic antidepressant treatments including fluvoxamine, fluoxetine (FLX), milnacepram, desipramine, venlafaxine, citalopram, among others by reducing the immobility behavior (Bekku et al., 2006; Estrada-Camarena et al., 2003; 2011; Molina-Hernández and Téllez-Alcántara, 2011; Recamier-Carballo et al., 2012). Usually in the FST, 10 mg/kg of FLX or desipramine are effective to reduce the immobility behavior in a sub-acute (3 doses) schedule or after 1.25-2.5 mg/kg given chronically for 14 or 21 days (Detke et al., 1997; Contreras et al., 2001; Estrada-Camarena et al., 2008).

Due to the fact that various factors may veil the synergism between estrogens and antidepressant (*vide supra*) in clinical trials, we and others have explored several combinations of antidepressants and estrogens in young and aged OVX rats. For example, when a single non-effective dose of E_2 (2.5 μg/rat) or EE_2 (1.25 μg/rat) was combined with a sub-effective dose of FLX (1.25 mg/kg), a significant reduction of the immobility behavior occurred (Estrada-Camarena et al., 2004, 2008).

One of the most interesting finding is that in spite that both estrogens were combined with the same FLX dose, the behavioral profile induced by each estrogenic compound differed, i.e. both combinations reduced immobility but E_2/FLX increased swimming, while EE_2 increased swimming and climbing, suggesting a different mechanism of action (Estrada-Camarena et al., 2004). A similar finding was observed when both E_2 and EE_2 were combined with the tricyclic antidepressant, desipramine (DMI).

In this case, DMI is mainly a noradrenergic reuptake inhibitor that typically decreases immobility and increases climbing. So when E_2 was combined with DMI, the effect on climbing prevails over that of E_2 on swimming; however, when combined with EE_2 both active behaviors tend to increase. In addition, E_2 also synergized with venlafaxine (VLX, Nowakowska and Kus, 2005; Estrada-Camarena et al., 2008) and citalopram (Estrada-Camarena et al., unpublished results) to produce antidepressant-like actions in the FST. These results suggest that the estrogens, E_2 and EE_2, effectively facilitate the antidepressant-like action of various antidepressants in young OVX rats.

After these data a question that remains unresolved is whether estrogens, in addition to potentiate, are also able to shorten the onset of action of antidepressants? In this sense, in another experiment we showed that E_2 drastically accelerates the onset of antidepressant-like action of FLX and DMI in the FST (Estrada-Camarena et al., 2008). In this case, the administration of a single non-effective dose of E_2 shortened to 24 or 72 hours the latency to observe the reduced immobility produced by a low dose of FLX or DMI which take at least 14 days to be observed (Estrada-Camarena et al., 2008).

Surprisingly, the combination of VLX with E_2 only produced a synergism within the first three days of treatment (Estrada-Camarena et al., 2008), which contrasted with the observations involving the combination of E_2 with FLX and DMI that lasted for at least two weeks (Estrada-Camarena et al., 2008). Despite the dual action of VLX on monoaminergic transporters (Owens et al., 1997; Bëique et al., 1998, 2000), the efficacy of combining E_2 with VLX was not better than when combining it with FLX. Furthermore, after a VLX-chronic treatment for 14 days, the addition of E_2 produced a pro-depressive behavior. From these data it is possible to suggest that estrogens potentiate and at the same time shorten the onset of action of particular antidepressants.

Thus, these observations indicate that the synergism between estrogens and antidepressants importantly depend upon the type of compound employed and may partly explain the controversial clinical data after such combinations.

3. SSRI's Effects of Age and Time of Intervention After Ovarian Loss

As previously reviewed few clinical trials analyze the antidepressant effects depending upon the women's menstrual condition: premenopausic, perimenopausic and postmenopausic. Furthermore, almost no study has considered as an important factor the lapse between the last menstruation and the initiation of treatment with HRT for its antidepressant effectiveness.

Interestingly, the antidepressant-like effect of estrogens reduces after several weeks post-OVX, which is in agreement with the lack of effect of ERT in advanced-aged post-menopausal women (Schneider et al., 2001). Thus, we observed that when E_2, but not EE_2, was injected 12 weeks after OVX, its antidepressant-like effect vanished (Estrada-Camarena et al., 2011), indicating that the '*beneficial window*' to observe an antidepressant action is not the same for all estrogens (Figure 1).

Further, EE_2 intervention appears to be more appropriate to induce an antidepressant-like action after 12 weeks post-OVX in young animals. Interestingly, the rats were unresponsive to both estrogens if the restitution was initiated 20 weeks post-OVX.

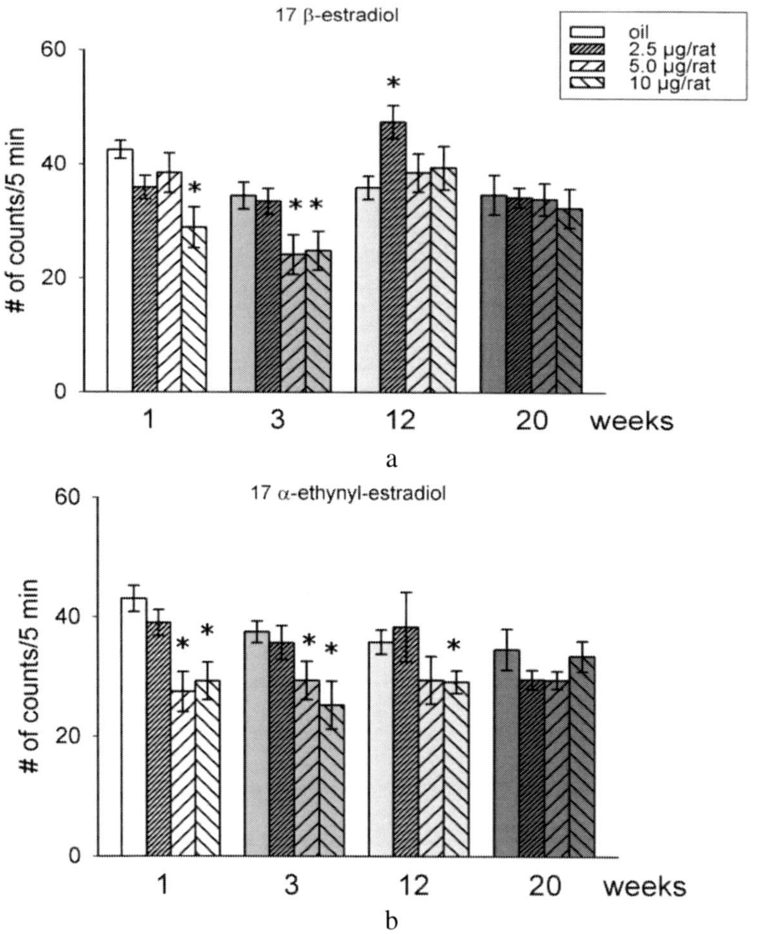

Holm-Sidack test. * p< 0.05 versus respective control group.

Figure 1. Effect of the post-OVX time on the antidepressant-like action of several doses of 17 β-estradiol (E_2; 2.5, 5.0 and 10 µg/rat, i.p,-48h; panel A) and 17 α-ethynyl-estradiol (EE_2; 1.25, 2.5, 5.0 µg/rat, s.c, -48h; panel B) in the forced swimming test (FST). Data are presented as mean ± S.E.M. of the number of immobilities in a 5 minutes test session. E_2 and EE_2 decreased the number of immobilites (antidepressant-like action) when administered at one and three weeks, but not at twelve respectively. Two way ANOVA test values for E_2 for post-OVX time $F{:}3,89=9.59$, $p<0.001$; for treatment $F{:}3,89=3.47$, $p=0.01$; and for interaction time X treatment $F{:}9,89=1.71$, $p=0.09$. For EE_2 for post-OVX time $F{:}3,95=0.65$, ns; for treatment F: $3,95=8.59$, $p<0.001$; and for interaction time X treatment $F{:}9;95=1.13$, ns.

These results agree with those reported by Walf et al. (2009) showing that female mice did not respond to chronic estradiol if the treatment was initiated 20 weeks post-OVX (Walf et al., 2009) and with clinical trials where ERT was effective to reduce or remit depressive symptomatology when given 5 to 7 years after menopause (Soares et al., 2003; Nagata et al., 2005; Kalay et al., 2007).

Little is known about the age factor in the antidepressant effect of HRT alone or combined with antidepressants. As reviewed, most clinical studies include women between 45-65 years old, but few analyze their findings considering age as a crucial factor. Moreover, in the studies where the authors did data adjustments according to the woman's age, the precise information regarding sample´s age and age of menopause onset are omitted. Therefore, it is necessary to do systematic studies that explore how this factor influences the putative beneficial effect of HRT. In this point basic studies showed that aged rats are less responsive than young rats. Our group is exploring the role of age in the antidepressant-like action of E_2, for this reason rats were OVX at 3, 12 or 15 months of age and were tested in the FST after a single injection of E_2. It is important to mention that 3 months old rats represent young females with regular estrous cycles, those aged 12 months represent peri-estropausic rats that mainly showed irregular cycles, reduced number of successful pregnancies and lower number of litter-mate; while those rats over 15 months old are in estropause, where a continuous estrous or diestrus vaginal cytology is observed (Walf et al., 2009; Olvera-Hernández and Fernández-Guasti, 2011). Consequently, it is considered that these ages represent different endocrine conditions at the moment when the ovaries were removed. Our results showed that young (3 months) and middle-aged (12 months) rats -but not those animals that were OVX at 15 months old- are responsive to the antidepressant-like actions of E_2. Interestingly the 12 months old animals required higher doses of E_2 to reduce the immobility behavior than their young counterpart (Figure 2), suggesting that the natural aging process modifies the estradiol-sensitivity.

Following this idea, it was expected that the antidepressant-like effect observed with the combination of estrogens and antidepressants also varies in function of the time of loss of ovarian function and/or aging. In this sense we tested the effect of the combination of E_2 and FLX in young (3 months) and middle-aged (11-14 months) rats which were OVX 3 weeks before testing. Noteworthy the antidepressant-like effect of the E_2/FLX combination was observed at the two ages selected in two animal models: FST and the chronic mild stress (Recamier-Carballo et al., 2012). Remarkably, a clear increase of depressive-like behavior was detected in both models in middle-age rats when compared with young animals (de Chaves et al., 2009; Recamier-Carballo et al., 2012). In contrast, when 15 months old rats were OVX and tested after several (around 7) weeks post-OVX, the antidepressant-like action of estradiol valerate and citalopram was absent, even both compounds alone, at effective doses, induced antidepressant-like effects (Romano-Torres and Fernández-Guasti, 2010). A similar finding was observed in 15 months old rats and the antidepressant-like action of EE_2 plus citalopram was tested after one or three weeks post-OVX. In this case, the synergism between EE_2 and citalopram was observed only one week after OVX (Estrada-Camarena, unpublished results). This lack of effect may be related with the limited antidepressant-like action of estrogens alone in 15 months old rats which is also restricted to one week post-OVX (Figure 3). These data taken together suggest specific estrogen sensitivity changes along aging that limit the antidepressant-like action of these steroids and that may also contribute to the divergent clinical findings.

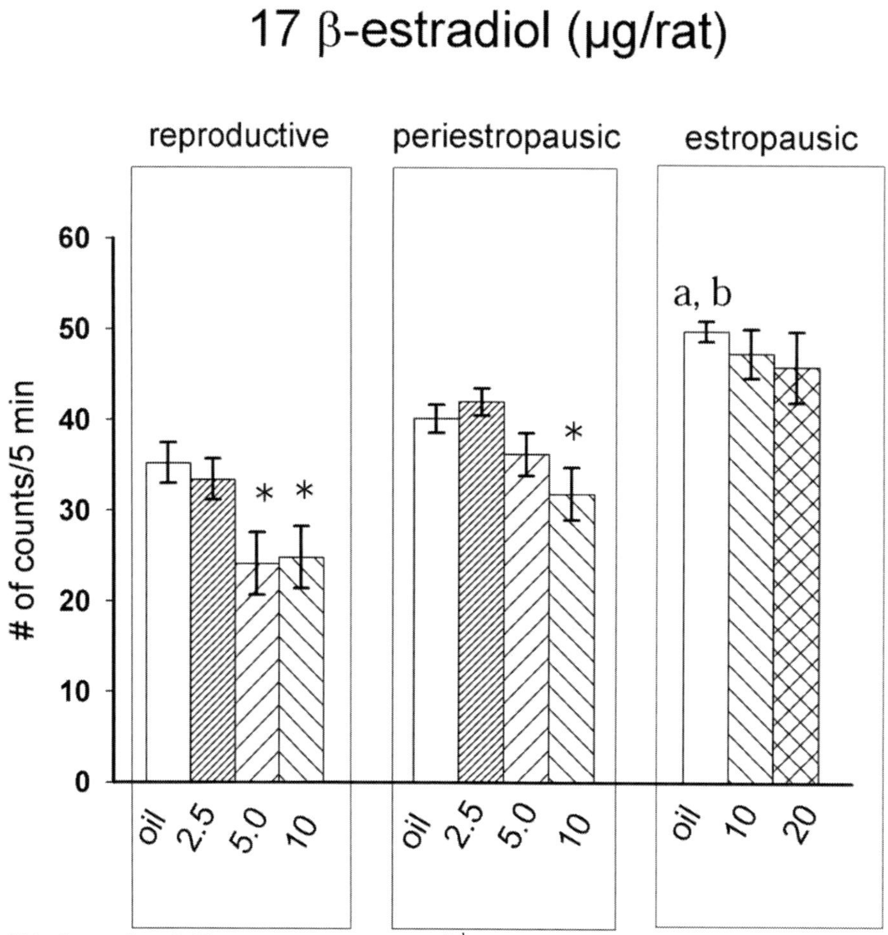

Holm-Sidack test *p <0.05 versus control group; [a, b] p<0.01 versus young adult and middle-aged rats, respectively.

Figure 2. Effect of ageing on the antidepressant-like action of several doses of 17 β-estradiol (E_2; 2.5, 5.0, 10 μg/rat for young adult and middle-aged animals; and 10 and 20 μg/rat for advanced-aged subjects; s.c, -48) in ovariectomized (OVX) rats tested in the forced swimming test at three weeks after OVX. Data are presented as mean ± S.E.M. of the number of immobilities in a 5 minutes test session. E_2 induced an antidepressant-like action in young adult and middle-aged but not in advanced aged rats. Also ageing increased the number of immobilities which is considered as a pro-depressive-like behavior (F:2,23= 21.27, $p<0.001$). One Way Anova test for young-adult F:3,25=4.3, $p<0.01$; for middle-aged F:3, 28=4.1, $p<0.01$ and advanced-aged rats F:2, 27=0.56, ns.

4. Mechanism of Action Involved in the Synergism between Estrogens and Antidepressants

The mechanism of action that underlies the antidepressant-like action of estrogens alone or in combination with antidepressants is not completely elucidated. A complex interaction between monoamine neurotransmitter systems (5-HT and catecholamines) and estrogens receptors has been described, but it is clear that other neurotransmitters could be involved (GABA and glutamate, among others) in both, the estrogens' and the antidepressants' effects.

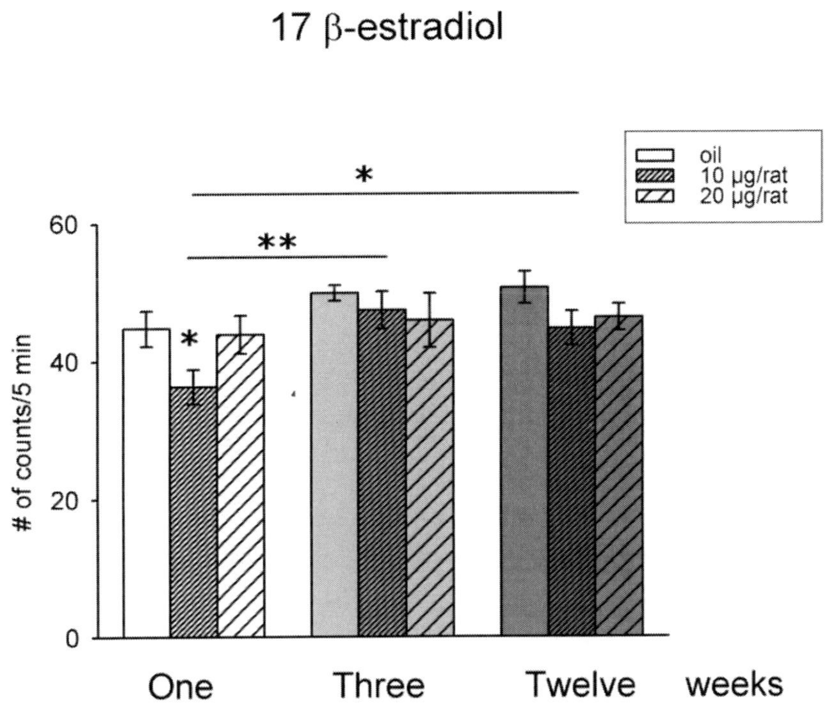

Holm-Sidack test, *p<0.05; ** p<0.001 versus their respective control group; lines indicate specific paired comparisons against groups tested at three or twelve weeks.

Figure 3. Effect of post-OVX time on the antidepressant-like action of 17-β estradiol (E_2; 10 and 20 μg/rat; s.c., -48h) in advanced-aged rats subjected to the forced swimming test. Data are presented as mean ± S.E.M. of the number of immobilities in a 5 minutes test session. E_2-restitution only decreased immobility one week post-OVX. Two Way Anova test values for post-OVX time $F{:}2,75=5.09$, $p=0.008$; for treatment $F{:}2,75=3.63$, $p=0.04$; and for the interaction time X treatment $F{:}\ 4,75=0.47$, ns.

For the scope of the present review only the relationship between estrogens and monoamines are discussed.

As mentioned above the antidepressant-like action of estrogenic compounds alone or in combination with antidepressants may involve different mechanisms. In the case of E_2, it is proposed the participation of the serotonergic system due to several evidences. First, E_2 induces a clear swimming increase in the FST (Estrada-Camarena et al., 2003), which is closely related to the 5-HT levels increase in some brain areas (Mikail et al., 2012; Kirby and Lucki 1997). Second, the antidepressant-like action of E_2 is blocked by the 5-HT1A receptor antagonist, WAY 100635 (Estrada-Camarena et al., 2006a) and most likely the receptor involved is post-synaptic since the administration of the specific 5-HT1A postsynaptic receptor antagonist, MM-77, canceled the E_2 antidepressant-like effects in the FST (López-Rubalcava et al., 2005). Third, other authors have shown that E_2 increases the expression of mRNA of the enzyme tryptophan hydroxylase and produces an antidepressant-like effect in the FST (Donner and Handa, 2009). Furthermore, the acute or chronic E_2 administration increases the 5-HT levels and its metabolite 5-hydroxy-indolacetic acid in the dorsal raphe nucleus and the hippocampus (Lubbers et al., 2010). Interestingly, human studies reported increased serotonin levels in postmenopausal women receiving ERT (Blum et al., 1996) and suggest that E_2 enhances 5-HT synthesis (O'Keane et al., 1991).

Other results suggest that the estrogenic actions on the serotonergic system require the estrogen receptor activation. For example, our research group found that RU58688, an estrogen receptor antagonist, blocked the E_2 antidepressant-like effect (Estrada-Camarena el al., 2006b); while the desensitization of postsynaptic 5-HT1A receptors located in the rat hippocampus requires the participation of a membrane estrogen receptor (Mize et al., 2001). In addition, it has been demonstrated that the membrane estrogen receptor, GPR30, is involved in the 5-HT1A receptor desensitization induced by estrogens in the rat hypothalamic paraventricular nucleus (Rossi et al., 2010). Moreover, recently it was shown that E_2 accelerates the FLX induced-desensitization of 5-HT1A receptors (Li et al., 2013). These authors showed that two days of combined treatment with E_2 and FLX produces an important desensitization of 5-HT1A receptors which is necessary to observe an antidepressant response (Li et al., 2013). Also two days of E_2 treatment prevented the FLX-increase of 5-HT1A receptor protein and reduced the levels of G-protein coupled to the estrogen receptor, GPR30 (Li et al., 2013). Noticeable is the coincidence between the time required to observe a synergism between low doses of FLX and E_2 in the FST: around 3 days (Estrada-Camarena et al., 2008) and that required for the 5-HT1A receptor desensitization and estrogen receptor changes reported by Li et al. (2013). Furthermore, these data also agree with the fact that both, the estrogen receptor antagonist as well the 5-HT1A receptor antagonist blocked the antidepressant-like action of the combination E_2 plus FLX (Estrada-Camarena et al., 2006b).

On the other side, the antidepressant-like action of EE_2 may involve the modulation of both the serotonergic and catecholaminergic systems. Evidence in support shows that EE_2 increased both swimming and climbing behaviors (Estrada-Camarena et al., 2003) and its antidepressant-like effect was blocked by the $\alpha 2$ adrenergic receptor antagonist, idazoxan (López-Rubalcava et al., 2007; Vega-Rivera et al., submitted). In addition, DSP4, a neurotoxin that selectively destroys noradrenergic nerve terminals blocked the antidepressant-like effect induced by EE_2 on swimming and climbing behavior (Vega-Rivera et al., submitted). Furthermore, in vitro studies showed that EE_2 inhibited the serotonin, noradrenaline and dopamine transporters (Hiemke et al., 1985). Additionally, the EE_2 antidepressant-like actions do not seem to be directly mediated by 5-HT1A receptors because WAY 100 635 did not blocked its effects (Estrada-Camarena et al., 2006a), but requires of 5-HT since the destruction of serotonergic terminals with 5,7-dyhydroxytryptamine prevented its antidepressant-like actions (Vega-Rivera et al., submitted). Interestingly, when the estrogen receptor was blocked by the antagonist, ICI 180, 780 the anti-immobility effect and the increased swimming after EE_2 was blocked, while its effects on climbing were not prevented (Vega-Rivera et al., submitted). Further, when non-effective doses of EE_2 and DMI were combined the immobility decrease was accompanied by an increase in both swimming and climbing. This behavioral profile was partially blocked with the $\alpha 2$-adrenergic receptor antagonist, idazoxan which canceled the combination effect on climbing while ICI 180, 780, the estrogen receptor antagonist, only blocked the swimming behavior increase (Figure 4). These results suggest a complex interaction between EE_2 and monoamines which requires a deep examination and reinforce the notion that different estrogenic compounds possess distinct mechanisms of action.

The observation that estrogens exert antidepressant-like effects after few hours (Estrada-Camarena et al., 2003), suggests that other mechanisms like neurogenesis and neuroplasticity parallel the monoaminergic modulation.

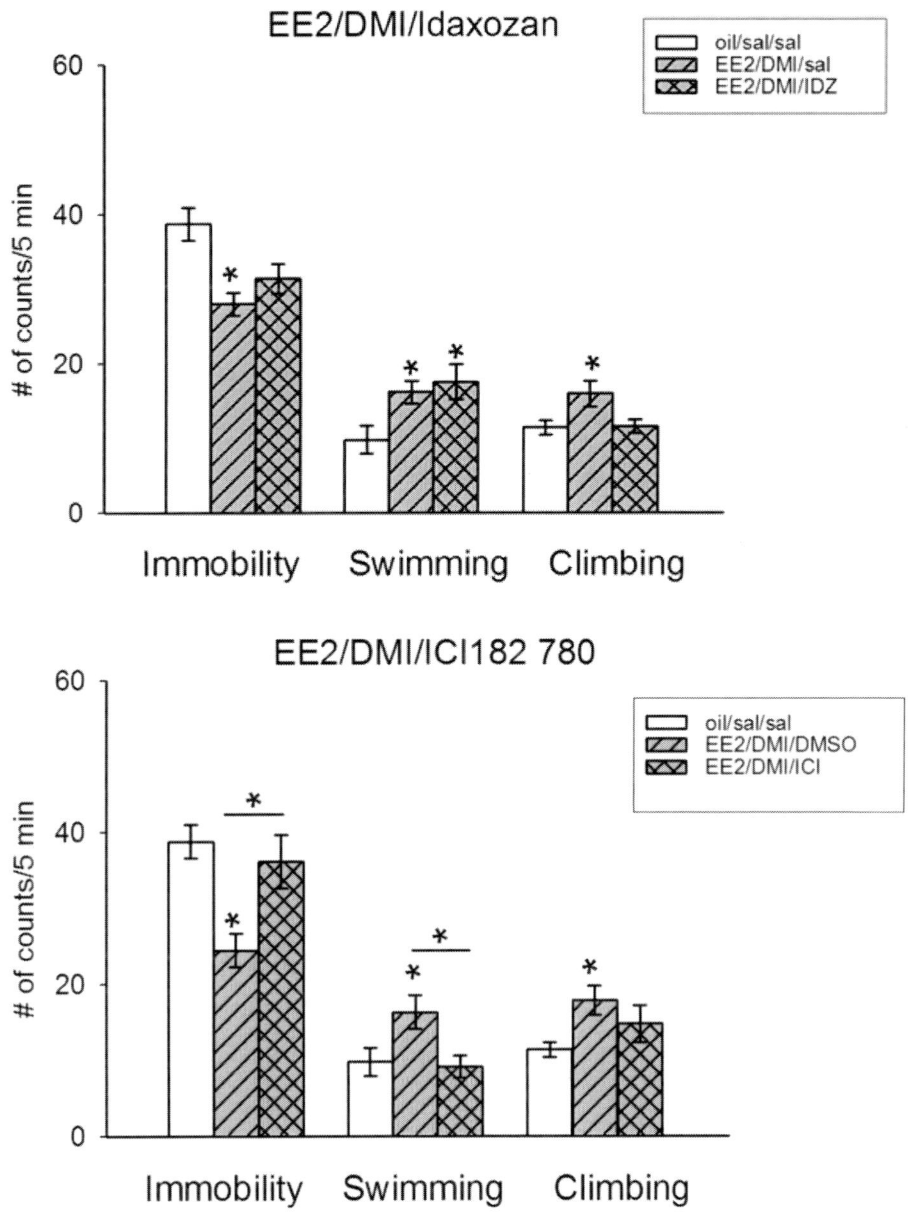

One Way Anova values followed by Holm-Sidack test. * $p<0.01$ versus control group, lines indicate specific paired comparisons against groups treated with the respective antagonist.

Figure 4. Effect of the idaxozan (1 mg/kg,i.p.-48 h; panel A) and ICI 182 780 (10 μg/rat, i.c.v, -1h before to EE_2, panel B) on the antidepressant-like action of the combination of 17 α-ethynyl-estradiol (1.25 μg/rat, s.c,-48h) plus desimpramine (0.625 mg/kg, i.p. -23,-5,-1h) in the forced swimming test. Data are presented as mean ± SEM of the number of immobilities in a 5 minutes test session. Idaxozan partially blocked the antidepressant-like action of the combination EE_2/DMI in contrast to ICI 182780, which completely blocked. Also, the α2-adrenergic antagonist canceled the increase in climbing behavior without affecting swimming, in contrast to the estrogen receptor antagonist that blocked the increase in swimming but not in climbing behavior.

Regarding neurogenesis it has been reported that OVX per se did not alter cell proliferation or survival of newborn cells in the brain (Tanapat et al., 2005; Vega-Rivera et al., 2013); however when OVX was combined with a stressful situation, as FST, a significant long-lasting reduction on cell survival was observed (Vega-Rivera et al., 2013). Additionally, it has been reported that the estrogen deficiency, natural in aging rats or induced by OVX, decreases the synaptic connectivity and reduces the dendritic arborization which is reverted after estrogen restitution (Kataria et al., 2010).

Taken together these data indicate that estrogens are modulating the neurogenic process in a similar manner than antidepressant drugs (Tanapat et al., 1999; Ormerod et al., 2004; Barker and Galea., 2008). Thus, for example it is well documented that after a chronic treatment various antidepressants increase several stages of the neurogenic process i.e, cell proliferation, survival and maturation (Malberg et al., 2000; 2003; Wang et al., 2008). Also, antidepressants augment synaptic connectivity and dendritic arborization after a chronic treatment (Norrholm et al., 2001).

In the interaction between estrogens and antidepressants it has been shown that the combination of low doses of FLX and E_2 increased the number of doublecortine (DCX) immuno-positive cells (a protein associated with neuronal differentiation and migration) (Plümpe et al., 2006; Ramírez-Rodriguez et al., 2011). Furthermore, such combination also increased the number of DCX-positive cells with mature appearance and more complex dendritic arborizations (Vega-Rivera et al., in preparation). A plausible mechanism through which estrogens shorten the onset of antidepressant-like effects may involve the stimulation of neuron maturation but naturally many more experiments are needed to support this novel mechanism of action.

Conclusion

Clinical and basic research findings provide evidence that estrogens facilitate the action of antidepressants for depression treatment associated to perimenopause, but these actions depend of several factors such as subject's age, time of menopause onset and type of estrogen and antidepressant. Ageing as well as the lapse after ovarian hormones loss (menopause or OVX) appear to decrease the estrogen sensitivity, thus reducing the efficacy of combining estrogens with antidepressants. All these factors should be taken into account before initiating an ERT alone or in combination with antidepressants.

In relation to the mechanism of action underlying the antidepressant effect of combining estrogens with antidepressants, basic research suggests a complex interaction involving monoaminergic systems, estrogen receptors and neuroplasticity, which seems specific to each particular drug-steroid combination.

Acknowledgments

This work was partially supported by CONACYT grant No. CB-104659 and INPRF NC-9380.1 to EE-C. NMVR received a fellowship from CONACYT (216658). Authors thank the editorial support of MSc Rebeca Reyes-Serrano.

References

Amsterdam, J., Garcia-España, F., Fawcett, J., Quitkin, F., Reimherr, F., Rosenbaum, J., Beasley, C., (1999). Fluoxetine efficacy in menopausal women with and without estrogen replacement. *J. Affect. Disord.* 55,11-17.

Barker, J. M., Galea, L. A., (2008). Repeated estradiol administration alters different aspects of neurogenesis and cell death in the hippocampus of female, but not male, rats. *Neuroscience* 152, 888-902.

Béïque, J. C., Lavoie, N., de Montigny, C., Debonnel, G., (1998). Affinities of venlafaxine and various reuptake inhibitors for the serotonin and norepinephrine transporters. *Eur. J. Pharmacol.* 349, 129-132.

Béïque, J. C., de Montigny Blier, P., Debonnel, G., (2000). Effects of sustained administration of the serotonin and norepinephrine reuptake inhibitor venlafaxine: I. in vivo electrophysiological studies in the rat. *Neuropharmacology* 39, 1800–1812.

Bekku, N., Yoshimura, H., Araki, H., (2006). Factors producing a menopausal depressive-like state in mice following ovariectomy. *Psychopharmacology (Berl.)* 187, 170-180.

Blum, I., Vered, Y., Lifshitz, A., Harel, D., Blum, M., Nordenberg, Y., Harsat, A., Sulkes, J., Gabbay, U., Graff, E., (1996). The effect of estrogen replacement therapy on plasma serotonin and catecholamines of postmenopausal women. *Isr. J. Med. Sci.* 32, 1158-62.

Burger, H. G., Hale, G. E., Dennerstein, L., Robertson, D. M., (2008). Cycle and hormone changes during perimenopause: the key role of ovarian hormones. *Menopause* 15, 603-612.

Chakraborty, T. R., Gore, A. C., (2004). Aging-related changes in ovarian hormones, their receptors, and neuroendocrine function. *Exp. Biol. Med. (Maywood)* 229, 977-987.

Chlebowski, R., Anderson, G., (2012). Changing Concepts: Menopausal Hormone Therapy and Breast Cancer. *J. Natl. Cancer Inst.* 104, 517–527.

Contreras, C. M., Rodriguez-Landa, J. F., Gutiérrez-García, A. G., Bernal-Morales, B., (2001). The lowest effective dose of fluoxetine in the forced swim test significantly affects the firing rate of lateral septal nucleus neurones in the rat. *J. Psychopharmacol.* 15, 231-236.

Cryan, J. F., Valentino, R. J., Lucki, I., (2005). Assessing substrates underlying the behavioral effects of antidepressants using the modified rat forced swimming test. *Neurosci. Biobehav. Rev.* 29, 547-569.

de Chaves, G., Moretti, M., Castro, A. A., Dagostin, W., da Silva, G. G., Boeck, C. R., Quevedo, J., Gavioli, E. C., (2009). Effects of long-term ovariectomy on anxiety and behavioral despair in rats. *Physiol. Behav.* 97, 420-425.

Detke, M. J., Johnson, J., Lucki, I., (1997). Acute and chronic antidepressant drug treatment in the rat forced swimming test model of depression. *Exp. Clin. Psychopharmacol.* 5,107-112.

Detke, M. J., Rickels, M., Lucki, I., (1995). Active behaviors in the rat forced swimming test differentially produced by serotonergic and noradrenergic antidepressants. *Psychopharmacology (Berl.).* 121, 66-72.

Dias, R. S., Kerr-Corrêa, F., Moreno, R. A., Trinca, L. A., Pontes, A., Halbe, H. W., Gianfaldoni, A., Dalben, I. S., (2006). Efficacy of hormone therapy with and without methyltestosterone augmentation of venlafaxine in the treatment of postmenopausal depression: a double-blind controlled pilot study. *Menopause* 13, 202-211.

Donner, N., Handa, R. J. (2009). Estrogen receptor beta regulates the expression of tryptophan-hydroxylase 2 mRNA within serotonergic neurons of the rat dorsal. *Neuroscience* 163, 705-18.

Estrada-Camarena, E., Fernández-Guasti, A., López-Rubalcava, C., (2003). Antidepressant-like effect of different estrogenic compounds in the forced swimming test. *Neuropsychopharmacology* 28, 830-838.

Estrada-Camarena, E., Fernández-Guasti, A., López-Rubalcava, C., (2004). Interaction between estrogens and antidepressants in the forced swimming test in rats. *Psychopharmacology (Berl.)* 173, 139-145.

Estrada-Camarena, E., López-Rubalcava, C., Hernández-Aragón, A., Mejía-Mauries, S., Picazo, O., (2011). Long-term ovariectomy modulates the antidepressant-like action of estrogens, but not of antidepressants. *J. Psychopharmacol.* 25,1365-1377.

Estrada-Camarena, E., Vega-Rivera, N. M., Berlanga, C., Fernández-Guasti, A., (2008). Reduction in the latency of action of antidepressants by 17 beta-estradiol in the forced swimming test. *Psychopharmacology (Berl.)* 201, 351-360.

Estrada-Camarena, E., Fernández-Guasti, A., López-Rubalcava, C., (2006a). Participation of the 5-HT1A receptor in the antidepressant-like effect of estrogens in the forced swimming test. *Neuropsychopharmacology* 31, 247-255.

Estrada-Camarena, E., López-Rubalcava, C., Fernández-Guasti, A., (2006b). Facilitating antidepressant-like actions of estrogens are mediated by 5-HT1A and estrogen receptors in the rat forced swimming test. *Psychoneuroendocrinology* 31, 905-914.

Freeman, E. W., Sammel, M. D., Lin, H., Nelson, D. B., (2006). Associations of hormones and menopausal status with depressed mood in women with no history of depression. *Arch. Gen. Psychiatry* 63, 375-382.

Galea, L. A, Wide, J. K., Barr, A. M., (2001). Estradiol alleviates depressive-like symptoms in a novel animal model of post-partum depression. *Behav. Brain Res.* 122:1–9.

Gurkan, L., Ekeland, A., Gautvik, K. M., Langeland, N., Ronningen, H., Solheim, L. F., (1986) Bone changes after castration in rats. A model for osteoporosis. *Acta Orthop. Scand.* 57, 67-70.

Hiemke, C., Bruder, D., Poetz, B., Ghraf, R., (1985). Sex-specific effects of estradiol on hypothalamic noradrenaline turnover in gonadectomized rats. *Exp. Brain Res.* 59, 68–72.

Joffe, H., Groninger, H., Soares, C. N., Nonacs, R., Cohen, L. S., (2001). An open trial of mirtazapine in menopausal women with depression unresponsive to estrogen replacement therapy. *J. Womens Health Gend. Based Med.* 10, 999-1004.

Kalay, A. E., Demir, B., Haberal, A., Kalay, M., Kandemir, O., (2007). Efficacy of citalopram on climacteric symptoms. *Menopause*. 14, 223-229.

Kalu, D. N., Liu, C. C., Hardin, R. R., Hollis, B. W., (1989). The aged rat model of ovarian hormone deficiency bone loss. *Endocrinology* 124, 7-16.

Kataria, S., Varshney, M. K., Kumar, P., Dhar, P., Mehra, R. J., (2010). Role of estrogen in regulation of morphology and synaptic connectivity in female rat subiculum. *J. Anat. Soc. Indian* 59, 144 - 149.

Kirby, L. G., Lucki, I., (1997). Interaction between the forced swimming test and fluoxetine treatment on extracellular 5-hydroxytryptamine and 5-hydroxyindoleacetic acid in the rat. *J. Pharmacol. Exp. Ther.* 282, 967-976.

Kobayashi, T., Tamura, M., Hayashi, M., Katsura, Y., Tanabe, H., Ohta, T., Komoriya, K., (2000). Elevation of tail skin temperature in ovariectomized rats in relation to menopausal hot flushes. *Am. J. Physiol. Regul. Integr. Comp. Physiol.* 278, 863-869.

Kornstein, S. G., Toups, M., Rush, A. J., Wisniewski, S. R., Thase, M. E., Luther, J., Warden, D., Fava, M., Trivedi, M. H., (2013). Do menopausal status and use of hormone therapy affect antidepressant treatment response? Findings from the Sequenced Treatment Alternatives to Relieve Depression (STAR*D) study. *J. Womens Health (Larchmt)* 22, 121-131.

Li, Q., Sullivan, N. R., McAllister, C. E., Van de Kar, L. D., Muma, N. A., (2013). Estradiol accelerates the effects of fluoxetine on serotonin 1A receptor signaling. *Psychoneuroendocrinology* 38, 1145-57.

López-Rubalcava, C., Mostalac-Preciado, C., Estrada-Camarena, E. (2009). The rat forced swimming test: an animal model for the study of the antidepressant drugs. In: *Models of neuropharmacology*. Rocha, L., Granados, V. (eds). Kenin, India. Transworld Res. Network. pp. 149-168, ISBN 978-81-7895-383-0.

López-Rubalcava, C., Oikawa-Sala, J., Chávez-Álvarez, K., Estrada- Camarena, E., (2005). Analysis of the participation of the serotonergic system in the antidepressant-like action of 17beta -estradiol in the forced swimming test (fst): presynaptic or postsynaptic actions. Program No. 67.12. *Abstract Viewer/Itinerary Planner.* Washington, DC: Society for Neuroscience.

López-Rubalcava, C., Vega Rivera, N. M., Cruz-Martínez, J. J., Estrada-Camarena, E., (2007). Participation of both estrogen and alpha2-adrenergic. Estrogens and monoamine receptors in the antidepressant-like actions of ethynil-estradiol in rats tested in the forced swimming test. *12th Biennial meeting of the European Behavioral Pharmacology Society.*

López-Rubalcava, C., Vega-Rivera, N. M., Páez-Martínez, N., Estrada-Camarena, E., (2012). Participation of the Monoaminergic System in the Antidepressant-Like Actions of Estrogens: A Review in Preclinical Studies. In Effects of Antidepressants. *In Tech.* First edition p.p 47-72.

Lubbers, L. S., Zafian, P. T., Gautreaux, C., Gordon, M., Alves, S. E., Correa, L., Lorrain, D. S., Hickey, G. J., Luine, V., (2010). Estrogen receptor (ER) subtype agonists alter monoamine levels in the female rat brain. *J. Steroid Biochem. Mol. Biol.* 122, 310-307.

Malberg, J. E., Duman, R. S., (2003). Cell proliferation in adult hippocampus is decreased by inescapable stress: reversal by fluoxetine treatment. *Neuropsychopharmacology* 28, 1562-1571.

Malberg, J. E., Eisch, A. J., Nestler, E. J., Duman, R. S., (2000). Chronic antidepressant treatment increases neurogenesis in adult rat hippocampus. *J. Neurosci.* 20, 9104-9110.

Martínez-Mota, L., Contreras, C. M., Saavedra, M., (1999). Progesterone reduces immobility in rats forced to swim. *Arch. Med. Res.* 30, 286-289.

Mikail, H. G., Dalla, C., Kokras, N., Kafetzopoulos, V., Papadopoulou-Daifoti, Z., (2012). Sertraline behavioral response associates closer and dose-dependently with cortical rather than hippocampal serotonergic activity in the rat forced swim stress. *Physiol. Behav.* 107, 201-206.

Mize, A. L., Poisner, A. M., Alper, R. H., (2001). Estrogens act in rat hippocampus and frontal cortex to produce rapid, receptor-mediated decreases in serotonin 5-HT(1A) receptor function. *Neuroendocrinology* 73, 166-174.

Molina-Hernández, M., Téllez-Alcántara, N. P., (2011). Fluoxetine, 17-β estradiol or folic acid combined with intra-lateral septal infusions of neuropeptide Y produced antidepressant-like actions in ovariectomized rats forced to swim. *Peptides* 32, 2400-2406.

Moretti, M., de Souza, A. G., de Chaves, G., de Andrade, V. M., Romao, P. R., Gavioli, E. C., Boeck, C. R., (2011). Emotional behavior in middle-aged rats: Implications for geriatric psychopathologies. *Physiol. Behav.* 102, 115-20.

Nagata, H., Nozaki, M., Nakano, H., (2005). Short-term combinational therapy of low-dose estrogen with selective serotonin re-uptake inhibitor (fluvoxamine) for oophorectomized women with hot flashes and depressive tendencies. *J. Obstet. Gynaecol. Res.* 31,107-114.

Norrholm, S. D., Ouimet, C. C., (2001). Altered dendritic spine density in animal models of depression and in response to antidepressant treatment. *Synapse* 42, 151-163.

Nowakowska, E., Kus, K., (2005). Antidepressant and memory affecting influence of estrogen and venlafaxine in ovariectomized rats. *Arzneimittelforschung* 55, 153-159.

Okada, M., Hayashi, N., Kometani, M., Nakao, K., Inukai, T., (1997). Influences of ovariectomy and continuous replacement of 17 beta-estradiol on tail-skin temperature and behavior in the forced swimming test in rats. *Jpn. J. Pharmacol.* 73, 93-96.

O'Keane, V., O'Hanlon, M., Webb, M., Dinan, T., (1991). d-fenfluramine/prolactin response throughout the menstrual cycle: evidence for an oestrogen-induced alteration. *Clin. Endocrinol. (Oxf.)* 34, 289-292.

Olvera-Hernández, S., Fernández-Guasti, A., (2011). Sex differences in the burying behavior test in middle-aged rats: Effects of diazepam. *Pharmacol. Biochem. Behav.* 99, 532-539.

Ormerod, B. K., Lee, T. T., Galea, L. A., (2004). Estradiol enhances neurogenesis in the dentate gyri of adult male meadow voles by increasing the survival of young granule neurons. *Neuroscience* 128, 645-654.

Owens, M. J., Morgan, W. N., Plott, S. J., Nemeroff, C. B., (1997). Neurotransmitter receptor and transporter binding profile of antidepressants and their metabolites. *J. Pharmacol. Exp. Ther.* 283, 1305-1322.

Pae, C. U., Mandelli, L., Kim, T. S., Han, C., Masand, P., Marks, D., Patkar, A., Steffens, D., De Ronchi, D., Serretti, A., (2009). Effectiveness of antidepressant treatments in premenopausal versus postmenopausal women: a pilot study on differential effects of sex hormones on antidepressant effects. *Biomed. Pharmacother.* 63, 228-235.

Parry, B. L., (2008). Perimenopausal depression. *Am. J. Psychiatry* 165, 23-27.

Payne, J. L., Roy, P. S., Murphy-Eberenz, K., Weismann, M. N., Swartz, K. L., McInnis, M. G., et al., (2007). Reproductive cycle-associated mood symptoms in women with major depression and bipolar disorder. *J. Affect. Disord.* 99, 221-229.

Picazo, O., Estrada-Camarena, E., Hernandez-Aragon, A., (2006) Influence of the post-ovariectomy time frame on the experimental anxiety and the behavioural actions of some anxiolytic agents. *Eur. J. Pharmacol.* 530, 88-94.

Plümpe, T., Ehninger, D., Steiner, B., Klempin, F., Jessberger, S., Brandt, M., Römer, B., Rodriguez, G. R., Kronenberg, G., Kempermann, G., (2006). Variability of doublecortin-associated dendrite maturation in adult hippocampal neurogenesis is independent of the regulation of precursor cell proliferation. *BMC Neurosci.* 5, 7:77.

Porsolt, R. D., Le Pichon, M., Jalfre, M., (1977). Depression: a new animal model sensitive to antidepressant treatments. *Nature* 266, 730-732.

Ramirez-Rodriguez, G., Ortíz-López, L., Domínguez-Alonso, A., Benítez-King, G. A., Kempermann, G., (2011). Chronic treatment with melatonin stimulates dendrite maturation and complexity in adult hippocampal neurogenesis of mice. *J. Pineal Res.* 50, 29-37.

Récamier-Carballo, S., Estrada-Camarena, E., Reyes, R., Fernández-Guasti, A., (2012). Synergistic effect of estradiol and fluoxetine in young adult and middle-aged female rats in two models of experimental depression. *Behav. Brain Res.* 233, 351-358.

Récamier-Carballo, S., Fernández-Guasti, A., (2012). Forced swimming and chronic mild stress as animal models of depression. En: *Behavioral animal models*. Cruz-Morales, S. E., Arriaga-Ramírez, J. C. (Eds). Research Signpost, Kerala, India, pp. 123–137, ISBN 978-81-308-0481-1.

Riecher-Rossler, A., de Geyter, C., (2007). The forthcoming role of treatment with oestrogens in mental health. *Swiss Med. Wkly* 137, 565-572.

Romano-Torres, M., Fernández-Guasti, A., (2010). Estradiol valerate elicits antidepressant-like effects in middle-aged female rats under chronic mild stress. *Behav. Pharmacol.* 21, 104-111.

Rossi, D. V., Dai, Y., Thomas, P., Carrasco, G. A., DonCarlos, L. L., Muma, N. A., Li, Q., (2010). Estradiol-induced desensitization of 5-HT1A receptor signaling in the paraventricular nucleus of the hypothalamus is independent of estrogen receptor-beta. *Psychoneuroendocrinology* 35, 1023-1033.

Rozenberg, S., Vandromme, J., Antoine, C., (2013). Postmenopausal hormone therapy: risks and benefits. *Nat. Rev. Endocrinol.* 9, 216–227.

Saavedra, M., Contreras, C. M., Azamar-Arizmendi, G., Hernández-Lozano, M., (2006). Differential progesterone effects on defensive burying and forced swimming tests depending upon a gradual decrease or an abrupt suppression schedules. *Pharmacol. Biochem. Behav.* 83, 130-135.

Schneider, L. S., Small, G. W., Clary, C. M., (2001). Estrogen Replacement Therapy and Antidepressant Response to Sertraline in Older Depressed Women. *Am. J. Geriatr. Psychiatry*. 9, 393-399.

Schneider, L. S., Small, G. W., Hamilton, S. H., Bystritsky, A., Nemeroff, C. B., Meyers, B. S., (1997). Estrogen replacement and response to fluoxetine in a multicenter geriatric depression trial. Fluoxetine Collaborative Study Group. *Am. J. Geriatr. Psychiatry* 5, 97-106.

Soares, C. N., (2010). Challenges and opportunities to manage depression during the menopausal transition and beyond. *Psychiatr. Clin. North Am.* 33, 295-308.

Soares, C. N., Cohen, L. S., (2001). The perimenopause depressive disorders and hormonal variability. *Sau Paolo Med. J.* 119, 78-83.

Soares, C. N., Poitras, J. R., Prouty, J., Alexander, A. B., Shifren, J. L., Cohen, L., (2003). Efficacy of citalopram as monotherapy or as an adjunctive treatment to estrogen therapy for perimenopausal and postmenopausal women with depression and vasomotor symptoms. *J. Clin. Psychiatry* 64, 473-479.

Soares, C. N., Zitek, B., (2008). Reproductive hormone sensitivity and risk for depression across the female life cycle: a continuum of vulnerability? *J. Psychiatry Neurosci.* 3, 331-343.

Studd, J. W., (2011). A guide to the treatment of depression in women by estrogens. *Climacteric* 14, 637-42.

Studd, J. W., Nappi, N. D., (2012). Reproductive depression. *Gynecol. Endocrinol. 28 Suppl.* 1 42-5.

Tanapat, P., Hastings, N. B., Gould, E., (2005). Ovarian steroids influence cell proliferation in the dentate gyrus of the adult female rat in a dose- and time-dependent manner. *J. Comp. Neurol.* 481, 252-265.

Tanapat, P., Hastings, N. B., Reeves, A. J., Gould, E., (1999). Estrogen stimulates a transient increase in the number of new neurons in the dentate gyrus of the adult female rat. *J. Neurosci.* 19, 5792-5801.

Vega-Rivera, N. M., Fernández-Guasti, A., Ramírez-Rodríguez, G., Estrada-Camarena, E., (2013). Acute stress further decreases the effect of ovariectomy on immobility behavior and hippocampal cell survival in rats. *Psychoneuroendocrinology* 38, 1407-1417.Walf, A. A., Paris, J. J., Frye, C. A., (2009). Chronic estradiol replacement to aged female rats reduces anxiety-like and depression-like behavior and enhances cognitive performance. *Psychoneuroendocrinology* 34, 909-916.

Wang, J. W., David, D. J., Monckton, J. E., Battaglia, F., Hen, R., (2008). Chronic Fluoxetine Stimulates Maturation and Synaptic Plasticity of Adult-Born Hippocampal Granule Cells. *J. Neurosci.* 28, 1374 –1384.

Willner, P., (1995). Animal models of depression: validity and applications. *Adv. Biochem. Psychopharmacol.* 49, 19-41.

Yin, W., Gore, A. C., (2006). Neuroendocrine control of reproductive aging: roles of GnRH neurons. *Reproduction* 131, 403-414.

In: Estradiol: Synthesis, Health Effects and Drug Interactions ISBN: 978-1-62808-962-2
Editors: Ricco Palmeri and Sal Grimaudo

Chapter 10

Estrogen and Nitric Oxide are the New Players in Diabetes Gastroparesis

M. Showkat Ali[1,*]*, Rebecca Smiley*[1]*, Kerry Preston*[1]*,*
Gengqing Song[2] *and Richard Mccallum*[2]
[1]Department of Clinical Investigation, William Beaumont Army Medical Center, Piedras Street, El Paso, TX, US
[2]Department of Internal Medicine, Texas Tech Health Science Center Paul L. Foster School of Medicine, El Paso, TX, US

Abstract

Diabetic gastroparesis, defined as delayed gastric emptying, is one of the most debilitating complications of both type 1 and type 2 diabetes. Normal gastric motility/emptying requires an integrated, coordinated interplay between sympathetic, parasympathetic, and intrinsic-gut (enteric) nervous systems, interstitial cells of Cajal, and gastrointestinal smooth muscle cells. Any disturbance in their interactions has the potential to alter gastric function, and ultimately affects gastric emptying. Multiple contributing factors, including depletion of interstitial cells of Cajal, oxidative stress, excitatory and inhibitory neuropeptides, estrogen, and the nitric oxide regulator of neuronal nitric oxide synthase activity (nNOSα), have been linked to the development of gastroparesis.

Gastroparesis is far more common in women (60-70%), suggesting a possible estrogen role in gastric emptying dysfunction. Several animal and human studies have demonstrated that estradiol-17β causes delayed gastric emptying. In one study, estrogen administration in overiectomized rats, as well as postmenopausal women receieving estrogen replacement therapy, resulted in delayed gastric emptying.

Nitric oxide is a major neurotransmitter in the gut and a key physiological mediator of non-adrenergic and non-cholinergic relaxation of gastrointestinal smooth muscle cells. There is a myriad of evidence suggesting that gastroparesis is associated with changes in

* Corresponding author: M. Showkat Ali Ph.D. Department of Clinical Investigation. William Beaumont Army Medical Center, 5005 N. Piedras Street, El Paso, TX 79920, E-mail: Mohammed.S.Ali@amedd.army.mil, Telephone: 915-742-6041.

gastric neuronal nitric oxide synthase (nNOSα) expression and its activation state, which directly regulates the bioavailability of nitric oxide. Taken together, these evidences suggest the estrogen's role in normal gastric emptying may be via a nitric oxide regulatory pathway. We recently developed an animal model of diabetic gastroparesis by injecting male and female rats with streptozotocin. Male diabetic rats without gastroparesis were subsequently injected with estrogen for 3 weeks and then evaluated for the development of gastroparesis. Although male diabetic gastroparetic (either streptozotocin- or estrogen-induced) rats exhibited similarity in disease pathology to that of females, the molecular mechanisms of development were different. Our results indicated that slow gastric emptying in both male diabetic groups was not associated with the level of expression and dimerization of nNOSα in gastric tissues. In contrast, females with diabetic gastroparesis demonstrated significantly impaired levels and dimerization of nNOSα in the antrum and pylorus. These results open new considerations for a potential role that estrogen may play in normal gastric emptying via a nitric oxide regulatory pathway.

Given the importance of nitric oxide in health and disease, studies on estrogen mediated regulation of nitric oxide will offer a better understanding of gastroparesis and potential development of new therapeutic interventions. In this article, we provide a synopsis of studies linking estrogen and nitric oxide to the development of gastroparesis. We discuss basic knowledge and our current understanding of mechanisms for gastroparesis development. Finally, perspectives on future directions of research on gastroparesis are discussed.

Introduction

According to the American Diabetes Association, approximately 8.3% of the US population is diabetic. A common gastrointestinal complication of both type 1 and type 2 diabetes is gastroparesis, and patients with gastroparesis may present with nausea, vomiting, bloating, early satiety, upper abdominal pain or postprandial fullness. Gastroparesis can develop in 20-55% of patients with type I diabetes and up to 30% of patients with type II diabetes (Adeghate et al., 2001; Smith et al., 2003). The other types of gastroparesis include postsurgical and idiopathic gastroparesis. Gastroparesis of unknown cause (idiopathic gastroparesis) is probably the most common form of gastroparesis. Diabetic and idiopathic gastroparesis in combination are estimated to affect up to 4% of the US population. A recent report estimated that inpatient costs for a patient with severe gastroparesis approach $7000/month (Cutts et al., 2005). Given that diabetes is pandemic and a silent killer, and that diabetics are at high risk for developing gastroparesis, which has high cost implications, studies to identify the developmental mechanisms involved are essential in future curbing of this debilitating disease and in facilitating effective therapy regimens, and may shed light on the molecular mechanisms of development for idiopathic and postsurgical gastroparesis.

The gastrointestinal wall contains smooth muscle, which allows for muscle constriction and dilation involved in the movement of food through the intestines. It also contains a local nervous system referred to as the enteric or intrinsic nervous system (ENS) involved in digestive tract motility. Networks of Interstitial Cells of Cajal (ICC) embedded in the musculature are pacemaker cells that generate spontaneous slow waves of muscle movement required for peristalsis, breakdown of food particles, and propulsion. Normal gastric motility/emptying requires an integrated, coordinated interplay between the sympathetic, parasympathetic, and intrinsic-gut (enteric) nervous systems, ICC and gastrointestinal smooth muscle cells. Disturbance at any level has the potential to alter gastric function, and, ultimately, to affect gastric emptying. The pathophysiological mechanisms involved in diabetic gastroparesis are complex, with multiple contributing factors including (1) loss of ICC; (2) oxidative stress and selective loss of heme oxygenase; (3) altered neuropeptide, chloride channel and androgen availability; (4) genomic and non-genomic effects of estrogen; (5) altered neuronal nitric oxide synthase (nNOS) activity, and (6) a pathogenic combination of estrogen and nitric oxide.

Loss of Interstitial Cells of Cajal (ICC)

ICCs are pacemaker cells that generate spontaneous electrical slow waves and transmit these waves to smooth muscle cells in the gut which generate phasic contractions and peristalsis. ICCs also regulate the motility of the ENS by transducing inputs from excitatory and inhibitory neurons. In the gut, the two main types of ICCs, myenteric (MY-ICC) and intramuscular (IM-ICC), transduce nitregic and cholinergic signals to smooth muscle cells and regulate the frequency and propagation of slow waves (Ward, 2000; Ward et al., 2000). Increasing evidence suggests that ICCs play a pivotal role in the pathogenesis of gastroparesis. For example, a study in nonobese diabetic mice (a mouse model of human type 1 diabetes) suggests that damage to both MY-ICCs and IM-ICCs is associated with a significant disruption in slow wave activity and delayed gastric emptying (Ordog, 2008; Yamamoto et al., 2008). Moreover, findings in db/db mice (a mouse model of type II diabetes carrying spontaneous deletion of the active form of the leptin receptor demonstrated that loss of ICCs and subsequent development of gastroparesis was not due to apoptosis or necrosis (Yamamoto et al., 2008). In human studies, histologic examination showed that ICC density was 60-100% lower in the stomachs of diabetic as compared to non-diabetic individuals (Lin et al., 2008; Wang et al., 2009a). Although the causes of diabetics and idiopathic gastroparesis are thought to differ, both conditions are characterized by ICC loss, with a clinical study indicating a similar extent of ICC loss in patients with either diabetic or idiopathic gastroparesis (Grover et al., 2011).

ICCs are defined by the expression of c-Kit, a membrane receptor with tyrosine kinase activity. Among the mechanisms implicated in ICC loss are loss of c-Kit (Sanders and Ward, 2007) , oxidative damage (Kashyap et al., 2010), and/or insulin signaling (He et al., 2001). Maintenance of ICCs in an organotypic cell culture study was found to require insulin or IGF-1, both of which are reduced or absent in diabetics (Horvath et al., 2005). The development and maintenance of ICC requires signaling via c-Kit. There is significant evidence that ICC loss is accompanied by loss of expression of c-Kit (Ordog, 2008; Ward, 2000). ICC development and maintenance were shown to depend on stem cell factor (SCF) (Horvath et al., 2006), a natural ligand for c-Kit involved in its activation. It was reported that the decrease in ICCs observed in patients with type II diabetes was accompanied by a reduction in SCF (Burns, 2007). There are two well established models of ICC deficiency, namely W/Wv mice and Ws/Ws rats. In both models, the deficiency was due to a mutation in the c-Kit gene. The significant reductions of IM-ICCs and MY-ICCs in W/Wv mice and Ws/Ws rats, respectively, were accompanied by an absence of active SCF (Sivarao et al., 2008; Wang et al., 2009b). Taken together, these findings indicate that alterations in SCF/c-Kit signaling may be responsible for several pathological processes causing loss and/or dysfunction of ICCs, and that ICCs are unique cell types with a central role in gut function.

Oxidative Stress and Selective Loss of Heme Oxygenase

Diabetes is associated with increased oxidative stress. Heme oxygenase (HO) is a ubiquitous enzyme that cleaves the α-methylene bridge of the heme ring (protoporphyrin ring attached to an iron atom) to produce carbon monoxide, bilirubin and iron. There are two main isoforms of HO: HO-1 is an inducible enzyme, whereas HO-2 is a constitutively expressed enzyme (Efimov et al., 2011). Induction of HO-1 has been identified as a powerful cellular defense mechanism against oxidative stress. The development of diabetes has been associated with an increased number of macrophages and an up-regulation of HO-1, whereas the onset of gastroparesis is accompanied by the selective loss of HO-1(Choi et al., 2010). In addition, HO-1 was recently shown to have a cytoprotective role in the pathophysiology of diabetic gastroparesis (Choi et al., 2008). Loss of c-Kit expression in a mouse model of gastroparesis was shown to be due to increased levels of oxidative stress caused by low HO-1 activity (Ndisang and Jadhav, 2009). Furthermore, it was demonstrated that reinduction of HO-1 expression resulted in the complete reversal of delayed gastric emptying (Choi et al., 2008), suggesting that HO-1 is an important regulator of gastric motility. Whether gastropareis development initiates loss of HO-1, or loss of HO-1 is a factor in gastroparetic development has not been reported.

Altered Neurotransmitters, Ca^{2+} Activated Cl^- Channel and Male Hormone

Normal gastric motility requires a balance between the release of excitatory neurotransmitters, such as substance P (SP), and inhibitory neurotransmitters, such as nitric oxide (NO). SP, which is expressed in ENS of the mammalian gut, has been shown to excite gastrointestinal motor activity in virtually all regions and layers of the mammalian gut (Adeghate et al., 2001). SP concentrations were found to be significantly lower in the plasma of patients with type I diabetes than in healthy controls (Kunt et al., 2000). Moreover, SP deficiency has been shown to result in a loss of ICCs in patients with type II diabetes (Iwasaki et al., 2006). These results suggest that SP might be an indispensable protective factor against diabetic gastropathy development.

Neuropeptide Y (NPY) is a 36-amino acid peptide which acts through a series of G-protein coupled receptors (NPY-Rs), which are found in the nerve plexuses and nerve fibers in the stomachs of all species examined. Both *in vivo* and *in vitro* studies have found that NPY inhibits glucose-stimulated insulin secretion (Adeghate et al., 2001; Satoh et al., 1999), which implies that NPY has an important pathophysiological role in diabetes. For example, plasma concentrations of NPY were shown to be higher in animal models and patients with type II diabetes than in their respective normal controls (El-Salhy and Spangeus, 2002; Ilhan et al., 2010). In diabetic rats up-regulation of NPY-R was accompanied by alterations in tissue levels of NPY (Fu et al., 2002). Genetic studies have shown that a leucine to proline polymorphism (Leu→Pro) at amino acid 7 of NPY was associated with accelerated atherosclerosis and type II diabetes (Ukkola and Kesaniemi, 2007). To our knowledge, however, the role of NPY in the development of diabetic gastroparesis has not been addressed.

The calcium-activated chloride channel anoctamin 1 (ANO1) is expressed abundantly and specifically in muscle layers of ICC. The ANO1 gene contains 26 exons and because of gene splicing, several isoforms have been reported to be expressed in ICC. These isoforms function as classical Ca^{2+} activated chloride channels. Mazzone *et al.* (Mazzone et al., 2011) have shown that expression of a novel variant of ANO1 with an alternative 5' end was increased 10-fold in patients with diabetic gastroparesis compared to matched controls. These authors hypothesized that this novel variant of ANO1 with altered electrophysiological properties might be responsible for the delayed gastric motility. These results were further substantiated by the observation that ANO1 knock-out mice exhibited abnormal ICC function and motility (Cole, 2011). Given the importance of Ca^{2+} activated chloride channel in maintaining the normal smooth muscle contraction, ANO1 might be a new molecular target for the future therapeutic treatment regimens.

Androgens exert effects on virtually all body tissues and have many physiological roles in maintaining health. A deficiency in testosterone, the predominant androgen in men (hypogonadism), leads to the development of diabetes (Pitteloud et al., 2005; Saad, 2009). Although the female sex hormone estrogen has been implicated in the development of gastroparesis (Chen et al., 1995; Gangula et al., 2007), there is no evidence to date of testosterone involvement in the development of gastroparesis. Due to the impact of both hormones on glucose homeostasis, the molecular pathways involved in diabetic gastropathy may be gender specific. We hypothesize that variations in testosterone concentrations may have significant effects on the development of diabetic gastroparesis in males. Substantiating our hypothesis, it was demonstrated that testosterone levels influenced the bioavailability of estrogen levels in the onset of diabetes (Maric, 2009). This observation might indicate that androgens' effect on estrogen indirectly affects the propensity for diabetic gastroparetic development, and that estrogen may have a more direct effect.

Genomic and Non-Genomic Effects of Estrogen

The female preponderance of gastroparesis suggests that estrogen may be involved in gastric emptying regulation. For example, estrogen replacement therapy in premenopausal women and postmenopausal women results in lower gastric emptying rates as compared to postmenopausal women who were not on hormone replacement therapy (Hutson et al., 1989; Sadik et al., 2003). These results are further substantiated by the observation that gastric emptying in menstruating women was significantly lower during the luteal phase of the cycle than in the follicular phase (Verrengia et al., 2011). While administration of estradiol and progesterone, in combination, or estradiol alone, to overiectomized rats slowed gastric emptying, progesterone alone enhanced gastric emptying (Chen et al., 1995). In contradiction, there is evidence that progesterone exerts its inhibitory effect on GI motility by changing plasma motilin levels (Wang et al., 2003). It is difficult to ascribe a direct role of progesterone in the development of gastroparessis, but there is persuasive evidence that the estrogen level is a critical determining factor for the disease pathology. This evidence was supported by our recent study that demonstrated that in both male and female rats elevated estrogen levels enhanced the development of gastroparesis (Showkat Ali et al., 2012)

The observed biological effects of estrogen as described above can be genomic, non-genomic, or both. The genomic and non-genomic effects of estrogen are mediated by estrogen receptor α (ERα) and β (ERβ). Although these two receptor subtypes share mechanistic similarities, they are functionally distinct and have different tissue distributions. For example, ERα knockout mice show a quite different phenotype as compared to ERβ knockout mice (Hewitt and Korach, 2003). Estrogen receptors are transcription factors that reside in the cytoplasm. After binding to the estrogen, these receptors dimerize and translocate to the nucleus. The dimerized receptor(s) can directly bind to their consensus target DNA sequence or interact with other nuclear proteins, and thereby enhance or repress gene activation. This has been referred to as a genomic effect. The non-genomic effects of estrogen involve interaction and modulation of functional activities of several cellular proteins. The net result is the activation of signaling pathways and rapid physiological responses in target tissues. Evidence for the genomic pathway responsible for the observed physiological effects in the gut in gastroparesis development is completely lacking. However, the role of an estrogen mediated non-genomic pathway in the development of gastroparesis is emerging. One of the well characterized non-genomic effects of estrogen is to regulate the production of NO, an important molecule in maintaining the healthy gut physiology.

Altered Neuronal Nitric Oxide Synthase Activity and Delayed Gastric Emptying

Nitric oxide (NO) is a major neuromodulator in the gut and a key physiological mediator of non-adrenergic, non-cholinergic (NANC) relaxation of gastrointestinal smooth muscle. NO is synthesized by a family of nitric oxide synthases (NOSs): neuronal NOS (nNOS or NOS I) and endothelial NOS (eNOS or NOS III), which are constitutive Ca2+ dependent isoforms, and one Ca^{2+} independent isoform, inducible NOS (iNOS or NOS II). All NOSs oxidize L-arginine in a process that consumes NADPH and oxygen, thus producing NO and L-citrulline. These enzymes have independent and distinct functions in maintaining the gut physiology. While nNOS controls the GI motility, eNOS regulates the vascular function of GI, and iNOS contributes to the development of inflammation in the GI (Toda and Herman, 2005). Given that nNOS plays a significant role in the development of gastroparesis, our discussion will be focused on nNOS, and more specifically, nNOSα, which is the only active nNOS isoform in the gut (Shah et al., 2004).

The nNOS gene is located on chromosome 12 and consists of 29 exons and 28 introns. This gene encodes a protein product of approximately 160 kDa. Among the NOSs, nNOS has the longest sequence with an N-terminal extension of 200 amino acids, which has been designated as the PDZ domain. The role of the PDZ domain is to interact with other proteins and to participate in the sub-compartmentalization of the nNOS protein in the cell. nNOS has a unique protein structure compared to other NOSs, and its function is tightly regulated by post-translational modifications. Among the posttranslational modifications is a site specific serine phosphorylation of NOSs that is associated with its activation/inactivation. For example, phosphorylation of nNOS at Ser^{847} reduces the catalytic activity and phoshorylation of at Ser^{1416} increases the catalytic activity (Luo and Zhu, 2011). There is also a report showing that nNOS is also phosphorylated at Ser^{741} and deregulates enzymatic activity (Song et al., 2004). The phosphorylations of these sites are reported to be catalyzed by serine kinases, including calcium-calmodulin protein kinase II, cyclic-AMP dependent protein kinase, AKT-kinase and protein kinase C (Zhou and Zhu, 2009). The identification of a specific kinase responsible for the phosphorylation of the specific serine sites on nNOS in enteric nerves and the mechanism of enzymatic activation remains to be determined. In addition to serine phosphorylation, nNOS has recently been reported to be modified by small ubiquitin-related modifier (SUMO), both *in vitro* and *ex vivo* (Watanabe and Itoh, 2011; Yeh, 2009). However, further studies are needed to support the hypothesis that SUMO-lyation is a major pathway regulating the synthesis of NO.

Interactions of nNOS with heterologous proteins have emerged as putative mechanisms by which activity and spatial distribution are governed. nNOS has been reported to interact with many proteins including post synaptic density protein-95 (Cui et al., 2007), CAPON (Chen et al., 2008), caveleon-1(Sato et al., 2004) , protein inhibitors of nNOS [PIN] (Rodriguez-Crespo et al., 1998) and NOS inertacting protein [NOSIP] (Dreyer et al., 2004). Available evidence suggests that interactions of PIN and NOSIP with nNOS inhibits the production of NO (Daff, 2010). Heat shock protein 90 (hsp90), a highly conserved molecular chaperone, associates with nNOS and is important for its proper folding and function (Peng et al., 2012) In many cases these interactions are mediated by the PDZ domain. The precise mechanism of these protein-protein interactions and the mechanism of regulation of NO production are not known. Similar to iNOS and eNOS, protein S-nitrosylation/denitrosylation is now recognized as another regulatory mechanism for the synthesis of NO by nNOS (Hess et al., 2005) .In summary, nNOS enzymatic activity is regulated by multiple mechanisms, including dimerization, post-translational modifications and protein-protein interactions. Considering the complexity of these mechanisms, there is no doubt that this area of research will remain very challenging and rewarding in the foreseeable future.

nNOS is predominantly expressed in neurons and plays a pivotal role in various parts of the GI tract. The first piece of evidence for a role for nNOS in the pathogenesis of gastroparesis came from the observation that $nNos^{-/-}$ mice have gastric dilation, gastric muscle thickening and delayed emptying of solids and liquids compared to wild type and eNOS deficient mice (Mashimo et al., 2000). Furthermore, the impairment of GI motility in $nNos^{-/-}$ mice has been shown to be linked with pyloric sphincter dysfunction (Sivarao et al., 2008). nNOS plays a pivotal role in the regulation of muscle tone in the lower esophagus, pylorus, sphincter of Oddi and antrum (Yamamoto et al., 2000). This important enzyme also regulates the accommodation reflex of the fundus and peristaltic reflex of the intestine (Takahashi, 2003).NO signaling involves the stimulation of guanylate cyclase activity, leading to cGMP generation and activation of protein kinase G (PKG). In this scenario, PKG emerged as the downstream effector molecule of NO signaling pathways. It was demonstrated that while $PKG^{-/-}$ mice did not recapitulate the exact phenotype of $nNos^{-/-}$ mice, they did develop marked gastric dilation and thickened pylorus (Huang et al., 1993). This study argues for the importance of the NO signaling pathway in pyloric relaxation. A study reported by the gastroparesis consortium sponsored by the National Institutes of Health demonstrated that nNOS expression was reduced more in patients with idiopathic gastroparesis compared to patients with diabetes gatsroparesis (Grover et al., 2011). The loss of expression of nNOS was accompanied by a similar loss of ICC and increase in CD45 and CD68 immunoreactivity in both groups of disorders. Consistent with this observation, it was demonstrated in animal studies that loss of nNOS is associated with the loss of smooth muscle relaxation (Goyal and Chaudhury, 2010), and thereby, development of delayed gastric emptying.

Because of 5'end splicing, nNOS mRNA results in the synthesis of different variants of nNOS, including nNOSα, nNOSβ and nNOSγ (Saur et al., 2000). Among these isoforms, nNOSα is the only catalytically active isoform in the gut (Shah et al., 2004). Altered expression and biological activity of nNOSα has been reported to be linked with several GI disorders, including achalaisa, hypertropic pyloric stenosis and diabetes gastroparesis (Boissel et al., 1998). Earlier reports are focused on elucidating the role of nNOS in a broad sense, but recent reports have focused more specifically on nNOSα. The catalytically active NOSs exist as homodimers and the dimerization creates binding sites for heme, tetrahydrobiopterin (BH4) and arginine, thus facilitating electron flow from one monomer to another, resulting in increased activity of the enzyme (Daff, 2010). Thus, another proposed mechanism in the pathophysiology of diabetes gastroparesis dysfunction is a decrease in dimerization of nNOSα in gastric tissues, and thereby, a decreased bioavailability of NO. For example, Gangula *et al.* (Gangula et al., 2007) reported the gender specific impairment of gastric nNOSα dimerization in rats with streptozotocin induced diabetes gastroparesis. BH4 is an essential co-factor for NOSs involved in stabilizing its dimeric structure and facilitating and enhancing binding of arginine. BH4 has been used as a therapeutically relevant tool to modulate nNOSα function in diabetes gastroparesis. For example, supplementation of BH4 to female rats with diabetic gastroparesis resulted in significant restoration of nNOSα expression and dimerization (Gangula et al., 2010). These results were further corroborated by a study showing that administration of sepiapterin, a precursor of BH4, has the same phenotypic effect as BH4 (Gangula et al., 2010). As a corollary, pharmacological inhibition of nNOSα in rodents delays gastric emptying (Smith et al., 2003). Collectively these findings suggest that nNOSα has emerged as the central point of interest for gastroparesis.

Estrogen and Nitric Oxide, A Pathogenic Duo

Because gastroparesis is far more common in women (60-70% of patients), and NO has emerged as a major protector of diabetic gastroparesis development, estrogen and/or progesterone may be involved in normal gastric emptying via a nitric oxide regulatory role. However, there are no reports to date indicating that estrogen exerts its effect by modulating the expression and activity of nNOS. In addition, most gastroparesis animal studies were done using male rats, which cannot implicate a direct estrogen role as male hormones are involved. Therefore there is substantial interest in the effects of estrogen on gastroparesis due to the marked gender difference in the incidence of this malady when comparing women with matched men. We hypothesized that estrogen mediated expression and activation of nNOSα, and post-translational modification of nNOSα are responsible for delayed gastric emptying commonly seen in diabetic women. To test this hypothesis, we developed an animal model of diabetic gastroparesis by injecting male and female rats with streptozotocin (Showkat Ali et al., 2012). Male diabetic rats without gastroparesis were subsequently injected with estrogen for 3 weeks and evaluated for the development of gastroparesis. Biochemical events associated with diabetes and gastroparetic dysfunction were analyzed in gastric tissues of these animals. Although male diabetic gastroparetic (either streptozotocin- or estrogen-induced) rats exhibited similarity in disease pathology to that of female diabetic gastroparesis, the molecular mechanisms of development were different. Our results indicated that slow gastric emptying in both groups of male diabetic gastroparetic rats was not associated with the level of expression of nNOSα in gastric tissues. In contrast, females with diabetic gastroparesis demonstrated significantly impaired levels of nNOSα in the antrum and pylorus (*data not shown*). It was previously reported that loss or reduced expression of nNOSα is associated with a loss of NO and thereby, impaired smooth muscle cell relaxation and development of gastroparesis (Smith et al., 2003).

Neuronal loss or degeneration and inhibition of nNOSα transcription by an unknown mechanism might be responsible for reduced expression of gastric nNOSα. However, in mouse models, this loss of nNOS expression does not reflect neuronal cell death (Sivarao et al., 2008). Increasing evidence suggests that estrogen may activate the ubiquitin proteasome degradation pathway (Tateishi et al., 2004), leading to degradation of the nNOSα protein, or it may modulate the translational regulation of the nNOSα gene. Studies with protease inhibitors support the former hypothesis that the steady state levels of nNOS may be regulated by a selective proteolytic process (Kamada et al., 2005). Furthermore, it was demonstrated that nNOS ubiquitination and proteasomal degradation is dependent on Hsp90/Hsp70-based chaperone machinery (Pratt et al., 2010). There are no reported studies of estrogen-mediated proteasomal degradation of nNOSα, as has been observed for eNOS (Schulz et al., 2005).

One proposed mechanism in the patho-physiology of diabetes and gastroparesis dysfunction postulates a decrease in the dimerization of nNOSα in gastric tissues and, thereby, a decrease in the bioavailability of NO (Burns, 2007). This potential mechanism led us to investigate whether estrogen had any effect on the dimerization of nNOSα in gastric tissues. We measured nNOSα levels and their dimerization state, which indicates the active form, in fundus, antrum and pylorus tissues from both male and female rats with diabetic gastroparesis. We found that dimerization was severely impaired both in antrum (*data not shown*) and pylorus (Figure-1) of female rats (DF+GP) exhibiting elevated estrogen levels, suggesting that estrogen may be affecting the bioavailability of NO in a tissue and gender-specific fashion in the female antrum and pylorus. The mechanism of estrogen's role in the reduced dimerization of nNOSα is unclear from the present study,however, as well as from published literature thus far.

NOSs have been described as highly controlled enzymes. Regulation of the NOSs has been described at all levels from gene transcription to modulation of protein-protein interactions and post-translational modification. We now provide evidence that post-translational modification might be the underlying mechanism responsible for the observed estrogen-mediated inactivation of nNOSα. Among the post-translational modifications, the site-specific serine phosphorylation of NOS enzymes is associated with their activation and inactivation. As discussed earlier, the phosphorylation of nNOS at Ser^{847} reduced the catalytic activity (Osuka et al., 2007), and phosphorylation at Ser^{1416} increased the catalytic activity (Adak et al., 2001). We therefore investigated whether the observed reduced dimerization of nNOSα in the antrum of diabetic and gastroparetic rats was due to increased phosphorylation of the inhibitory site (Ser^{847}) or reduced phosphorylation of the activation site (Ser^{1416}) using the respective phospho-specific antibodies (Zhou and Zhu, 2009). Western blot analysis demonstrated a significant decrease in Ser^{1416} phosphorylation in diabetic gastroparetic antrum tissue, suggesting that the inhibition of the activating phosphorylation site might be a possible mechanism for the inactivation of nNOSα.

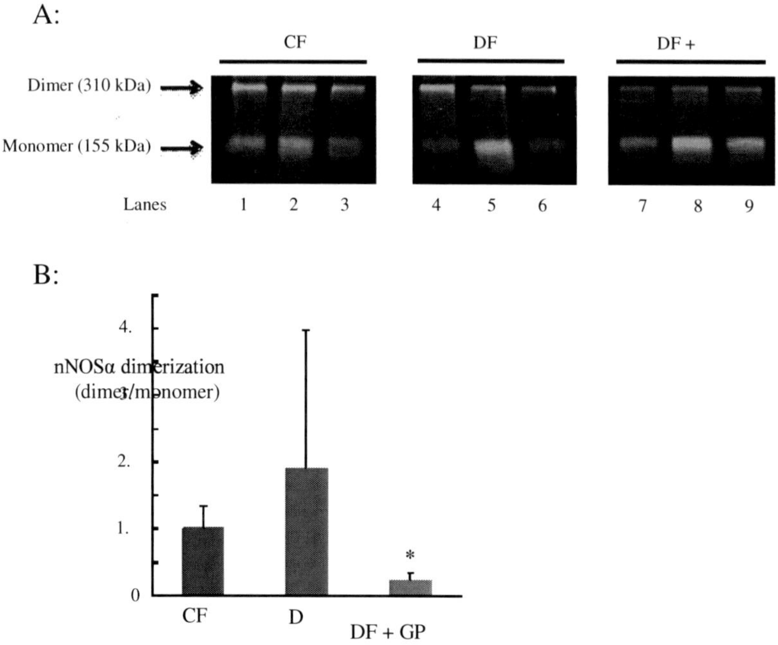

CF: normal rats, *DF:* STZ-diabetic rats and *DF + GP:* STZ-diabetic and gastroparetic rats. The experimental conditions were same as described previously (*Digestive Diseases and Sciences, 57:* 2814-2825).

A: Representative immunoblot showing the formation of dimer (310 kDa) and monomer (155 kDa) in various groups of female pylori. *B:* Densitometric analysis data for nNOSα dimerization expressed as the dimer to monomer ratio. *p <0.05. Data are expressed as the mean ± SE of 3 animals per group.

DF + GP rats showed significantly decreased ratio of dimer and monomer (p <0.016). *Female rat groups is defined as :* 1. Control (CF); 2. Diabetic after STZ treatment (DF), and 3. Diabetic and gastroparetic after STZ treatment (DF + GP). The pathophysiology of disease development in these animals is described in Figures 1 and 2 of the manuscript: *Digestive Diseases and Sciences, 57*: 2814-2825. *This figure is adapted from the principal author's publication: Showkat Ali et al. (2013): *Digestive Diseases and Sciences, 57:* 2814-2815.

Figure 1. Dimerization of nNOSα in the gastric pylorus of female rats*.

The precise mechanism of the observed changes in the phosphorylation of the activation site and subsequent impairment of dimerization, however, remains obscure and needs further investigation.

There are currently conflicting reports in the literature regarding the role of estrogen in the regulation of expression and activation of nNOSα. Many of the earlier reports have shown that NO production and total NOS expression are increased by estradiol in a variety of tissues. Shah *et al.* (Shah et al., 2000) reported that increased release of NO is responsible for the development of delayed gastric emptying in rats in late stage of pregnancy when the estrogen is at peak levels. Contrastingly, a recent study reported by Ravella *et al.* (Ravella et al., 2013) demonstrated that there was increased dimerization of nNOSα in the follicle stimulating hormone receptor (FSH-R) knock out mouse. FSH-R gene deletion in these mice causes complete loss of ovarian estrogen production, suggesting a possible role of estrogen in down-regulating the activition of nNOSα, as reported by us and other investigators (Gangula et al., 2007; Saito et al., 1999; Showkat Ali et al., 2012).

In summary, these results support the emerging hypothesis that increased levels of estrogen as observed in female gastroparetic patients is associated with decreased nitrergic activities. Together, estrogen and NO form a pathogenic duo which might be a predominant molecular mechanism involved in the development of gastroparesis.

Current Concept and Future Perspectives

Several factors have limited the physiological and therapeutic applications thus far for diabetic gastroparesis.The role of endogenous NO in the gut is being investigated using NOS inhibitors, animal model, estrogen supplementation in post menopausal women and mice that lack nNOS gene. Human studies are limited by the small number of participants and logistical difficulties in obtaining tissue samples. Pharmacological studies use inhibitors of questionable specificity,.nNOS deficient mice (nNos$^{-/-}$) have an apparently compensatory mechanism by other NOS (iNOS and eNOS). While human studies are cumbersome, phenotypic changes between genetically engineered triple negative mice n/i/eNOS$^{-/-}$ and singly gene deleted mice (nNos$^{-/-}$, eNos$^{-/-}$ and/or iNos$^{-/-)}$ might be ideal for addressing the experimental limitations.

The risk factors for the development of gastroparesis in men and women are different. The female GI tract develops a more favorable physiological condition than males for this malady. Although the development of disease pathology is multi-factorial, there is ample evidence that estrogen and NO might be among the main players.The development of gastroparesis in males is not known. We hypothesize that male development of gastroparesis may involve mechanisms other than the bioavailability of NO, such as loss of ICC, HO-1 activity, level of the excitatory neurotransmitters SP and NPY, and testosterone. There is an ongoing debate as to how applicable results derived from animal models are to human gastroparesis. Although data is limited, the most reproducible and convincing results from animal model to humans include depletion of ICC (Grover et al., 2011), loss of some of the neurotransmitters (Holmes, 2012), gender and estrogen specific development of disease pathology (Oh and Pasricha, 2013; Ravella et al., 2012) and bioavailability of NO (Adak et al., 2001; Gangula et al., 2007; Ravella et al., 2012; Showkat Ali et al., 2012). Recent advances in genomics and proteomics will allow for more studies using human subjects that will increase our understanding of the pathogenesis of gastroparesis.

Current studies have identified single nucleotide polymorphisms (SNP) that are associated with diabetes (Fagerholm et al., 2012; Staiger et al., 2009). It is well established that SNPs are associated with epigenetic changes in genes.Thus, genetic variants can alter epigenetic features and epigenetic changes can result in distinct phenotypes. Such an experimental approach has become a powerful tool and has never been applied for diabetes gastroparesis. Particularly in the era of personalized medicine, there is an increasing need for studies related to gene polymorphisms and epigenetic changes. By doing so, we will identify novel mechanisms of potential therapeutic utility in both men and women.

References

Adak, S., Santolini, J., Tikunova, S., Wang, Q., Johnson, J.D., and Stuehr, D.J., 2001. Neuronal nitric-oxide synthase mutant (Ser-1412 --> Asp) demonstrates surprising connections between heme reduction, NO complex formation, and catalysis. *J. Biol. Chem.,* 276, 1244-52.

Adeghate, E., Ponery, A.S., Pallot, D.J., and Singh, J., 2001. Distribution of vasoactive intestinal polypeptide, neuropeptide-Y and substance P and their effects on insulin secretion from the in vitro pancreas of normal and diabetic rats. *Peptides,* 22, 99-107.

Boissel, J.P., Schwarz, P.M., and Forstermann, U., 1998. Neuronal-type NO synthase: transcript diversity and expressional regulation. *Nitric Oxide*, 2, 337-49.

Burns, A.J., 2007. Disorders of interstitial cells of Cajal. *J. Pediatr. Gastroenterol. Nutr.,* 45 Suppl 2, S103-6.

Chen, M., Cheng, C., Yan, M., Niu, S., Gao, S., Shi, S., Liu, H., Qin, Y., and Shen, A., 2008. Involvement of CAPON and nitric oxide synthases in rat muscle regeneration after peripheral nerve injury. *J. Mol. Neurosci.,* 34, 89-100.

Chen, T.S., Doong, M.L., Chang, F.Y., Lee, S.D., and Wang, P.S., 1995. Effects of sex steroid hormones on gastric emptying and gastrointestinal transit in rats. *Am. J. Physiol.,* 268, G171-6.

Choi, K.M., Gibbons, S.J., Nguyen, T.V., Stoltz, G.J., Lurken, M.S., Ordog, T., Szurszewski, J.H., and Farrugia, G., 2008. Heme oxygenase-1 protects interstitial cells of Cajal from oxidative stress and reverses diabetic gastroparesis. *Gastroenterology,* 135, 2055-64, 2064 e1-2.

Choi, K.M., Kashyap, P.C., Dutta, N., Stoltz, G.J., Ordog, T., Shea Donohue, T., Bauer, A.J., Linden, D.R., Szurszewski, J.H., Gibbons, S.J., and Farrugia, G., 2010. CD206-positive M2 macrophages that express heme oxygenase-1 protect against diabetic gastroparesis in mice. *Gastroenterology,* 138, 2399-409, 2409 e1.

Cole, W.C., 2011. ANO1-ther brick in the wall--role of Ca2+-activated Cl- channels of interstitial cells of Cajal in cholinergic motor control of gastrointestinal smooth muscle. *J. Physiol.,* 589, 4641-2.

Cui, H., Hayashi, A., Sun, H.S., Belmares, M.P., Cobey, C., Phan, T., Schweizer, J., Salter, M.W., Wang, Y.T., Tasker, R.A., Garman, D., Rabinowitz, J., Lu, P.S., and Tymianski, M., 2007. PDZ protein interactions underlying NMDA receptor-mediated excitotoxicity and neuroprotection by PSD-95 inhibitors. *J. Neurosci.,* 27, 9901-15.

Cutts, T.F., Luo, J., Starkebaum, W., Rashed, H., and Abell, T.L., 2005. Is gastric electrical stimulation superior to standard pharmacologic therapy in improving GI symptoms, healthcare resources, and long-term health care benefits? *Neurogastroenterol. Motil.,* 17, 35-43.

Daff, S., 2010. NO synthase: structures and mechanisms. *Nitric. Oxide,* 23, 1-11.

Dreyer, J., Schleicher, M., Tappe, A., Schilling, K., Kuner, T., Kusumawidijaja, G., Muller-Esterl, W., Oess, S., and Kuner, R., 2004. Nitric oxide synthase (NOS)-interacting protein interacts with neuronal NOS and regulates its distribution and activity. *J. Neurosci.,* 24, 10454-65.

Efimov, I., Basran, J., Thackray, S.J., Handa, S., Mowat, C.G., and Raven, E.L., 2011. Structure and reaction mechanism in the heme dioxygenases. Biochemistry 50, 2717-24.

El-Salhy, M., and Spangeus, A., 2002. Gastric emptying in animal models of human diabetes: correlation to blood glucose level and gut neuroendocrine peptide content. *Ups. J. Med. Sci.,* 107, 89-99.

Fagerholm, E., Ahlqvist, E., Forsblom, C., Sandholm, N., Syreeni, A., Parkkonen, M., McKnight, A.J., Tarnow, L., Maxwell, A.P., Parving, H.H., Groop, L., Groop, P.H., and FinnDiane Study, G., 2012. SNP in the genome-wide association study hotspot on chromosome 9p21 confers susceptibility to diabetic nephropathy in type 1 diabetes. *Diabetologia,* 55, 2386-93.

Fu, M., Li, X., Zhang, M., and Xian, Y., 2002. Increased expression of neuropeptide Y and its mRNA in STZ-diabetic rats. *Chin. Med. J.,* (Engl) 115, 690-5.

Gangula, P.R., Maner, W.L., Micci, M.A., Garfield, R.E., and Pasricha, P.J., 2007. Diabetes induces sex-dependent changes in neuronal nitric oxide synthase dimerization and function in the rat gastric antrum. *Am. J. Physiol. Gastrointest Liver Physiol.,* 292, G725-33.

Gangula, P.R., Mukhopadhyay, S., Ravella, K., Cai, S., Channon, K.M., Garfield, R.E., and Pasricha, P.J., 2010. Tetrahydrobiopterin (BH4), a cofactor for nNOS, restores gastric emptying and nNOS expression in female diabetic rats. *Am. J. Physiol. Gastrointest Liver Physiol.,* 298, G692-9.

Goyal, R.K., and Chaudhury, A., 2010. Mounting evidence against the role of ICC in neurotransmission to smooth muscle in the gut. *Am. J. Physiol. Gastrointest Liver Physiol.,* 298, G10-3.

Grover, M., Farrugia, G., Lurken, M.S., Bernard, C.E., Faussone-Pellegrini, M.S., Smyrk, T.C., Parkman, H.P., Abell, T.L., Snape, W.J., Hasler, W.L., Unalp-Arida, A., Nguyen, L., Koch, K.L., Calles, J., Lee, L., Tonascia, J., Hamilton, F.A., Pasricha, P.J., and Consortium, N.G.C.R., 2011. Cellular changes in diabetic and idiopathic gastroparesis. *Gastroenterology,* 140, 1575-85 e8.

He, C.L., Soffer, E.E., Ferris, C.D., Walsh, R.M., Szurszewski, J.H., and Farrugia, G., 2001. Loss of interstitial cells of cajal and inhibitory innervation in insulin-dependent diabetes. *Gastroenterology,* 121, 427-34.

Hess, D.T., Matsumoto, A., Kim, S.O., Marshall, H.E., and Stamler, J.S., 2005. Protein S-nitrosylation: purview and parameters. *Nat. Rev. Mol. Cell Biol.,* 6, 150-66.

Hewitt, S.C., and Korach, K.S., 2003. Oestrogen receptor knockout mice: roles for oestrogen receptors alpha and beta in reproductive tissues. *Reproduction,* 125, 143-9.

Holmes, G.M., 2012. Upper gastrointestinal dysmotility after spinal cord injury: is diminished vagal sensory processing one culprit? *Front Physiol.,* 3, 277.

Horvath, V.J., Vittal, H., and Ordog, T., 2005. Reduced insulin and IGF-I signaling, not hyperglycemia, underlies the diabetes-associated depletion of interstitial cells of Cajal in the murine stomach. *Diabetes,* 54, 1528-33.

Horvath, V.J., Vittal, H., Lorincz, A., Chen, H., Almeida-Porada, G., Redelman, D., and Ordog, T., 2006. Reduced stem cell factor links smooth myopathy and loss of interstitial cells of cajal in murine diabetic gastroparesis. *Gastroenterology,* 130, 759-70.

Huang, P.L., Dawson, T.M., Bredt, D.S., Snyder, S.H., and Fishman, M.C., 1993. Targeted disruption of the neuronal nitric oxide synthase gene. *Cell,* 75, 1273-86.

Hutson, W.R., Roehrkasse, R.L., and Wald, A., 1989. Influence of gender and menopause on gastric emptying and motility. *Gastroenterology,* 96, 11-7.

Ilhan, A., Rasul, S., Dimitrov, A., Handisurya, A., Gartner, W., Baumgartner-Parzer, S., Wagner, L., Kautzky-Willer, A., and Base, W., 2010. Plasma neuropeptide Y levels differ in distinct diabetic conditions. *Neuropeptides,* 44, 485-9.

Iwasaki, H., Kajimura, M., Osawa, S., Kanaoka, S., Furuta, T., Ikuma, M., and Hishida, A., 2006. A deficiency of gastric interstitial cells of Cajal accompanied by decreased expression of neuronal nitric oxide synthase and substance P in patients with type 2 diabetes mellitus. *J. Gastroenterol.,* 41, 1076-87.

Kamada, Y., Jenkins, G.J., Lau, M., Dunbar, A.Y., Lowe, E.R., and Osawa, Y., 2005. Tetrahydrobiopterin depletion and ubiquitylation of neuronal nitric oxide synthase. *Brain Res. Mol. Brain Res.,* 142, 19-27.

Kashyap, P.C., Choi, K.M., Dutta, N., Linden, D.R., Szurszewski, J.H., Gibbons, S.J., and Farrugia, G., 2010. Carbon monoxide reverses diabetic gastroparesis in NOD mice. *Am. J. Physiol. Gastrointest Liver Physiol.,* 298, G1013-9.

Kunt, T., Forst, T., Schmidt, S., Pfutzner, A., Schneider, S., Harzer, O., Lobig, M., Engelbach, M., Goitom, K., Pohlmann, T., and Beyer, J., 2000. Serum levels of substance P are decreased in patients with type 1 diabetes. *Exp. Clin. Endocrinol. Diabetes,* 108, 164-7.

Lin, Z., Hou, Q., Sarosiek, I., Forster, J., and McCallum, R.W., 2008. Association between changes in symptoms and gastric emptying in gastroparetic patients treated with gastric electrical stimulation. *Neurogastroenterol. Motil.,* 20, 464-70.

Luo, C.X., and Zhu, D.Y., 2011. Research progress on neurobiology of neuronal nitric oxide synthase. *Neurosci. Bull.,* 27, 23-35.

Maric, C., 2009. Sex, diabetes and the kidney. Am J Physiol Renal Physiol 296, F680-8.

Mashimo, H., Kjellin, A., and Goyal, R.K., 2000. Gastric stasis in neuronal nitric oxide synthase-deficient knockout mice. *Gastroenterology,* 119, 766-73.

Mazzone, A., Bernard, C.E., Strege, P.R., Beyder, A., Galietta, L.J., Pasricha, P.J., Rae, J.L., Parkman, H.P., Linden, D.R., Szurszewski, J.H., Ordog, T., Gibbons, S.J., and Farrugia, G., 2011. Altered expression of Ano1 variants in human diabetic gastroparesis. *J. Biol. Chem.,* 286, 13393-403.

Ndisang, J.F., and Jadhav, A., 2009. Heme oxygenase system enhances insulin sensitivity and glucose metabolism in streptozotocin-induced diabetes. *Am. J. Physiol. Endocrinol. Metab.,* 296, E829-41.

Oh, J.H., and Pasricha, P.J., 2013. Recent advances in the pathophysiology and treatment of gastroparesis. *J. Neurogastroenterol. Motil.,* 19, 18-24.

Ordog, T., 2008. Interstitial cells of Cajal in diabetic gastroenteropathy. *Neurogastroenterol. Motil.,* 20, 8-18.

Osuka, K., Watanabe, Y., Usuda, N., Atsuzawa, K., Aoshima, C., Yamauchi, K., Takayasu, M., and Yoshida, J., 2007. Phosphorylation of neuronal nitric oxide synthase at Ser847 in the nucleus intermediolateralis after spinal cord injury in mice. *Neuroscience,* 145, 241-7.

Peng, H.M., Morishima, Y., Pratt, W.B., and Osawa, Y., 2012. Modulation of heme/substrate binding cleft of neuronal nitric-oxide synthase (nNOS) regulates binding of Hsp90 and Hsp70 proteins and nNOS ubiquitination. *J. Biol. Chem.,* 287, 1556-65.

Pitteloud, N., Hardin, M., Dwyer, A.A., Valassi, E., Yialamas, M., Elahi, D., and Hayes, F.J., 2005. Increasing insulin resistance is associated with a decrease in Leydig cell testosterone secretion in men. *J. Clin. Endocrinol. Metab.,* 90, 2636-41.

Pratt, W.B., Morishima, Y., Peng, H.M., and Osawa, Y., 2010. Proposal for a role of the Hsp90/Hsp70-based chaperone machinery in making triage decisions when proteins undergo oxidative and toxic damage. *Exp. Biol. Med.,* (Maywood) 235, 278-89.

Ravella, K., Yang, H., and Gangula, P.R., 2012. Impairment of gastric nitrergic and NRF2 system in apolipoprotein E knockout mice. *Dig Dis. Sci.,* 57, 1504-9.

Ravella, K., Al-Hendy, A., Sharan, C., Hale, A.B., Channon, K.M., Srinivasan, S., and Gangula, P.R., 2013. Chronic Estrogen Deficiency Causes Gastroparesis by Altering Neuronal Nitric Oxide Synthase Function. *Dig. Dis. Sci.,*

Rodriguez-Crespo, I., Straub, W., Gavilanes, F., and Ortiz de Montellano, P.R., 1998. Binding of dynein light chain (PIN) to neuronal nitric oxide synthase in the absence of inhibition. *Arch. Biochem. Biophys.,* 359, 297-304.

Saad, F., 2009. The role of testosterone in type 2 diabetes and metabolic syndrome in men. *Arq. Bras. Endocrinol. Metabol.,* 53, 901-7.

Sadik, R., Abrahamsson, H., and Stotzer, P.O., 2003. Gender differences in gut transit shown with a newly developed radiological procedure. *Scand. J. Gastroenterol.,* 38, 36-42.

Saito, S., Aras, R.S., Lou, H., Ramwell, P.W., and Foegh, M.L., 1999. Effects of estrogen on nitric oxide synthase expression in rat aorta allograft and smooth muscle cells. *J. Heart Lung Transplant., 18*, 937-45.

Sanders, K.M., and Ward, S.M., 2007. Kit mutants and gastrointestinal physiology. *J. Physiol.,* 578, 33-42.

Sato, Y., Sagami, I., and Shimizu, T., 2004. Identification of caveolin-1-interacting sites in neuronal nitric-oxide synthase. Molecular mechanism for inhibition of NO formation. *J. Biol. Chem.,* 279, 8827-36.

Satoh, C., Satoh, F., Takahashi, K., Murakami, O., Sone, M., Totsune, K., Yabe, T., Ohneda, M., Fukuda, M., Sugimura, K., Ogawa, S., Nagakubo, H., Sato, T., and Mouri, T., 1999. Elevated plasma immunoreactive neuropeptide Y concentrations and its increased urinary excretion in patients with advanced diabetic nephropathy. *Endocr. J.,* 46, 139-46.

Saur, D., Paehge, H., Schusdziarra, V., and Allescher, H.D., 2000. Distinct expression of splice variants of neuronal nitric oxide synthase in the human gastrointestinal tract. *Gastroenterology,* 118, 849-58.

Schulz, E., Anter, E., Zou, M.H., and Keaney, J.F., Jr., 2005. Estradiol-mediated endothelial nitric oxide synthase association with heat shock protein 90 requires adenosine monophosphate-dependent protein kinase. *Circulation,* 111, 3473-80.

Shah, S., Hobbs, A., Singh, R., Cuevas, J., Ignarro, L.J., and Chaudhuri, G., 2000. Gastrointestinal motility during pregnancy: role of nitrergic component of NANC nerves. *Am. J. Physiol. Regul. Integr. Comp. Physiol.,* 279, R1478-85.

Shah, V., Lyford, G., Gores, G., and Farrugia, G., 2004. Nitric oxide in gastrointestinal health and disease. *Gastroenterology,* 126, 903-13.

Showkat Ali, M., Tiscareno-Grejada, I., Locovei, S., Smiley, R., Collins, T., Sarosiek, J., and McCallum, R., 2012. Gender and estradiol as major factors in the expression and dimerization of nNOSalpha in rats with experimental diabetic gastroparesis. *Dig. Dis. Sci.,* 57, 2814-25.

Sivarao, D.V., Mashimo, H., and Goyal, R.K., 2008. Pyloric sphincter dysfunction in nNOS-/- and W/Wv mutant mice: animal models of gastroparesis and duodenogastric reflux. *Gastroenterology,* 135, 1258-66.

Smith, D.S., Williams, C.S., and Ferris, C.D., 2003. Diagnosis and treatment of chronic gastroparesis and chronic intestinal pseudo-obstruction. *Gastroenterol. Clin. North. Am.,* 32, 619-58.

Song, T., Hatano, N., Horii, M., Tokumitsu, H., Yamaguchi, F., Tokuda, M., and Watanabe, Y., 2004. Calcium/calmodulin-dependent protein kinase I inhibits neuronal nitric-oxide synthase activity through serine 741 phosphorylation. *FEBS Lett.,* 570, 133-7.

Staiger, H., Machicao, F., Fritsche, A., and Haring, H.U., 2009. Pathomechanisms of type 2 diabetes genes. *Endocr. Rev.,* 30, 557-85.

Takahashi, T., 2003. Pathophysiological significance of neuronal nitric oxide synthase in the gastrointestinal tract. *J. Gastroenterol.,* 38, 421-30.

Tateishi, Y., Kawabe, Y., Chiba, T., Murata, S., Ichikawa, K., Murayama, A., Tanaka, K., Baba, T., Kato, S., and Yanagisawa, J., 2004. Ligand-dependent switching of ubiquitin-proteasome pathways for estrogen receptor. *EMBO J.,* 23, 4813-23.

Toda, N., and Herman, A.G., 2005. Gastrointestinal function regulation by nitrergic efferent nerves. *Pharmacol. Rev.,* 57, 315-38.

Ukkola, O., and Kesaniemi, Y.A., 2007. Leu7Pro polymorphism of PreproNPY associated with an increased risk for type II diabetes in middle-aged subjects. *Eur. J. Clin. Nutr.,* 61, 1102-5.

Verrengia, M., Sachdeva, P., Gaughan, J., Fisher, R.S., and Parkman, H.P., 2011. Variation of symptoms during the menstrual cycle in female patients with gastroparesis. *Neurogastroenterol. Motil.,* 23, 625-e254.

Wang, F., Zheng, T.Z., Li, W., Qu, S.Y., and He, D.Y., 2003. Action of progesterone on contractile activity of isolated gastric strips in rats. *World J. Gastroenterol.,* 9, 775-8.

Wang, X.Y., Huizinga, J.D., Diamond, J., and Liu, L.W., 2009a. Loss of intramuscular and submuscular interstitial cells of Cajal and associated enteric nerves is related to decreased gastric emptying in streptozotocin-induced diabetes. *Neurogastroenterol. Motil.,* 21, 1095-e92.

Wang, X.Y., Alberti, E., White, E.J., Mikkelsen, H.B., Larsen, J.O., Jimenez, M., and Huizinga, J.D., 2009b. Igf1r+/CD34+ immature ICC are putative adult progenitor cells, identified ultrastructurally as fibroblast-like ICC in Ws/Ws rat colon. *J. Cell Mol. Med.,* 13, 3528-40.

Ward, S.M., 2000. Interstitial cells of Cajal in enteric neurotransmission. Gut 47 Suppl 4, iv40-3; discussion iv52.

Ward, S.M., Beckett, E.A., Wang, X., Baker, F., Khoyi, M., and Sanders, K.M., 2000. Interstitial cells of Cajal mediate cholinergic neurotransmission from enteric motor neurons. *J. Neurosci.,* 20, 1393-403.

Watanabe, M., and Itoh, K., 2011. Characterization of a novel posttranslational modification in neuronal nitric oxide synthase by small ubiquitin-related modifier-1. *Biochim. Biophys. Acta.,* 1814, 900-7.

Yamamoto, I., Fujimura, M., Kihara, N., Kumano, K., Yamada, T., Yamamoto, H., and Fujimiya, M., 2000. Nitric oxide formation in the dog sphincter of Oddi from nitric oxide donors as measured with in vivo micro-dialysis. *Aliment. Pharmacol. Ther.,* 14, 1095-101.

Yamamoto, T., Watabe, K., Nakahara, M., Ogiyama, H., Kiyohara, T., Tsutsui, S., Tamura, S., Shinomura, Y., and Hayashi, N., 2008. Disturbed gastrointestinal motility and decreased interstitial cells of Cajal in diabetic db/db mice. *J. Gastroenterol. Hepatol.,* 23, 660-7.

Yeh, E.T., 2009. SUMOylation and De-SUMOylation: wrestling with life's processes. *J. Biol. Chem.,* 284, 8223-7.

Zhou, L., and Zhu, D.Y., 2009. Neuronal nitric oxide synthase: structure, subcellular localization, regulation, and clinical implications. *Nitric. Oxide.,* 20, 223-30.

In: Estradiol: Synthesis, Health Effects and Drug Interactions ISBN: 978-1-62808-962-2
Editors: Ricco Palmeri and Sal Grimaudo

Chapter 11

Estradiol Synthesis after Ovarian Tissue Cryopreservation and Transplantation

***Sanghoon Lee*[1] *and Seung Yup Ku*[2,*]**
[1]Department of Obstetrics and Gynecology,
Korea University College of Medicine, Seoul, Korea
[2]Department of Obstetrics and Gynecology,
Seoul National University College of Medicine, Seoul, Korea

Abstract

Fertility preservation is an effort to help cancer patients retain their fertility and an emerging discipline that now plays a central role in the care of reproductive women with cancer. An increasingly larger number of women are surviving with cancer because of improvement in diagnostic and therapeutic strategies. As a result, quality-of-life issues, including issues involving fertility preservation, have gained significant importance in cancer care. Breast cancer is the most common cancer in reproductive women in the US. Most women with breast cancer require the adjuvant chemotherapy including cyclophosphamide.

Cytotoxic treatment such as chemotherapy and/or radiotherapy can cause severe gonadal damages resulting in premature ovarian failure and infertility in female. Adjuvant chemotherapy particularly with alkylating agents such as cyclophosphamide is gonadotoxic and induces premature ovarian failure. The American Society of Clinical Oncology issued practice guideline update for fertility preservation options in cancer patients. Several well established methods for fertility preservation were introduced such as embryo and oocyte cryopreservation, gonadal shielding during radiotherapy, trachelectomy, and ovarian transposition. For fertility preservation, ovarian stimulation with gonadotropins for embryo or oocyte cryopreservation results in excessive levels of estrogen production. To reduce the estrogen exposure during ovarian stimulation in

[*] Corresponding author: Seung Yup Ku MD, PhD. Email: jyhsyk@snu.ac.kr.

hormone dependent cancer, a novel protocol using letrozole (aromatase inhibitor) and gonadotropins was developed.

Ovarian tissue cryopreservation and transplantation is a main option to preserve their fertility in cancer patients who need cancer treatments without delay or do not want to undergo ovarian stimulation. For prepubertal girls diagnosed with cancer, ovarian tissue freezing is the only option for fertility preservation. Based on the site of transplantation of cryopreserved ovarian tissue, transplantation can be divided into two different types as orthotopic and heterotopic transplantation.

In a recent review of 60 cases of frozen-thawed ovarian transplantation, all ovarian tissue were frozen with the slow-freezing method and the restoration of ovarian activity was observed in at least 92.9%. In all cases, it took 3.5–6.5 months after transplantation before a rise in E2 and a decrease in FSH were detected (mean 4.5 months). To date, a total of 24 live births and 4 ongoing pregnancies have been reported worldwide from ovarian tissue cryopreservation and transplantation. Based on our review, we believe that ovarian cryopreservation and transplantation before cancer treatments is an effective option to preserve their fertility and to restore gonadal endocrine function including estradiol synthesis.

Keywords: Estradiol, Ovary, Cryopreservation, Transplantation, Fertility, and Preservation

Introduction

An increasingly larger number of women are surviving with cancer because of improvement in diagnostic and therapeutic strategies. More than 790,000 new female cancer cases were diagnosed in 2012 in the United States [1]. Approximately 10% of these patients occur under the age of 45 years. From 2002 to 2012, 83% of women younger than 45 years diagnosed with cancer survived [2]. As a result, quality-of-life, including future pregnancies, has gained a significant importance in the care of women with cancer.

Fertility preservation is an effort to help cancer patients retain their fertility and an emerging discipline that now plays a central role in the care of reproductive women with cancer. Indications for fertility preservation include childhood cancers, breast cancers, gynecologic cancers, hematologic cancers such as leukemia and lymphoma, those who need hematopoietic stem cell transplantation or pelvic irradiation for other diseases, and those with a high risk of premature ovarian failure (or primary ovarian insufficiency). Since several departments are involved in fertility preservation treatment, collaborating as a team with several specialists who take part in the initial cancer diagnosis and treatment is necessary to manage cancer patients.

Ovarian tissue cryopreservation and transplantation is a main option to preserve their fertility in cancer patients who need cancer treatments without delay or do not want to undergo ovarian stimulation. For prepubertal girls with cancer, ovarian tissue freezing is the only option for fertility preservation. Oktay et al. reported the first case of human ovarian tissue cryopreservation and auto-transplantation in 1999 [3]. To date, a total of 24 live births and 4 ongoing pregnancies have been reported worldwide from ovarian tissue cryopreservation and transplantation [4].

Human ovarian tissue transplantation is still considered as an investigational method since there are many uncertainties and unanswered questions including the restoration of ovarian function after transplantation. Thus, in this chapter, we would like to review the concepts and methods of fertility preservation, and endocrine function including estradiol synthesis after ovarian tissue cryopreservation and transplantation.

Cytotoxic Treatment induced Gonadal Damage

Cytotoxic treatment such as chemotherapy and/or radiotherapy can cause severe gonadal damages resulting in premature ovarian failure and infertility in female. Adjuvant chemotherapy particularly with alkylating agents such as cyclophosphamide is gonadotoxic and induces premature ovarian failure. The drugs are generally classified as low risk (e.g., methotrexate, 5-fluorouracil, vincristine, bleomycin, and actinomycin D), intermediate risk (e.g., cisplatin, and adriamycin), and high risk (e.g., cyclophosphamide, chlorambucil, melphalan, busulfan, nitrogen mustard, and procarbazine) [5]. The degree of chemotherapy-induced ovarian damage is dependent on the patient's age, the drug used, and the dosage of the drugs. Since most cancer patients are treated with multi-agent chemotherapy protocols, it is not easy to assess the degree of gonadal damage caused by a single specific agent. Radiotherapy-induced follicular damage resulting in a high risk of prolonged amenorrhea in women can occur when exposed by pelvic or whole abdominal radiation dose ≥6 Gy in adult women, ≥10 Gy in postpubertal girls, and ≥15 Gy in prepubertal girls [6-10]. The radiation dose of concurrent chemoradiation therapy (CCRT) for patients with advanced stage cervical cancer is usually about 50 Gy. Thus gynecologic oncologists should consider a possibility of post-treatment infertility in patients who undergo CCRT.

Patients should be referred to fertility preservation specialists before chemotherapy; however, many of those who do not have this opportunity may develop infertility and may be referred for post-chemotherapy assisted reproduction [11]. Because the likelihood of the success of assisted reproductive techniques after chemotherapy is significantly diminished [12], it is extremely important to understand the factors that determine the access to fertility preservation and early referral. In a previous study, we evaluated the socioeconomic, demographic, and medical factors that influence early referral to fertility preservation before cancer treatment versus delayed referral to post-chemotherapy assisted reproduction in 314 women with breast cancer. Factors favoring referrals for fertility preservation were older age, early stage breast cancer, cancer care at an academic center, and family history of breast cancer [13]. This information has revealed the barriers against accessing early fertility preservation care.

Value of Early Referral to Fertility Preservation

Oncologists should recognize the importance of fertility preservation and early referral to specialists. Both embryo and oocyte freezing for fertility preservation require ovarian stimulation with gonadotropins. Since ovarian stimulation requires approximately two weeks for completion, early referral is crucial to avoid delay in chemotherapy. The author's previous study concluded that early referral prior to breast surgery enables women with breast cancer to initiate a fertility preservation cycle sooner and to undergo multiple cycles of oocyte or embryo freezing, when desired. Referral prior to breast surgery results in the initiation of chemotherapy on average 3 weeks earlier in single fertility preservation cycles, as well as when the data from double cycles are included, compared to those referred after breast surgery. This additional time allows patients to undergo multiple cycles of fertility preservation. Women who can undergo multiple cycles are likely to be at an advantage for fertility preservation because of the additional number of eggs or embryos generated [14].

A recent study, however, indicated that still less than half of physicians routinely refer cancer patients of childbearing age to reproductive specialists [15]. Another recent study reported that while most oncologists recognize the importance of discussing infertility risks after cancer treatment, few actually discuss fertility preservation with their patients [16]. In addition, Armuand *et al.* [17] reported that there have been sex differences in access to fertility-related information and the use of fertility preservation treatment. Only half of the women had discussed fertility issues with a health care professional, although the majority of men had received information about fertility preservation such as sperm cryopreservation [17]. Potential explanations are that sperm banking for men is an easy and well established method, and that the delay is negligible compared to the required duration of ovarian stimulation for embryo or oocyte cryopreservation.

Oncologists play a key role in understanding patients' concerns regarding fertility. Fertility preservation specialists should make an effort to publicize the significance of fertility preservation for reproductive women with cancer and should provide appropriate education for both associated physicians and cancer patients who wish to preserve their fertility. As important as it is to encourage oncologists to refer young people with cancer to fertility preservation counseling, it is just as important to emphasize referral as early in the process as possible to maximize the likelihood of success.

Fertility Preservation Options in Females

Recently, the American Society of Clinical Oncology (ASCO) has issued practice guideline update for fertility preservation options in cancer patients [18]. Several well established methods of FP have been introduced, including both embryo and oocyte cryopreservation, gonadal shielding during radiotherapy, trachelectomy, and ovarian transposition. (Table 1)

Table 1. Fertility preservation options in females: ASCO Clinical Practice Guideline Update

Standard methods	Embryo cryopreservation Oocyte cryopreservation * Gonadal shielding during radiation therapy Ovarian transposition (oophoropexy) Trachelectomy Other conservative gynecologic surgery
Experimental methods	Ovarian cryopreservation and transplantation Ovarian suppression with GnRH analogs or antagonists

* Note that oocyte cryopreservation was newly accepted as an established method for fertility preservation in 2013 ASCO Clinical Practice Guideline Update.

Embryo cryopreservation is a well-established technique and the current live-birth rate per transfer using frozen thawed embryos is 35.6% in US women under 35-year-old (http://www.sart.org, 2008). Embryo freezing should initially be considered for fertility preservation treatment if there is adequate time for ovarian stimulation and a partner or donor sperm.

Success rates for cryopreservation of unfertilized oocytes have improved significantly, and it is no longer considered experimental by the American Society of Reproductive Medicine. Because of the improvements in advanced technologies including freezing-thawing methods, oocyte cryopreservation is included as an established method. Some reproductive specialty centers have reported success rates comparable to those obtained using unfrozen eggs, especially in younger women. Like embryo cryopreservation, this technique also requires ovarian stimulation and ultrasound-guided oocyte retrieval. Oocyte cryopreservation is of particular importance for women who do not have a male partner or prefer not to use donor sperm.

Gonadal shielding during radiotherapy should be considered if radiotherapy is required for cancer treatment. For example, radiation plays an important role in the management of breast cancer, which can be classified into four categories: 1) Primary radiotherapy in breast-conserving treatment for early breast cancer, 2) Adjuvant radiotherapy after mastectomy for high-risk patients, 3) Radiotherapy after neo-adjuvant chemotherapy in locally-advanced breast cancers, and 4) Palliative radiotherapy for metastatic disease [19].

Trachelectomy is also an accepted method for the surgical management of early stage cervical cancer in women who wish to preserve their fertility. Cervical cancer is one of the most common cancers in women younger than 40 along with breast cancer, non-Hodgkin's lymphoma, and leukemia [20]. Indications for trachelectomy are as follows: 1. Women who desire to preserve fertility (age<40-45) 2. Stage Ia1 (with lymph vascular space involvement), Ia2, Ib1 3. Lesion size ≤2 cm 4. Histologically squamous, adeno-, or adenosquamous carcinoma 5. No upper cervical canal involvement of cancer 6. No evidence of lymph node metastasis

Plante *et al.* [21] reported their experience with 125 patients who underwent vaginal radical trachelectomy. The recurrence rate of cervical cancer after trachelectomy was less than 5% and the death rate was less than 2%. Having lesions sized >2 cm was a strong risk factor for recurrence. A total of 58 women out of 125 conceived a total of 106 pregnancies, and of those, 73% of pregnancies reached the third trimester, of which, in turn, 75% gave birth at term. Overall, 13.5% of patients were associated with fertility problems.

Ovarian transposition can be performed not only for preservation of fertility but also for prevention of premature ovarian failure in cervical cancer patients who require radiotherapy. It is necessary for gynecologic oncologists to understand the field of radiotherapy to prepare for ovarian transposition. Usually, standard fields are used with the upper field border on the fourth/fifth lumbar vertebra [22]. It is widely accepted that surgical transposition should be at least 3 cm above the upper border of the radiation field [23]. Hwang *et al.* [24] reported that a location for the transposed ovary higher than 1.5 cm above the iliac crest is recommended to avoid ovarian failure after primary or adjuvant pelvic radiotherapy in cervical cancer.

Breast Cancer and Estradiol

Breast cancer is the most common cancer in women of reproductive age in the US [25]. Most women with breast cancer require adjuvant chemotherapy including cyclophosphamide. At an average age of 40, administration of cyclophosphamide, methotrexate, and 5-Fluorouracil (CMF) or Adriamycin, cyclophosphamide and Taxol (AC+T) resulted in amenorrhea in 20% to 100% or 37% to 77% of patients followed up for 1 year after adjuvant chemotherapy, respectively [26].

For fertility preservation, ovarian stimulation with gonadotropins for embryo or oocyte cryopreservation results in excessive levels of estrogen production. To reduce estrogen exposure during ovarian stimulation in hormone-dependent cancer, a novel protocol using letrozole (a third generation aromatase inhibitor) and gonadotropins was developed by Dr. Oktay [27]. Use of aromatase inhibitors became increasingly common in the treatment of breast cancer [28]. They have also recently been introduced for ovulation induction. When compared to clomiphene cycles, they produce comparable peak estradiol levels or those even lower than the natural cycle. Because of their dual effects, they can be used in breast and endometrial cancer patients for ovulation induction. Tamoxifen cannot be used in those women during ovarian stimulation as it is antagonistic to the endometrium.

Aromatase inhibitors are generally well tolerated and known side effects are hot flushes, nausea/vomiting, headache, back pain, and leg cramps [29-31]. These adverse effects were reported in older breast cancer patients who were given the drugs on a daily basis over several months in Phase III trials. Very few withdrew from the trials because of drug-related adverse effects [32, 33]. In the clinical experience, using a short course of aromatase inhibitor for induction of ovulation in young healthy women had fewer side effects than with clomiphene citrate [27, 34].

Ovarian stimulation for embryo or oocyte cryopreservation should be started within the first four days of the menstrual cycle. In urgent settings, random-start ovarian stimulation is emerging as a new technique for the purpose of fertility preservation without compromising oocyte yield and maturity [35]. Although newly developed protocols are effective in inducing controlled ovarian stimulation and obtaining suitable number of oocytes/embryos, only a small number of the patients have undergone thawing and embryo transfer. Thus, there are not enough reliable data reported to evaluate the implantation and pregnancy outcomes of these new protocols. Depending on whether the referral is made before or after breast surgery, usually no more than one or two cycles of ovarian stimulation can be performed without delaying chemotherapy in women with breast cancer [14]. This delay is generally acceptable as multiple studies have shown no effect on survival or recurrence in breast cancer patients if chemotherapy had been initiated as late as 12 weeks after breast surgery [36, 37].

In fertility preservation cycles, since there is limited time available prior to the onset of chemotherapy in breast cancer patients [14], ovarian stimulation is often performed with higher doses of gonadotropins to maximize the number of embryos or oocytes cryopreserved, and to increase the likelihood of future pregnancies. In the previous study, we compared a low dose FSH start (=150 IU) with a high dose (>150 IU) in women with breast cancer undergoing fertility preservation with letrozole and found that the higher dose FSH stimulation in letrozole cycles did not improve pregnancy outcomes, and may be associated with a lower live birth rate [38]. Thus we concluded that higher dose FSH stimulation with letrozole in women with breast cancer did not improve reproductive outcomes and may be associated with lower live birth rates. In addition, it may increase estrogen exposure as well as the costs of fertility preservation.

Ovarian tissue Cryopreservation and Transplantation

The first ovarian transplant with cryopreserved ovarian tissue was performed by Kutluk Oktay in 1999 [3, 39]. In 2004, Dr. Donnez reported the first successful birth from slow, or controlled rate, frozen ovarian tissue [40]. In 1997, samples of ovarian cortex were taken from a woman with Hodgkin's lymphoma and cryo-preserved in a rate freezer and stored in liquid nitrogen. After chemotherapy the patient had premature ovarian failure. In 2003, after freeze-thawing, orthotopic autotransplantation of ovarian cortical tissue was done by laparoscopy and five months after transplantation signs indicated recovery of regular ovulatory cycles. A viable intrauterine pregnancy was confirmed eleven months after transplantation that resulted in a live birth.

The first case report of nonautologous orthotopic transplantation of fresh ovarian tissue was from one monozygotic twin sister to the other, who had suffered from premature ovarian failure [41]. The procedure resulted in a live birth. These investigators have repeated this procedure in 10 sets of monozygotic twins [42], and successfully transplanted an intact fresh ovary [43]. Others have reported a live birth after allografting of ovarian cortex between monozygotic twins with Turner mosaic and discordant ovarian function [44].

Human ovarian tissues have been xenotransplanted to immunodeficient mice, with subsequent ovulation [45-47]; however, aberrant microtubule organization and chromatin patterns observed during the maturation process are of significant concern [48, 49]. The risk of contamination with trans-species retroviral infections also needs to be addressed prior to testing this experimental approach clinically.

Successful pregnancies after ovarian tissue cryopreservation followed by transplantation have been reported in some human studies [50-53]. Transplantation of cryopreserved ovarian tissue has shown to be a potential method for recovery of ovarian function [3]. Advantages of ovarian tissue transplantation are not only preservation of fertility but also restoration of endocrine function in young women after cancer treatment.

Ovarian tissue cryopreservation and transplantation is a main option for preserving the fertility of cancer patients who need cancer treatments without delay or do not want to undergo ovarian stimulation. For prepubertal girls diagnosed with cancer, ovarian tissue freezing is the only option for FP. To date, a total of 24 live births and 4 ongoing pregnancies have been reported worldwide from ovarian tissue cryopreservation and transplantation [4]. Based on the site of transplantation of cryopreserved ovarian tissue, transplantation can be classified into two different types: orthotopic (e.g., to remaining ovarian tissue or pelvic peritoneum) and heterotopic(e.g., in the abdominal wall, forearm, and chest wall) transplantation.

Ovarian function Restoration after Ovarian Transplantation

Transplantation of cryopreserved ovarian tissue has shown to be a potential method for recovery of ovarian function [3, 54]. Advantages of ovarian tissue transplantation are not only preserving fertility but also restoring endocrine function in young women after cancer treatment. In a review of successful orthotopic frozen-thawed ovarian transplantation, restoration of ovarian activity was shown to be between 3.5 and 6.5 months after transplantation [55]. Oktay et al. [3, 56] reported the first case of laparoscopic transplantation of frozen-thawed ovarian tissue into the pelvic sidewall with subsequent ovulation and subcutaneous ovarian transplantation to the forearm, which resulted in preserved endocrine function and follicular development. Approximately 10 weeks after ovarian transplantation to the forearm, endocrine function was restored with decreased FSH and LH levels, and cyclical variation of peripheral estradiol levels [56]. Silber reported the recovery of ovarian function in terms of recovery of menstrual cycles and hormone levels (FSH) approximately 80 to 140 days after transplantation from their fresh and frozen transplant cases [54].

1. Ovarian Function after Auto-transplantation

Recently, a review of 60 cases of reimplantation was reported from Donnez's group, Andersen's group, and Pellicer's group [4]. All ovarian tissue were frozen with the slow-freezing method and the restoration of ovarian activity was observed in at least 92.9% (52 cases among the [4]. In all cases, it took 3.5–6.5 months after transplantation before a rise in E2 and a decrease in FSH were detected (mean 4.5 months). The time to the E2 peak, concomitant with the FSH decrease, was longer (5.5–6.5 months) in patients who had received chemotherapy before cryopreservation than in those who had not (3.5–4.5 months).

2. Ovarian Function after Iso-transplantation

Dr. Silber reported his novel experience about the nine identical twin pairs discordant for premature ovarian failure that underwent their orthotopic ovarian isotransplantation between 2004 and 2008 [41]. All of these fresh ovary transplants were successful, resulting in 11 healthy babies in 7 of the 9 recipients. The same surgical techniques were then applied to 3 frozen ovary tissue transplants, up to 14 years after the ovary had been frozen, resulting in 3 more healthy babies [42, 43].

Silber *et al.* reported that the first rise in estradiol was observed 71 days after implantation of fresh tissue [41]. In their published series, the time to first menses after transplantation ranged between 65 to 93 days [42]. Recipients routinely resumed ovulatory menstrual cycles and normal Day 3 serum FSH levels by 4.5 months. Most conceived naturally (three of them twice or three times from the same graft). The duration of function of fresh ovarian grafts indicated minimal oocyte loss from ischemia period. Grafts of just modest portions of ovarian tissue have lasted >7 years. *In vitro* studies suggest that vitrification of ovarian tissue may be an improvement over the 70% oocyte viability loss from slow freeze [43].

This newly favorable experience is not limited just to one center [4, 55]. Equally robust results are being experienced in Brussels, Paris, Spain, Denmark and Israel. Frozen ovarian grafts with the slow freeze technique in Denmark are lasting over 5 years and many spontaneous pregnancies have been reported without IVF techniques or other adjuvant treatment. To date, 35 healthy babies have been born from ovarian tissue grafting including fresh/frozen ovarian tissue transplantation, and most involved no IVF, and resulted from just regular intercourse without any other treatment [3, 4].

3. Ovarian Function after Allo-Transplantation

Dr. Donnez reported three cases of ovarian transplantation between two genetically non-identical sisters in 2010 [57]. The three recipient patients presented with iatrogenic premature ovarian failure due to chemotherapy and radiotherapy. The recipients had all received ovarian tissue from their HLA-compatible sisters in each case. Premature ovarian failure was confirmed by very high FSH and LH levels, very low estradiol concentrations and the absence of follicles in large biopsies removed from the patients' atrophic ovaries during transplantation. For the first time, successful restoration of ovarian function after transplantation of ovarian cortex between genetically different sisters was reported.

The time interval between implantation of ovarian tissue and follicular development was found to be between 3.5 and 6 months, consistent with the previous study by Silber *et al.* [41]. The time interval of 6 months observed in patients 1 was associated with a low follicular reserve in the donor (aged 32 years), and a delay for the primordial follicles development. In Patients 2 and 3, the follicular density of the donor ovarian specimen was high and recovery of ovarian activity occurred 3.5 months after transplantation, as observed in the series of Silber and Gosden [42], who also observed an interval of 3.5 months after transplantation of fresh ovarian cortex between monozygotic twins. In addition, the ischemic period was recently estimated to be between 3 and 5 days by van Eyck *et al.* [58, 59].

Longevity of Ovarian Transplantation

Dr. Kim reported the longevity of ovarian grafts in five cancer patients who underwent heterotopic autotransplantation of frozen-thawed ovarian tissue between 2001 and 2011 [60]. The age of patients at the time of ovarian transplantation was between 30 and 40. Cryopreserved ovarian tissue (for 1–10 years) was rapidly thawed and transplanted into the space between the rectus sheath and muscle. Endocrine function was measured by monthly blood tests (FSH, LH, E_2, progesterone and testosterone) and ultrasound after transplantation. The monitoring was continued until the cessation of endocrine function had been confirmed by consecutive blood tests (E_2<20 pg/mL; FSH≥35 IU/L).

Endocrine function was restored in all patients between 12–20 weeks after ovarian tissue transplantation. Four patients required the second transplantation one to two years after the first transplantation. The duration of endocrine function after the second transplantation was much longer (9–84 months). The longest duration of endocrine function was observed in a patient who underwent ovarian transplantation in 2003 and 2004 after radiotherapy for cervical cancer. Even for more than seven years after transplantation, endocrine function had not ceased (FSH 9.5 IU/L, E_2 108 pg/mL). She underwent three IVF cycles which resulted in four embryos.

The longevity of grafted ovarian tissue has been debated for many years. The duration of endocrine function after frozen-thawed ovarian tissue transplantation is still uncertain. Dr. Kim described that the endocrine function lasting for seven years can be established with heterotopic transplantation of cryobanked human ovarian tissue. This information will benefit young cancer survivors with premature ovarian failure.

In the UK, researchers indicated that the duration of graft life is greater than 7 years [61].Undoubtedly, the length of time the grafts function will depend on several factors [60, 61].

Table 2. Factors associated with the longevity of grafted ovarian tissue

1. Age at the time of cryopreservation
2. Baseline ovarian reserve
3. History of cancer treatment
4. Techniques of ovarian tissue preparation
5. Freezing-thawing protocols
6. Number of cortical tissue grafted
7. Techniques and sites of transplantation
8. Degree of ischemia after transplantation
9. Number of follicles in the ovarian grafts

One of the most important factors may be the number of eggs' survival during the freezing-thawing and revascularization process. If one makes an assumption that one third of an ovary is transplanted into the patient (the proportion quoted in the linked report), and that during revascularization two thirds of the immature eggs are lost,[62, 63] then we can calculate how many immature eggs are likely to survive the freeze/thaw and revascularization process to ensure that >1000 non-growing follicles are successfully transplanted (the number present at the menopause) [64, 65]. It has been estimated that at age 36.9 years insufficient non-growing follicles will remain after cryopreservation to sustain ovarian function in 40% of the healthy population. At age 40 years we estimate that 60% of healthy women will be unlikely to benefit from ovarian cryopreservation.

We need to assess the indications and risk-benefit analysis carefully for future patients. The value of ovarian cryopreservation to preserve fertility for young cancer survivors may be proven, however the indications for those who should be offered this new technology are not yet established.

Pregnancy Outcomes after Ovarian Tissue Cryopreservation and Transplantation

Recent data from the three different groups, including a total of 60 patients who underwent orthotopic transplantation reported that eleven patients became pregnant including two ongoing pregnancies at 24 and 30 weeks, and six of these women have already delivered

12 healthy babies [4]. Approximately, the success rate of pregnancy after ovarian tissue cryopreservation and transplantation has been reached 18.3% (11 cases out of 60 patietns). The slow-freezing procedure was used in all cases. The fact that more than 50% of women were able to conceive naturally constitutes a good argument in favor of orthotopic reimplantation. The age of patients at the time of cryopreservation is a predictive factor, as previously mentioned. The majority of pregnant women were under 30 years old. Although all pregnancies were obtained from the slow-freezing technique, vitrification results in experimental models are considering increasingly promising.

Based on the site of reimplantation of cryopreserved ovarian tissue, transplantation can be divided into two different types as orthotopic (into the pelvic cavity or onto the ovarian medulla or peritoneal window) and heterotopic (to the abdominal wall, forearm, rectus muscle, etc.) transplantation [66]. The clinical value of heterotopic reimplantation remains questionable due to the lack of pregnancy with this approach compared with the 24 live births obtained after ortothopic transplantation. Heterotopic sites may not provide an optimal environment for follicular development. There may be differences in temperature, pressure, paracrine factors, and blood supply. However, endocrine function restoration has been reported consistently after heterotopic ovarian transplantation [56]. Oktay et al. [56, 66] and Kim [60] indiacated that the advantages of heterotopic ovarian tissue transplantation include: 1) avoidance of invasive procedures; 2) easy recovery of oocytes; 3) cost-effective technology when repeated transplantation is required; and 4) feasibility even in case of severe pelvic adhesions that preclude orthotopic transplantation

Medical Ovarian Suppression to Preserve Fertility

Given the current evidence, both the efficacy and safety of the use of GnRH agonists or antagonists during chemotherapy for prevention of gonadal damage are controversial. Several studies have suggested a decreased incidence of amenorrhea with the use of GnRH agonists throughout chemotherapy; however, most have been non-randomized or small sample sized studies. Only five randomized trials have been completed.

Badawy *et al.* [67] and Del Mastro *et al.* [68] demonstrated the positive effect of GnRH agonists on the resumption of menses and ovulation; however, Leonard *et al.* [69], Gerber *et al.* [70], and Munster *et al.* [71] revealed that there was no impact of GnRH agonists on the prevention of early menopause or ovarian function.

Recently, Partidge [72] reported that women who are interested in future fertility and the providers who are assisting them should not depend on GnRH agonist treatment during chemotherapy for preservation of menstrual and ovarian function or fertility. There is one randomized ongoing study by the Southwest Oncology Group, called the Prevention of Early Menopause Study, a large international multicenter trial. This study will provide additional complementary information including biomarkers of ovarian reserve and rates of long-term amenorrhea or premature ovarian failure in women with or without ovarian suppression throughout treatment period.

Given the current state of knowledge about these agents, GnRH agonist is not an effective method of fertility preservation. Additionally, complete ovarian suppression is not achieved for several weeks after GnRH agonist administration. However, there may be other potential benefits such as inhibiting menses during intensive chemotherapy, thus preventing complications such as menorrhagia. This class of drugs also has adverse effects such as hot flashes and bone loss [18].

Conclusion

Based on our review, we believe that ovarian cryopreservation and transplantation in women diagnosed with cancer before cancer treatments is an effective option to preserve their fertility and to restore gonadal endocrine function. Restoration of ovarian activity in terms of estrogen production was observed in almost all cases of ovarian transplantation. All pregnancies were reported from the orthotopic autotransplantation, but none from the heterotopic autotransplantation. Restoration of endocrine function has been demonstrated consistently in both methods, although heterotopic sites may not provide an optimal environment for pregnancy. Physicians should consider the life span and the time period for the initiation of estrogen production of transplanted ovarian tissue in order to provide an exact data, especially when counseling and making a treatment plan for cancer survivors.

References

[1] American Cancer Society. Cancer facts and figures 2012. Atlanta: American Cancer Society. Available at: http://www.cancer.org/research/cancerfactsfigures/cancerfactsfigures/cancer-facts-figures-2012; 2012. Accessed December 16, 2012.

[2] Howlader N, Noone AM, Krapcho M, Neyman N, Aminou R, Waldron W, et al. (eds.). *SEER cancer statistics review,* 1975–2009 (vintage 2009 populations). Bethesda, MD: National Cancer Institute. Available at: http: //seer.cancer.gov/csr/ 1975_ 2009_pops09/. Accessed December 16, 2012.

[3] Oktay K, Karlikaya G. Ovarian function after transplantation of frozen, banked autologous ovarian tissue. *NEngl J Med.* 2000;342:1919.

[4] Donnez J, Dolmans MM, Pellicer A, Diaz-Garcia C, Serrano MS, Schmidt KT, et al. Restoration of ovarian activity and pregnancy after transplantatoin of cyopreserved ovarian tissue : a review of 60 cases of reimplantation. *Fertil Steril* 2013 ;99:1503-13.

[5] Rodriguez-Wallberg KA, Oktay K. Options on fertility preservation in female cancer patients. *Cancer Treat Rev* 2012;38:354-61.

[6] Sklar C. Maintenance of ovarian function and risk of premature menopause related to cancer treatment. *J Natl Cancer Inst Monogr* 2005:25-7.

[7] Wallace WH, Thomson AB, Saran F, Kelsey TW. Predicting age of ovarian failure after radiation to a field that includes the ovaries. *Int J Radiat Oncol Biol Phys* 2005;62:738-44.

[8] Wo JY, Viswanathan AN. Impact of radiotherapy on fertility, pregnancy, and neonatal outcomes in female cancer patients. *Int J Radiat Oncol Biol Phys* 2009;73:1304-12.

[9] Green DM, Sklar CA, Boice JD Jr, Mulvihill JJ, Whitton JA, Stovall M, et al. Ovarian failure and reproductive outcomes after childhood cancer treatment: results from the Childhood Cancer Survivor Study. *J Clin. Oncol* 2009;27:2374-81.

[10] Chemaitilly W, Mertens AC, Mitby P, Whitton J, Stovall M, Yasui Y, et al. Acute ovarian failure in the childhood cancer survivor study. *J Clin Endocrinol Metab* 2006;91:1723-8.

[11] Oktem O, Oktay K. Fertility preservation for breast cancer patients. *Semin Reprod Med* 2009;27:486-92.

[12] Azim A, Rauch ER, Ravich M, Witkin S, Oktay K. Ovarian reserve is impaired in cancer patients with normal baseline FSH who previously received chemotherapy as determined by response to controlled ovarian stimulation and anti-mullerian hormone measurements: a controlled study. *Fertil Steril* 2006;86 (Suppl 2):S123-S4.

[13] Lee S, Heytens E, Moy F, Ozkavukcu S, Oktay K. Determinants of access to fertility preservation in women with breast cancer. *Fertil Steril* 2011;95:1932-6.

[14] Lee S, Ozkavukcu S, Heytens E, Moy F, Oktay K. Value of early referral to fertility preservation in young women with breast cancer. *J Clin Oncol* 2010;28:4683-6.

[15] Quinn GP, Vadaparampil ST, Lee JH, Jacobsen PB, Bepler G, Lancaster J, et al. Physician referral for fertility preservation in oncology patients: a national study of practice behaviors. *J Clin Oncol* 2009;27:5952-7.

[16] Forman EJ, Anders CK, Behera MA. Pilot survey of oncologists regarding treatment-related infertility and fertility preservation in female cancer patients. *J Reprod Med* 2009;54:203-7.

[17] Armuand GM, Rodriguez-Wallberg KA, Wettergren L, Ahlgren J, Enblad G, Hoglund M, et al. Sex differences in fertility-related information received by young adult cancer survivors. *J Clin Oncol* 2012;30:2147-53.

[18] Loren AW, Mangu PB, Beck LN, Brennan L, Magdalinski BA, Partridge AH, et al. Fertility Preservation for Patients With Cancer:American Society of Clinical Oncology Clinical Practice Guideline Update. *J ClinOncol* 2013 May 28 [Epub ahead of print]

[19] Suh CO. Radiotherapy for breast cancer. *J Korean Med Assoc* 2003;46:503-11.

[20] Jemal A, Murray T, Ward E, Samuels A, Tiwari RC, Ghafoor A, et al. Cancer statistics, 2005. *CA Cancer J Clin* 2005;55:10-30.

[21] Plante M, Gregoire J, Renaud MC, Roy M. The vaginal radical trachelectomy: an update of a series of 125 cases and 106 pregnancies. *Gynecol Oncol* 2011;121:290-7.

[22] Marnitz S, Kohler C, Schneider A, Seiler F, Hinkelbein W. Interindividual variability of lymph drainages in patients with cervical cancer. Implication on irradiation planning. *Strahlenther Onkol* 2006;182:80-5.

[23] Martin JR, Kodaman P, Oktay K, Taylor HS. Ovarian cryopreservation with transposition of a contralateral ovary: a combined approach for fertility preservation in women receiving pelvic radiation. *Fertil Steril* 2007;87:189 e5-7.

[24] Hwang JH, Yoo HJ, Park SH, Lim MC, Seo SS, Kang S, et al. Association between the location of transposed ovary and ovarian function in patients with uterine cervical cancer treated with (postoperative or primary) pelvic radiotherapy. *Fertil Steril* 2012;97:1387-93 e2.

[25] American Cancer Society: Cancer Facts & Figures 2009. [Internet]. Atlanta: American Cancer Society Inc.; c2009 [2012 Jun 27]. Available from: http://www.cancer.org/acs/groups/content/@nho/documents/document/500809webpdf.pdf.

[26] Sonmezer M, Oktay K. Fertility preservation in young women undergoing breast cancer therapy. *Oncologist* 2006;11:422-34.

[27] Azim AA, Costantini-Ferrando M, Oktay K. Safety of fertility preservation by ovarian stimulation with letrozole and gonadotropins in patients with breast cancer: a prospective controlled study. *J Clin Oncol* 2008;26:2630-5
[28] Goss PE, Ingle JN, Martino S, Robert NJ, Muss HB, Piccart MJ, et al. A randomized trial of letrozole in postmenopausal women after five years of tamoxifen therapy for early-stage breast cancer. *N Engl J Med* 2003;349:1793-802.
[29] Winer EP, Hudis C, Burstein HJ, et al. American Society of Clinical Oncology technology assessment on the use of aromatase inhibitors as adjuvant therapy for women with hormone receptor-positive breast cancer: status report 2002. *J ClinOncol* 2002; 20(15):3317-3327.
[30] Buzdar A, Jonat W, Howell A, et al. Anastrozole, a potent and selective aromatase inhibitor, versus megestrol acetate in postmenopausal women with advanced breast cancer: results of overview analysis of two phase III trials. Arimidex Study Group. *J Clin Oncol* 1996; 14:2000-2011.
[31] Marty, M, Gershanovich, M, Campos, B, Romien, G, et al. Aromatase inhibitors, a new potent, selective aromatase inhibitor superior to aminoglutethimide in postmenopausal women with advanced breast cancer previously treated with antioestrogens. *Proc Am Soc Clin Oncol* 1997; 16:156.
[32] Hamilton A, Piccart M. The third-generation non-steroidal aromatase inhibitors: a review of their clinical benefits in the second-line hormonal treatment of advanced breast cancer. *Ann Oncol* 1999; 10:377-384.
[33] Goss PE. Risks versus benefits in the clinical application of aromatase inhibitors. *Endocr Relat Cancer* 1999; 6:325-332.
[34] Oktay K. Further evidence on the safety and success of ovarian stimulation with letrozole and tamoxifen in breast cancer patients undergoing in vitro fertilization to cryopreserve their embryos for fertility preservation. *J Clin Oncol* 2005;23:3858-3859.
[35] Cakmak H, Rosen MP. Ovarian stimulation in cancer patients. *Fertil Steril* 99:1476-84,2013.
[36] Lohrisch C, Paltiel C, Gelmon K, Speers C, Taylor S, Barnett J, et al. Impact on survival of time from definitive surgery to initiation of adjuvant chemotherapy for early-stage breast cancer. *J Clin Oncol* 2006;24:4888-94.
[37] Cold S, During M, Ewertz M, Knoop A, Moller S. Does timing of adjuvant chemotherapy influence the prognosis after early breast cancer? Results of the Danish Breast Cancer Cooperative Group (DBCG). *Br J Cancer* 2005;93:627-32.
[38] Lee S, Oktay K. Does higher starting dose of FSH stimulation with letrozole improve fertility preservation outcomes in women with breast cancer. *Fertil Steril* 2012 ;98 :961-4.
[39] Oktay K, Oktem O. Ovarian cryopreservation and transplantation for fertility preservation for medical indications: report of an ongoing experience. *Fertil. Steril.* 2008;93(3): 762–8.
[40] Donnez J, Dolmans MM, Demylle D, et al. Livebirth after orthotopic transplantation of cryopreserved ovarian tissue. *Lancet* 2004;364:1405-10.
[41] Silber SJ, Lenahan KM, Levine DJ, et al. Ovarian transplantation between monozygotic twins discordant for premature ovarian failure. *N Engl J Med* 2005; 353:58.

[42] Silber SJ, Gosden RG. Ovarian transplantation in a series of monozygotic twins discordant for ovarian failure. *N Engl J Med* 2007; 356:1382.

[43] Silber SJ, Grudzinskas G, Gosden RG. Successful pregnancy after microsurgical transplantation of an intact ovary. *N Engl J Med* 2008; 359:2617.

[44] Donnez J, Dolmans MM, Squifflet J, et al. Live birth after allografting of ovarian cortex between monozygotic twins with Turner syndrome (45,XO/46,XX mosaicism) and discordant ovarian function. *Fertil Steril* 2011; 96:1407.

[45] Oktay K, Newton H, Mullan J, Gosden RG. Development of human primordial follicles to antral stages in SCID/hpg mice stimulated with follicle stimulating hormone. *Hum Reprod* 1998; 13:1133.

[46] Oktay K, Newton H, Gosden RG. Transplantation of cryopreserved human ovarian tissue results in follicle growth initiation in SCID mice. *Fertil Steril* 2000;73:599.

[47] Gook DA, McCully BA, Edgar DH, McBain JC. Development of antral follicles in human cryopreserved ovarian tissue following xenografting. *Hum Reprod* 2001; 16:417.

[48] Lucifero D, Mertineit C, Clarke HJ, et al. Methylation dynamics of imprinted genes in mouse germ cells. *Genomics* 2002; 79:530.

[49] Kim SS, Kang HG, Kim NH, et al. Assessment of the integrity of human oocytes retrieved from cryopreserved ovarian tissue after xenotransplantation. *Hum Reprod* 2005; 20:2502.

[50] Donnez J, Dolmans MM, Demylle D, et al. Livebirth after orthotopic transplantation of cryopreserved ovarian tissue. *Lancet* 2004;364:1405-10.

[51] Meirow D, Levron J, Eldar-Geva T, et al. Pregnancy after transplantation of cryopreserved ovarian tissue in a patient with ovarian failure after chemotherapy. *N Engl J Med* 2005;353:318-21.

[52] Demeestere I, Simon P, Emiliani S, et al. Fertility preservation: successful transplantation of cryopreserved ovarian tissue in a young patient previously treated for Hodgkin's disease. *Oncologist* 2007;12:1437-42.

[53] Andersen CY, Rosendahl M, Byskov AG, et al. Two successful pregnancies following autotransplantation of frozen/thawed ovarian tissue. *Hum Reprod* 2008;23:2266-72.

[54] Sibler SJ. Ovarian cryopreservation and transplantation for fertility preservation.*Mol Hum Reprod 2012*;18:59-67.

[55] Donnez J, Silber S, Andersen CY, Demeestere I, Piver P, Meirow D, et al. Children born after autotransplantation of cryopreserved ovarian tissue. a review of 13 live births. *Ann Med* 2011;43:437-50.

[56] Oktay K, Economos K, Kan M, Rucinski J, Veeck L, Rosenwaks Z. Endocrine function and oocyte retrieval after autologous transplantation of ovarian cortical strips to the forearm. *JAMA* 2001;286:1490-3.

[57] Donnez J, Squifflet J, Pirard C, Jadoul P, Dolmans MM. Restroration of ovarian function after allografting of ovarian cortex between genetically non-identical sisters. *Hum Reprod* 2010;25:2489-2495.

[58] Van Eyck AS, Jordan B, Gallez B, Heilier JF, Van Langendonckt A, Donnez J.Electron paramagnetic resonance as a tool to evaluate human ovariantissue reoxygenation after xenografting. *Fertil Steril* 2009;92:374–381.

[59] Van Eyck AS, Bouzin C, Feron O, Romeu L, Van Langendonckt A,Donnez J, Dolmans MM. Both host and graft vessels contribute torevascularization of xenografted human ovarian tissue in a murinemodel. *Fertil Steril* 2010;93:1676–1685.
[60] Kim SS. Assessment of long term endocrine function after transplantation of frozen-thawed human ovarian tissue to the heterotopic site: 10 year longitudinal follow-up study. *J Assist Reprod Genet.* 2012;29:489-493.
[61] Wallace WH, Kelsey TW, Anderson RA. Ovarian cryopreservation: experimental or established and a cure for the menopause? *Reprod Biomed Online* 2012;25:93-95.
[62] Baird, D.T., Webb, R., Campbell, B.K., Harkness, L.M., Gosden,R.G. Long-term ovarian function in sheep after ovariectomyand transplantation of autografts stored at -196°C. *Endocrinology* 1999;140: 462–471.
[63] Demirci, B., Lornage, J., Salle, B., Frappart, L., Franck, M.,Guerin, J.F., 2001. Follicular viability and morphology ofsheep ovaries after exposure to cryoprotectant and cryopreservationwith different freezing protocols. *Fertil. Steril.* 2001;75:754–762.
[64] Faddy, M.J., Gosden, R.G. A model conforming the decline infollicle numbers to the age of menopause in women. *Hum Reprod.* 1996;11:1484–1486.
[65] Wallace, W.H., Kelsey, T.W. Human ovarian reserve fromconception to the menopause. *PLoS One* 2010;5:e8772.
[66] Rodriguez-Wallberg KA, Oktay K. Recent advances in oocyte and ovarian tissue cryopreservation and transplantation. *Best Pract Res Clin Obstet Gynaecol* 2012;26:391–405.
[67] Badawy A, Elnashar A, El-Ashry M, Shahat M. Gonadotropin-releasing hormone agonists for prevention of chemotherapy-induced ovarian damage: prospective randomized study. *Fertil Steril* 2009;91:694-7.
[68] Del Mastro L, Boni L, Michelotti A, Gamucci T, Olmeo N, Gori S, et al. Effect of the gonadotropin-releasing hormone analogue triptorelin on the occurrence of chemotherapy-induced early menopause in premenopausal women with breast cancer: a randomized trial. *JAMA* 2011;306:269-76.
[69] Leonard RC, Adamson D, Anderson R, Ballinger R, Bertelli G, Coeman RE, et al. The OPTION trial of adjuvant ovarian protection by goserelin in adjuvant chemotherapy for early breast cancer [abstract 590]. *J ClinOncol* 2010;28 (Suppl 15):89s.
[70] Gerber B, von Minckwitz G, Stehle H, Reimer T, Felberbaum R, Maass N, et al. Effect of luteinizing hormone-releasing hormone agonist on ovarian function after modern adjuvant breast cancer chemotherapy: the GBG 37 ZORO study. *J Clin Oncol* 2011;29:2334-41.
[71] Munster PN, Moore AP, Ismail-Khan R, Cox CE, Lacevic M, Gross-King M, et al. Randomized trial using gonadotropin-releasing hormone agonist triptorelin for the preservation of ovarian function during (neo)adjuvant chemotherapy for breast cancer. *J Clin Oncol* 2012;30:533-8.
[72] Partridge AH. Ovarian suppression for prevention of premature menopause and infertility: empty promise or effective therapy? *J Clin Oncol* 2012;30:479-81.

In: Estradiol: Synthesis, Health Effects and Drug Interactions ISBN: 978-1-62808-962-2
Editors: Ricco Palmeri and Sal Grimaudo

Chapter 12

Estradiol-Mediated Overmodulation of the Neuroendocrine Hormone Dopamine is Central to the Pathophysiology of Restless Legs Syndrome During Pregnancy

***Jose Carlos Pereira Jr.*[*1], *Ingrid Ramos Rocha e Silva*[2] and *Marcia Pradella-Hallinan*[3]**

[1]Faculdade de Medicina de Jundiaí, Rua Francisco Telles, Jundiaí, São Paulo, Brazil

[2]Faculdade de Medicina da Universidade de São Paulo, Brazil

[3]Universidade Federal de São Paulo, Instituto do Sono, Departamento de Psicobiologia, São Paulo, SP, Brazil

Abstract

A large corpus of evidence points to an imbalance between the classical thyroid gland hormone (TH) and the neuroendocrine hormone dopamine (DA, [IMBTH/DA]) as the main derangement underpinning the pathophysiology of restless legs syndrome (RLS). DA is released by the hypothalamus into the portal blood circulation of the pituitary stalk, where it modulates the release of thyrotropin by the pituitary: DA inhibits the synthesis of the two component subunits of thyrotropin, alpha and beta. Furthermore, the dopaminergic system enhances the activity of the cytochrome P450 superfamily of enzymes via mesolimbic and tuberoinfundibular pathways. As nearly 20% of thyroid hormone is metabolized in these pathways, when DA activity increases, TH activity decreases. TH is essential for somatosensory system physiology, including the sensitivity of somatosensory receptors deep in the legs. When the thresholds of these somatic receptors are diminished, or when their signaling to the sensory cortex is too strongly transmitted, RLS may ensue. One action of TH is to positively influence the sensitivity of

* Email: jcpereirajr@uol.com.br.

the receptors and the strength of their signal transmission to the sensory cortex. DA modulates this TH activity, and when DA is diminished, TH is increased, which may result in IMBTH/DA and RLS. RLS is more common in pregnant than in non-pregnant women, and during pregnancy, TH activity increases to meet the augmented metabolic necessities of pregnancy. Estradiol during pregnancy increases exponentially, and one of the effects of estradiol is the inhibition of DA release in the pituitary stalk. Furthermore, estradiol also increases thyrotropin release by increasing the sensitivity of thyrotrophic cells in the pituitary to thyrotropin-releasing hormone from the hypothalamus. It is known that estradiol levels in RLS pregnant women are higher than those in non-RLS pregnant women. In this chapter, we present evidence that suggests that excessive estradiol-mediated modulation of DA is central to the pathophysiology of RLS during pregnancy.

Introduction

Restless legs syndrome (RLS), also called Willis-Ekbom disease, is a common sensorimotor disorder affecting approximately 5 to 15 percent of the population [1, 2]. Prevalences vary widely depending upon the population studied and the severity of the symptoms required for diagnosis. RLS has been reported to be moderately or severely distressing by 2,7-percent of the population [3]. RLS is more common in pregnant (up to 26%) than in non-pregnant women [4, 5]. RLS may severely impair sleep and the quality of life of the affected patients.

RLS is a typical "case-description" disease, that is, the establishment of a diagnosis requires the fulfillment of some criteria. The four criteria described by the International Restless Legs Syndrome Study group (IRLSSG) are the following: 1) symptoms begin when the patient is at rest; 2) symptoms include an almost irresistible desire to move the legs that is accompanied (in most cases) or unaccompanied by annoying paresthesias; 3) relief is obtained while the patient continues to move; and 4) the symptoms only appear in the evening/night or are worse in the evening/night [6]. There are other features that can be supportive of the diagnosis and may guide clinical judgments when diagnoses are not straightforward: 1) there are one or more cases of RLS in the family of the patient; 2) the patient presents with periodic movements (PLM) during sleep (up to 90% of RLS patients present with PLM) and may also present with PLM during wakefulness; and 3) nearly all patients report amelioration of symptoms after treatment with dopamine agonists, at least initially. This latter finding supports the diagnosis, and its absence makes the diagnosis unlikely. RLS may be primary (idiopathic) or secondary to other disease conditions [6, 7].

For the majority of scholars who study RLS, its comprehensive pathophysiology is currently uncertain. Nonetheless, some topics have reached consensus among researchers: 1) a dopaminergic dysfunction is involved, as dopamine agonists ameliorate symptoms in the majority of affected patients; and 2) iron deficiency (or deranged iron physiology) plays a role, as iron-deficient patients are more predisposed to RLS, and frequently, iron administration relieves symptoms [7]. However, the medical literature contains overwhelming evidence supporting the idea that an imbalance between the dopaminergic system and the thyroid axis (IMBDA/TH) is the derangement underlying RLS pathophysiology (8). One function of the neurohormone dopamine (DA) is the modulation of the classical hormone of the thyroid gland (TH) (9, 10), and one function of TH is the enhancement of receptivity to stimuli from the peripheral sensory system (PSS) that enhances signaling to the somatosensory cortex (11).

When DA activity is insufficient to counteract TH, the PSS receptors deep inside the legs have lower thresholds for stimuli that result in enhanced signaling to the sensory cortex, which may precede RLS (12, 13) (Figure 1). Much circumstantial evidence favors the IMBDA/TH theory as the causative factor of RLS [8]; in the following, we will cite these lines of evidence by topic.

1) DA agonists alleviate RLS symptoms, meaning that the DA *dysfunction* hypothesis involves a *decline* in DA activity [7].
2) TH is essential for the somatosensory system (11); when TH activity is augmented, peripheral sensations are strongly transmitted to the sensory cortices, and an inhibition in transmission occurs when TH activity is diminished [11, 14].
3) DA is an inhibitor of prolactin and thyrotropin [9, 10]; through inhibition of thyrotropin, DA decreases the release of TH by the TH gland, which diminishes the sensitivity and strength of signaling of the PSS receptors (which would be felt as RLS sensations) [12]. DA agonists decrease TH activity *via* enhancing DA activity [12, 13].
4) DA also induces increased activity of the enzyme CYP4503A4 isoform [15, 16], through which some TH is metabolized [17]; when CYP3A4 is inhibited, TH levels increase, and RLS symptoms may ensue [8]. The great majority of drugs that inhibit CYP3A4 worsen RLS symptoms, and many drugs that ameliorate RLS enhance CYP3A4 activity. Additionally, DA-antagonist drugs frequently cause secondary RLS [18] (Table 1).
5) The fourth IRLSSG criterion for WED (worsening of the symptoms at night) [6] occurs concomitantly with a steep increase in thyrotropin levels in the evening, which represent the highest levels of TH during wakefulness [13, 19].
6) Iron deficiencies may play a role in triggering RLS symptoms in some subjects or worsening existant RLS [7]. Iron is a component of the enzyme tyrosine hydroxylase, which catalyzes the conversion of L-tyrosine into L-DOPA; this reaction is the rate-limiting step in the production of DA [14]. When iron levels are insufficient, tyrosine hydroxylase may not be fully expressed and DA synthesis may be decreased [8]. Figuratively, we can say that the *iron* hypothesis for RLS is actually the same as the *DA* hypothesis; that is, both are related to a decline in DA activity.
7) Iron is also a component of CYP3A4 [14]; as such, the expression of this enzyme may be reduced when iron is lacking. In these circumstances, CYP3A4 activity is diminished, which consequently diminishes TH degradation, resulting in increased levels of TH. DA may not sufficiently increase to adequately counteract TH. Therefore, iron scarcity may play a dual role in favoring IMBDA/TH, that is, it diminishes DA and increases TH (Figure 2).
8) In Grave's disease (hyperthyroidism) patients, RLS-like symptoms are much more common than in normal subjects (8,8% versus 0,9%). However, in all of these patients, RLS presents without the fourth IRLSSG criterion (worsening at night), which may preclude Grave's disease subjects from receiving a definite RLS diagnosis [20]. Notwithstanding, in Grave's disease, TH release does not follow any circadian rhythmicity; TSH-receptor antibodies bind to the thyrotropin-receptor in a

continued, non-pulsatile and non-chaotic fashion (21). As the fourth criterion for RLS cases is secondary to the thyrotropin evening surge (as discussed above), most Grave's disease patients who concomitantly present RLS do not fulfill all of the IRLSSG criteria for an RLS diagnosis.

9) Pramipexole, an effective treatment for WED, is a typical DA agonist with a selective affinity for the D2 receptor subfamily [22]. Pramipexole induces the expression of many CYP450 enzymes through the tuberoinfundibular and mesolimbic dopaminergic pathways [15, 16], thus increasing TH metabolism. Furthermore, pramipexole decreases thyrotropin release [10].
10) It is known from clinical settings that intravenous administration of dopamine diminishes TH levels [23, 24].
11) From clinical studies of RLS, sleep deprivation is known to worsen its symptomatology [25]. One of the most conspicuous endocrine alterations occurring during sleep deprivation is a striking increase in thyrotropin levels [26]), which causes an IMBDA/TH.
12) Recently, it has been observed (2013) that a side effect of domperidone, a DA antagonist, is the worsening of RLS severity. This is in contrast to what was accepted before [27]. Previously, it was believed that domperidone was not able to cross the blood brain barrier (BBB) and would thus not be harmful to RLS patients, in contrast to other DA antagonists that do cross the BBB [7]. "This unexpected finding suggests that dopaminergic neurons outside of the BBB may be important in RLS pathophysiology" [27]. The DA tuberoinfundibular pathway is the only DA system that modulates thyrotropin release through inhibiting the synthesis of the two subunits (alpha and beta) that constitute this thyroid-stimulating hormone [10]. DA neurons in the arcuate nucleus of the hypothalamus project to the median eminence (outside the BBB) and release the neurohormone DA, which then reaches the blood portal system of the pituitary stalk. Thereafter, DA inhibits thyrotropin (and prolactin) release, which results in a diminished TH secretion by the TH gland [14, 28]. Domperidone has strong affinities for the DA2 and DA3 dopamine receptors, which are found outside of the BBB, and it is a specific blocker of these receptors [29]. Domperidone, by blocking the DA receptors present in the lactotroph and thyrotroph cells of the pituitary, increases prolactin and thyrotropin release. Domperidone does not affect DA systems inside the BBB, and prolactin is not recognized to have a role in RLS pathophysiology.Therefore, the DA antagonist action of domperidone on thyrotrophs provides strong evidence that when the thyroid axis is not appropriately modulated, RLS may ensue.

In sum, there are many ways in which IMBDA/TH may be induced, and most of them are due to increasing the activity of the TH axis. However, incrementing TH activity alone will not cause RLS.

To trigger RLS symptoms, impairment of the neurohormone DA in its function of TH modulation is required; this condition is more likely to occur in the evening and at night. Primary RLS is due to idiopathic changes in DA activity that intrinsically diminish TH activity, and secondary RLS is due to abnormal conditions that enhance TH activity and/or the impairment of DA activity by exogenous DA antagonists (e.g., metoclopramide) or endogenous antagonists (e.g., estradiol) [8, 13].

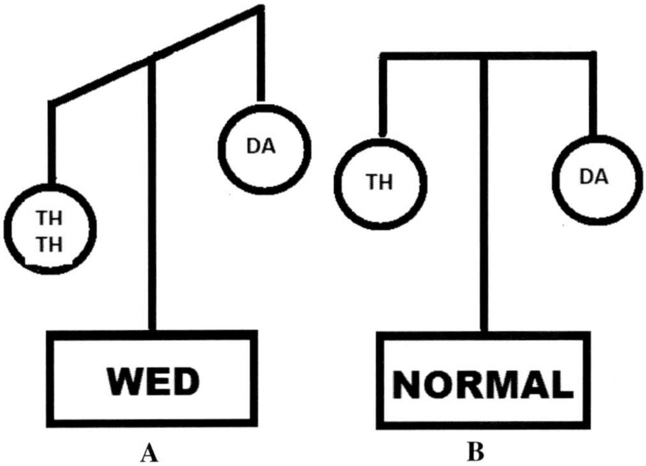

Figure 1. (A) A representation of how Willis-Ekbom syndrome (Restless legs syndrome) symptoms may occur when the "weight" of the TH axis is magnified compared to DA. (B) The "weight" of DA is sufficient to counterbalance the excitatory effects of TH. WED= Willis-Ekbom syndrome; TH = thyroid hormone; DA = dopamine.

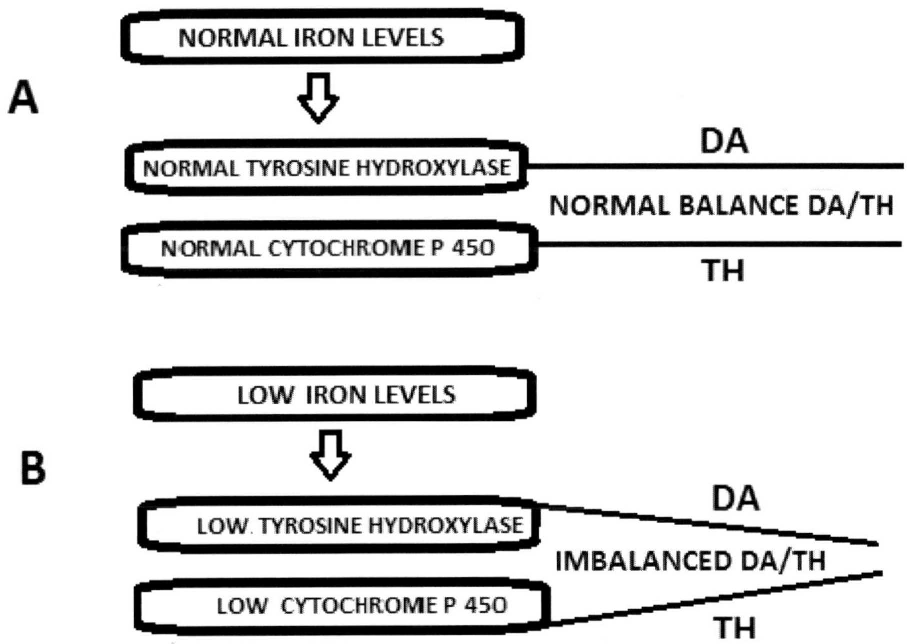

Figure 2. (A) Normal levels of iron correspond to normal expression of tyrosine hydroxylase and cytochrome P450, which result in normal DA synthesis and TH breakdown. (B) Low levels of iron correspond to diminished expression of tyrosine hydroxylase and cytochrome P450, which leads to diminished DA synthesis and TH breakdown. This effect causes an imbalance in the interaction between TH and DA. DA = dopamine; TH = thyroid hormone.

Table 1. Suggested mechanisms by which some drugs aggravate WED. The drugs listed in Table 1 affect WED by interfering with CYP3A4, as these drugs are substrates and/or inhibitors of CYP3A4, and thus, decrease TH metabolism. In addition, some drugs may cause a direct decline in dopaminergic system signaling

Class of drugs	Examples	CYP3A4 substrates	CYP3A4 inhibitors	Effects on DA system
Calcium channel blockers	Verapamil Diltiazem	Yes +++ Yes +++	Yes ++ Yes ++	No
Selective serotonin reuptake inhibitors	Fluoxetine Paroxetine Sertraline Citalopram Escitalopram Fluvoxamine	Yes + No Yes + Yes +++ Yes +++ No	Yes + Yes + Yes ++ No No Yes +	No
Neuroleptics	Haloperidol Chlorpromazine Clozapine Pimozide Quetiapine	Yes +++ Yes + Yes + Yes +++ Yes +++	Yes ++ No Yes + Yes + No	Yes: block DA D2 receptors
Anti-nausea agents	Metoclopramide Domperidone	No	No	Yes: block DA D2 receptors
Lipid-lowering agents	Atorvastatin Lovastatin Simvastatin	Yes +++ Yes +++ Yes +++	Yes + Yes + No	No
Non-steroidal anti-inflammatory drugs	Diclofenac	Yes +	Yes ++	No
Stimulants	Caffeine	Yes +	Yes ++	No

Thyroid Actions That Are Noteworthy for the Theory That Imbalance between Thyroid Hormone and Dopamine Cause Restless Legs Syndrome

TH is involved in the regulation of nearly every organ system and is responsible for the optimal development and function of all body tissues. TH acts through genomic (e.g., protein synthesis) and non-genomic (e.g., boosting of synaptic transmission) mechanisms [14, 30, 31]. TH genomic effects occur slowly and with long durations [14]. TH non-genomic actions are rapid and occur through TH's actions on mitochondria [19]. TH actions on mitochondria [14, 30, 31] make TH suitable to play an important role in circadian rhythms and synaptic neurotransmission [14, 19]. Mitochondria are the organelles responsible for adenosine triphosphate (ATP) production, and TH increases their number and activity [14]. Neurons depend on neurotransmitter synthesis in axon terminals, which is dependent on ATP production for signaling activities. Mitochondria have receptors for TH on their surfaces that enable very quick responses that increase ATP production [14, 30, 31]. Burnstock introduced the concept of purinergic neurotransmission (1972), which has been evolving, and it is currently generally accepted that the multifunctional nucleoside ATP is also a neurotransmitter. ATP acts mainly as an excitatory neurotransmitter [32, 33]. ATP is now recognized to have roles in a wide range of nervous system activities, including pain and mechanosensory transduction [32]. Ionotropic purinergic receptors are widely distributed throughout the nervous system, and they play an important role in sensory nerves. ATP is also present in the neurons of the dorsal root ganglia as an excitatory neurotransmitter. These neurons have an axon connected to PSS receptors [32-34]. Thus, by enhancing ATP production, TH increases the velocity of PSS receptor signaling to the somatosensory cortex. If modulation of this vital process, for instance, by GABA, glycine, or DA systems [14, 33], does not occur, IMBTH/DA may ensue and may result in consequent RLS symptoms [8]. From clinical settings, it is known that the drugs gabapentin (a GABA analog) and pramipexole (a dopaminergic agonist) are efficient in ameliorating RLS symptoms [7]. There is strong evidence that the dopaminergic system plays an important role in the modulation of the sensory inputs that come from the PSS receptors on their pathway to the sensory cortex [8, 35, 36]. Notably, it is known that RLS severity is greater in the evening and night [6], when thyroid axis activity is also more intense [37, 38].

Neural Basis of the Generation of Willis–Ekbom Disease Symptoms

Clinical correlates of RLS and the reasoning based on somatosensory system (SS) physiology point to the peripheral somatosensory system as the site at which RLS symptoms are generated. RLS symptoms born in the somatosensory cortex itself would actually be, in some sense, hallucinations. Indeed, sensations that are felt to come from the periphery but do not actually come from the periphery are hallucinations. It is not reasonable to assume that RLS symptoms are hallucinations because, for example, leg massages can alleviate the symptoms and cold pads frequently alleviate symptoms as well; thus, it is improbable that such common-place non-pharmacological measures would alleviate RLS symptoms if they were generated centrally. Movement of the legs brings relief to RLS patients (indeed, this is one criterion for an RLS case description). It is difficult to imagine a mechanism by which movement of the periphery would dissipate sensations born within the sensory cortex itself. There are other insights into the clinical presentation of RLS that should also be considered: patients who have undergone limb amputation above the knee may feel RLS symptoms that are restricted to the amputated leg (phantom RLS). Karl A. Ekbom, who initiated the modern era of studies (1945) of RLS [1, 2], was also one of the first researchers to describe RLS in amputees (1961). In his paper [39], and with clear and logical reasoning, he hypothesized that RLS symptoms were generated in the periphery of the nervous system. Furthermore, patients who have undergone total knee arthroplasty may feel RLS symptoms that are restricted to the leg that was operated on [12].

The exclusion of the possibility that RLS symptoms are generated centrally prompts the reasoning that they cannot prescind from the normal mechanisms of the somatosensory system physiology to be felt. As such, we assume that the PSS receptors deep inside the legs have lowered stimulation sensitivity thresholds due to the lack of appropriate DA modulation of TH actions, which enhances the strength of signaling to the sensory cortex. The dorsal sensory ganglia axons contain a number of receptors, including proprioceptors, thermoreceptors, nociceptors, mechanoreceptors, and combinations of these receptor families. We assume that the hyper-stimulation of various types of tegument receptors can cause a variety of different sensations experienced by RLS patients [14, 40]. By stretching or moving their legs, patients stretch muscles with PSS receptors, and massage produces effective relief. Patients learn that movement brings relief, and the urge to move becomes a conditioned reflex. PLMs during sleep and wakefulness [7] can be interpreted as spinal reflexes that follow the same mechanism of over-sensitivity in the PSS receptors and enhanced signaling transmission. As such, there would be a failure in the suprasegmental inhibition of the spinal cord reflexes either by the pyramidal tract or higher centers as suggested by some authors [41]. This hypothesis is plausible, as the sleep state can lead to the disinhibition of spinal cord reflexes. It is known from neurology semiology that the Babinski reflex can be found in normal subjects during sleep [34]. Our hypothesis is the following: once the receptors have been activated, their signals in the spinal cord might not be sufficiently modulated, and PLMs occur due to spinal reflexes. For RLS symptoms to occur it is necessary that the patient is awake because "higher centers" are the site of the unpleasant perceptions; and for PLM it is necessary that the patient is asleep because "higher centers" are their (PLM) inhibitors during wakefulness.

Restless Legs Syndrome during Pregnancy

RLS is more prevalent in pregnant women than in non-pregnant women; the reported prevalences of RLS in pregnant women vary from 12% to 26% [4, 5, 42, 43], implying that the physiological and biochemical changes during pregnancy influence the development of RLS [13]. Many maternal physiologic changes occur, and metabolic demands are greatly increased during pregnancy. To attend to the increased metabolic demands of pregnancy, it is necessary to enhance the TH axis; this enhancement is achieved by over-stimulation of the thyroid gland, which leads to elevated TH levels [44, 45]. Human chorionic gonadotropin (HCG) is produced by the placenta and has a direct stimulating effect on the thyroid gland [44, 45]. This stimulation is responsible for much of the TH increase in the first trimester of pregnancy. HCG production by the placenta rises exponentially until the tenth gestational week and then declines gradually until term [44, 45]. Beginning a few weeks after conception, gestational RLS prevalence increases with time, and in the third trimester, when human chorionic gonadotropin production has already declined, the prevalence of RLS reaches its highest point [4, 5, 42, 43]. As with every RLS condition, IMBTH/DA underlies the pathophysiology of RLS in pregnancy [8]. Most likely, during the initial weeks of pregnancy, the IMBDA/TH is a consequence of the direct stimulation of the TH gland by HCG. RLS develops in some but not all pregnant women, indicating that in the affected women, the production of DA neurohormone by DA neurons of the arcuate nucleus is not sufficient to counteract TH activity. During the third gestational trimester, levels of HCG decline. As RLS is more common in the third trimester, some factor other than HCG must be the prevailing cause of IMBDA/TH [13]. From the time of conception, progesterone and cortisol levels rise until term [45]. It is known that levels of the fetoplacental estrogens, estriol, estradiol, and estrogen, peak near term [45]. Notably, higher levels of estradiol have been observed in pregnant women with RLS compared to pregnant women without RLS [46]. Estradiol strongly inhibits the neurohormone DA; thus, elevated levels of estradiol in the third trimester of gestation place the effects of this hormone squarely within the core time course of the pathophysiology of RLS during pregnancy [13, 46]. DA is a tonic inhibitor of prolactin release from pituitary lactotrophs; as such, DA is also frequently called the prolactin inhibitor factor [47]. With the progression of pregnancy, the mammary glands must prepare for milk production after birth. Because prolactin is essential for this event, its level and activity must increase significantly [45]. One of the most powerful hormones that counteract DA to enable the liberation of prolactin is estradiol [45]. Estradiol inhibits DA in the tuberoinfundibular dopaminergic pathway, which enables prolactin levels to rise to respond to the physiological needs of the mammary glands for breastfeeding [48-51]. As DA release declines, DA inhibition of the two subunits (alpha and beta) that constitute the thyrotropin hormone [10] declines; this process results in increased stimulation of the TH gland and increased production and release of TH, which may lead to an IMBDA/TH. Furthermore, estradiol enhances the sensitivity of thyrotrophs to thyrotropin releasing hormone (TRH); women have stronger responses to TRH than do men, and pre-treatment with estradiol in men increases their induced TRH-thyrotropin response [9]. Therefore, it is notable that estradiol may have a dual role in causing IMBDA/TH during pregnancy: it may increase thyrotropin and decrease DA. However, estrogen replacement therapy has not been found to increase the incidence of RLS [7]. In 2013, it has been observed that domperidone; a DA blocking agent that does not cross the blood brain barrier worsens RLS symptoms of patients that make use of the drug. Of the four main DA systems, the tuberoinfundibular is the only one that is located outside the blood brain barrier, as such the only DA that domperidone may antagonize is that one of this system. It is possible to state that domperidone, in a certain manner, acts as the same the estradiol does: counteracting the action of the neurohormone DA inhibition function on thyrotrophic cells of the pituitary [52].

Other variables may also contribute to the high prevalence of RLS during pregnancy. For instance, peripheral venous distension progressively increases in pregnant women; and the peripheral vascular resistance decreases [45]. These changes may cause an increase in the pressure of the tissues surrounding the peripheral somatosensory system receptors, thus lowering their stimulus sensitivity thresholds. Iron deficiency is common during pregnancy [5, 53] and may also play a role in triggering RLS symptoms as explained in the introductory part of this chapter. Folate deficiencies may also be a factor that predisposes women to acquire RLS during pregnancy [53].

Folate is important in the production of tetrahydrobiopterin, a co-factor compound for the hydroxylation of the amino acids phenylalanine and tryptophan. These hydroxylation reactions are known to be the rate-limiting step in the synthesis of DA, norepinephrine, and serotonin [54].

Regarding treatment for RLS during pregnancy, the risk of harm to the fetus is a concern. However, small case studies have suggested that levodopa/decarboxylase inhibitor, or dopamine agonists (pramipexole) are not harmful to the fetus [55, 56], and larger studies of 650 pregnant women given cabergoline, a dopaminergic agonist effective in the treatment of RLS, reported no harm to the fetuses. Therefore, dopamine agonists have been proposed for the treatment of RLS during pregnancy [56, 57].

Conclusion

The pathophysiology of transient RLS during pregnancy may be mediated by alterations in the normal balance between TH and DA. The importance of the role of DA as a TH modulator has not yet been fully appreciated. However, acceptance of the importance of TH for the appropriate function of the somatosensory system, along with the realization that such a vital biological function must have regulatory systems, such as DA, suggests that an imbalance between TH and DA may cause RLS pathophysiology. The maintenance of normal iron and folic acid levels is important for pregnant woman because deficiencies may derange the normal balance of TH and DA. Whenever possible, the normal activity of the cytochrome P3A4 enzyme isoform should be preserved, as its inhibition may reduce the breakdown of TH and result in elevated TH levels. Some practical issues may arise for WED patients. For example, it may not be advisable for these patients to consume grapefruit juice, which is popular in the United States, because grapefruit juice is a strong inhibitor of the cytochrome P4503A4 isoform and may increase the severity of RLS symptoms. Caffeine is also a moderate inhibitor of cytochrome P4503A4. Thus, it may be advisable that WED patients do not drink coffee during the whole day because there is a possibility that the resulting cytochrome P450 inhibition will remain well beyond the average half-life of caffeine. In pregnant women, sleep and quality of life can be concomitantly and severely affected by RLS; thus, all efforts should be made to relieve the RLS symptoms of pregnant women.

References

[1] Ekbom K-A. Restless legs: a clinical study. *Acta Med. Scand.* 1945; 158:1–122.

[2] Ekbom Jr K, Ulfberg J. Restless legs syndrome. *J. Intern. Med.* 2009; 266(5):419–31.

[3] Allen RP, Walters AS, Montplaisir J, et al. Restless legs syndrome prevalence and impact: REST general population study. *Arch. Intern. Med.* 2005; 165:1286.

[4] Alves DA, Carvalho Morais JF, Prado GF. Restless legs syndrome during pregnancy in Brazilian women. *Sleep Med.* 2010; 11(10):1049–54.

[5] Manconi M, Govoni V, De Vito A, et al. Restless legs syndrome and pregnancy. *Neurology* 2004; 63 (6):1065–9.

[6] Allen RP, Picchietti D, Hening WA, et al. Restless legs syndrome: diagnostic criteria, special considerations, and epidemiology. A report from the restless legs syndrome diagnosis and epidemiology workshop at the National Institutes of Health. *Sleep Med.* 2003; 4:101.

[7] Allen RP. Restless Legs Syndrome (Willis-Ekbom's Disease) and Periodic limb Movement Disorder. In, Carney PR, Geyer JD, and Berry RB, editors: Clinical sleep Disorders, second edition. Wolters Kluwer/ Lippincot Williams&Wilkins; Philadelphia, 2012. Pgs 203-218.

[8] Pereira Jr JC, Pradella-Hallinan M, Lins Pessoa JH. Imbalance between thyroid hormones and the dopaminergic system might be central to restless legs syndrome pathophysiology: a hypothesis. *Clinics* 2010;65(5):547–54.

[9] Aron DC, Findling JW, and Tyrrell. Hypothalamus & Pituitary Gland. In Gardner DG, and Shoback D, editors: Greenspan's Basic & Clinical Endocrinology, eighth edition, 2004. McGrawHill, New York. Pgs 101-56.
[10] Shupnik MA, Greenspan SL, Ridgway EC. Transcriptional regulation of thyrotropin subunit by thyrotropin-releasing hormone and dopamine in pituitary cell culture. *J. Biol. Chem.* 1986; 261(12):675–9.
[11] Nunez J, Celi FS, Ng L, Forrest D. Multigenic control of thyroid functions in the nervous system. *Mol. Cell Endocrinol.* 2008; 287(1-2):1–12.
[12] Pereira Jr JC, Silva Neto JLP, Pradella-Hallinan. Restless legs syndrome in subjects with knee prosthesis: evidence that symptoms are generated in the periphery. *Clinics* 2011; 66(11):1955–9.
[13] Pereira JC Jr, Rocha e Silva IR, Pradella-Hallinan M. Transient Willis-Ekbom's disease (restless legs syndrome) during pregnancy may be caused by estradiol-mediated dopamine overmodulation. *Med. Hypotheses*. 2013 Feb; 80(2):205-8.
[14] Guyton AC. Textbook of medical physiology. 7th ed. WB Saunders Company 1981.
[15] Wójcikowski J, Daniel WA. The brain dopaminergic system as an important center regulating liver cytochrome P450 in the rat. *Expert Opin Drug Metab. Toxicol.* 2009;5 (6):631–45.
[16] Wójcikowski J, Golembiowska K, Daniel WA. Regulation of liver cytochromeP450 by activation of brain dopaminergic system: physiological and pharmacological implications. *Biochem. Pharmacol.* 2008; 12:675–9.
[17] Visser TJ. Pathways of thyroid hormone metabolism. *Acta Med Austriaca* 1996; 23:10-16.
[18] Pereira Jr JC, Alves RC, Pradella-Hallinan M. Saint John's Wort, an herbal inducer of the cytochrome P4503A4 isoform, may alleviate Willis–Ekbom's disease symptoms. Presented in the 21st congress of the European sleep research society, Paris, France; Sep 4–8; 2012 (requests to jcpereirajr@uol.com.br).
[19] Pereira Jr JC, Alves RC. The ''forbidden zone for sleep'' might be caused by the evening thyrotropin surge and its biological purpose is to enhance survival: a hypothesis. *Sleep Sci.* 2011; 4(2):1–5.
[20] Tan EK, Ho SC, Eng P, et al. Restless legs symptoms in thyroid disorders. *Parkinsonism Relat Disord* 2004; 10:149–51.
[21] Schuppert F, Diegelmann B, Geest T, et al. Loss of variability in Graves' disease stimulatory TSH-receptors antibodies bind to the TSH-receptor in a continued non pulsatile and non-chaotic fashion. *Chronobiologia* 1994; 21:21–32.
[22] Antonini A, Calandrella D. Pharmacokinetic evaluation of pramipexole. *Expert Opin Drug Metab. Toxicol.* 2011; 7 (10): 1307-14.
[23] G Delitala. Dopamine and TSH secretion in man. *The Lancet.* 1977; 310:760-1.
[24] Kaptein EM, Spencer CA, Kamiel MB, and Nicoloff JT. Prolonged dopamine administration and thyroid hormone economy in normal and critically ill subjects. *J. Clin. Endocrinol. Metab.* 1980; 51:387-393.
[25] Becker PM. Restless Legs Syndrome. In Lee-Chiong TL, editor. Sleep a Comprehensive Handbook. Willey-Liss, Hoboken; 2006. Pgs 473-81.
[26] Parker DC, Rossman LG, Pekary AE, et AL. Effect of 64-hour sleep deprivation on the circadian waveform of thyrotropin (TSH): further evidence of sleep-related inhibition of TSH release. *J. Clin. Endocrinol. Metab.* 1987;64: 157-61.

[27] Rios Romenets S, Dauvilliers Y, Cochen De Cock V, et al. Restless legs syndrome outside the blood-brain barrier--exacerbation by domperidone in Parkinson's disease.Parkinsonism Relat Disord. 2013 19(1):92-4. doi: 10.1016/j.parkreldis. 2012.07.019. Epub 2012 Aug 24.PMID:22922159.

[28] Gore A. Neuroendocrine Systems. In: Squire LR, Berg D, Bloom DS, et al., editors. Fundamental Neuroscience, 3rd edition. Elsevier Inc, San Diego. 2008; 905-30.

[29] DrugBank, Open Data Drug & Drug Target Database.David Wishart, Departments of Computing Science&Biological Sciences, University of Alberta. (Accessed in March/10/2013).

[30] Lys CV, Verstreken P. Mitochondria at the synapse. *Neuroscientist.* 2006; 12 (4):291-9.

[31] Goglia F, Moreno M, Lanni A. Action of thyroid hormones at the cellular level: the mitochondrial target. *FEBS Lett.* 1999; 452(3):115-20.

[32] Burnstock G, Krugel U, Abbracchio MP, and Illes P. Purinergic signaling: From normal behaviour to pathological brain function. *Progress in Neurobiology*, 2011; 95: 229-274.

[33] Purves D, Augustine GJ, Fitzpatrick D, et al. Neuroscience. 4th ed. Sunderland, MA, USA: Sinauer Associates Inc.; 2008.

[34] Ropper AH, Samuels MA. Adams and Victor's Principles of Neurology, 9th edition, 2009. McGraw Hill. New York.

[35] Lindvall O, Bjorklund A, and Scargerberg G. Dopamine-containing neurons in the spinal cord: Anatomy and some functional aspects. *Annals of Neurology*, 1983; 14 (3): 255-60.

[36] Clemens S, Rye D, and Hochman S. Restless legs syndrome. Revisiting the dopamine hypothesis from the spinal cord perspective. *Neurology,* 2006; 67: 125-30.

[37] Scanlon MF, Weetman AP, Lewis M, et al. Dopaminergic modulation of circadian thyrotropin rhythm and thyroid hormone levels in euthyroid subjects. *J. Clin. Endocrinol. Metabol.* 1980; 51:1251–6.

[38] Brabant G, Prank K, Ranft U, et al. Physiological regulation of circadian and pulsatile thyrotropin secretion in normal man and woman. *J. Clin. Endocrinol. Metab.*, 1990; 70: 403-9.

[39] Ekbom KA. Restless legs in amputees. *Acta Med. Scand.* 1961; 169: 419-21.

[40] Hendry S, Hsiao S. Somatosensory System. In: Squire LR, Berg D, Bloom DS, et al., editors. Fundamental Neuroscience, 3rd edition. Elsevier Inc, San Diego. 2008; 581-608.

[41] Bara-Jimenez W, Aksu M, Graham B, et al. Periodic limb movements in sleep: state-dependent excitability of the spinal flexor reflex. *Neurology*, 2000; 54; 1609-16.

[42] Ko H, Shin J, Kim MY, et al. Sleep disturbances in Korean pregnant and postpartum women. *J. Psychosom. Obstet. Gynaecol*. 2012; 33(2): 85-90.

[43] Hübner A, Krafft A, Gadient S, et al. Characteristics and determinants of restless legs syndrome in pregnancy: A prospective study. *Neurology*. 2013, 19; 80(8):738-42.

[44] Glinoer D. The regulation of thyroid function during normal pregnancy: importance of the iodine status. *Best Pract. Res. Clin. Endocrinol. Metab.* 2004:133–52.

[45] Taylor RN, Lebovic DI. The endocrinology of pregnancy. In: Gardner DG, Shoback D, editors. Greenspan's basic & clinical endocrinology. McGraw Hill; 2007. p. 641–59.

[46] Dzaja A, Wehrle R, lancel M, Pollmacher T. Elevated estradiol plasma levels in women with restless legs during pregnancy. *Sleep* 2009; 32:169–74.

[47] Ben-Jonathan N, Hnasco R. Dopamine as a prolactin (PRL) inhibitor. *Endocr. Rev.* 2001; 22(6):724–63.

[48] Shaw-Bruha CM, Happe HK, Murrin LC, Rodriguez-Sierra JF, Shull JD. 17beta-Estradiol inhibits the production of dopamine by the tuberoinfundibular dopaminergic neurons of the male rat. *Brain Res. Bull* 1996; 40(1):33–6.

[49] Cramer OM, Parker Jr RC, Porter JC. Estrogen inhibition of dopamine release into hypophysial portal blood. *Endocrinology* 1979; 104 (2):419–22.

[50] MohanKumar BS, Kasturi BS, Shin AC, et al. Chronic estradiol exposure induces oxidative stress in the hypothalamus to decrease hypothalamic dopamine and cause hyperprolactinemia. *Am. J. Physiol. Regul Integr. Comp. Physiol.* 2001; 300 (3):693–9.

[51] Rios Romenets S, Dauvilliers Y, Cochen De Cock V, et al. Restless legs syndrome outside the blood brain barrier - exacerbation by domperidone in Parkinson´s disease. *Parkinsonism Relat. Disord.* 2013 Jan;19(1):92-4.

[52] Peters LL, Hoefer MT, Ben-Jonathan. The posterior pituitary: regulation of anterior pituitary prolactin secretion. *Science* 1981; 213 (4508): 659–61.

[53] Lee KA, Zafke ME, Baratte-Beebe K. Restless legs syndrome and sleep disturbance during pregnancy: the role of folate and iron. *J. Women Health Gend. Based Med.* 2001;10 (4):335–41.

[54] Coppen A, Bailey J. Enhancement of the antidepressant action of fluoxetine by folic acid: a randomised, placebo controlled trial. *J. Affect Disord.* 2000; 60 (2):121–30.

[55] Dostal M, Weber-Schoendorfer C, Sobesky J, Schaefer C .Pregnancy outcome following use of levodopa, pramipexole, ropinirole and rotigotine for restless legs syndrome during pregnancy: a case series. *Eur. J. Neurol.* 2012; doi:10.1111/ene.12001. [Epub ahead of print].

[56] Trenkwalder C. Emergencycall from gynecologists: how to treatrestlesslegs syndrome during pregnancy? *Eur. J. Neurol.* 2013 Jan 7. doi: 10.1111/ene.12047. [Epub ahead of print].

In: Estradiol: Synthesis, Health Effects and Drug Interactions ISBN: 978-1-62808-962-2
Editors: Ricco Palmeri and Sal Grimaudo

Chapter 13

Estrogen Modulation of Oxidative Stress and Synaptic Plasticity in the Dorsal Hippocampus

V. Beltrán-Campos, E. Gómez-Padilla, G. I. Medina-Aguirre, S. A. Castro-Chavira and S. Díaz-Cintra
Instituto de Neurobilogía, Universidad Nacional Autónoma de México, Mexico

Abstract

Estrogens are important for antioxidant mechanisms, maintenance of synaptic plasticity, and modulation of zinc content in the hippocampus of young and senile animals. The female brain is influenced by multiple factors including the decrease in estrogen levels, with that commonly accompanies stress and aging. However, plasticity in the hippocampus in pre- and postsynaptic sites, such as the mossy fiber system and dendritic spines, responds to the neuroprotective and antioxidant actions of hormone supplementation. Furthermore, in hippocampus, the ovariectomy produces spine pruning in pyramidal cells of CA1, a reduction of the mossy fiber area in CA3, a decrease of the zinc level in the whole hippocampus and an increase in oxidative stress. Following supplementation with a minimal dose of 17β-estradiol, these effects are reversed and these parameters have values similar to those observed during the proestrus stage of the estrous cycle, which is associated with a better performance in learning and memory in female rats. These studies confirm the roles of estrogen in protecting the hippocampus before oxidative stress and maintaining its synaptic plasticity.

Introduction

Estrogens are known to have broad effects on hippocampus synaptic plasticity which is also affected by oxidative stress and aging (Foy, 2010). Multiple lines of evidence suggest that loss of estrogens in the aging brain may play a role in the cognitive decline associated with Alzheimer´s disease (Janicki &, Schupf, 2010; Barron & Pike, 2012). The hippocampus has steroid receptors (Spencer-Segal et al., 2012) that make it sensitive to the interaction between antioxidant defense systems and sex steroids. This effect is shown in studies of estrogen deprivation which increases the vulnerability to injury of granule cells in the adult hippocampus and may predispose to neurological diseases and deficits in working memory occurring after menopause (Liu et al., 2001). Estrogen can prevent oxidative stress in neurons (Behl et al., 1997, 2003), and in the hippocampus they can act as an antioxidant agent to modulate lipid oxidation, thereby regulating oxidative phosphorylation (Yao et al., 2011). It has been demonstrated that estrogens produce a neurotrophic effect that prevents neuronal damage in the adult brain, protecting and supporting synaptic connections which are essential for signaling and neural survival (Maggi et al., 2004; Yao et al., 2011; Srivastava, 2012). This mechanism regulates pre- and postsynaptic proteins such as synaptophysin, syntaxin, and spinophilin in CA1 pyramidal cells (Brake et al., 2001; Prange-Kiel et al., 2006). These synaptic changes in hippocampal pyramidal cells are also related to spatial behavioral experience (Ramírez-Amaya et al., 1999; 2001; Beltrán Campos et al., 2010).

In the hippocampus of the adult rat, mossy fiber (MF) axons from dentate granule cells converge in the dentate hilus and run through a narrow area called the *stratum lucidum* (CA3) forming excitatory glutamatergic synapses. The well-documented synaptic rearrangement of MF is associated with several factors like learning, memory, temporal lobe epilepsy (Koyama et al., 2004), malnutrition (Díaz-Cintra et al., 1991; 1997; 2007), stress and neurotrophic factors. The idea that levels of circulating estrogens are also important for cognition is supported by animal studies in which ovariectomy produces acquisition deficits in Morris water maze (MWM) task (Xu & Zhang, 2006; Sarkaki et al., 2008).

Here, the main objetives were to study the protective effects of estrogens before oxidative stress and the pre- and postsynaptic dorsal hippocampal plasticity (MF and spines, respectively) involved in the regulation of spatial memory. Our experiments were performed in female Sprague-Dawley rats which were treated in accordance with the NIH Guide for Care and Use of Laboratory Animals. The experimental protocols were approved by the local Animal Care and Use Committee.

1. Estrogen Modulation of Hippocampal Oxidative Stress

Oxidative stress (OS), together with inflammatory processes and the aggregation of oxidized products of aberrant proteins in the brain, induces apoptosis and autophagy (Caballero & Coto-Montes, 2012). Biological aging is associated with neurodegeneration due to the presence of lipid peroxidation products, protein oxidation, and oxidative modifications in nuclear and mitochondrial DNA (Richwine et al., 2005; Zhu et al., 2006; Poon et al., 2006). In addition, the decrease of sexual steroid levels due to aging can have an impact on brain functions; thus, therapies to replace these hormones may reduce this impact, which is supported by evidence in experimental animals (Green & Simpkins, 2000; Garcia-Segura et al., 2001; Lee & McEwen, 2001; Feng, 2005). To test if the interaction between antioxidant defense systems and sex steroids affects the antioxidant activity in the hippocampus of young and senile animals, we evaluated lipid peroxidation in five experimental groups, each containing 10 animals: young proestrus (Pro), young ovariectomized (OvxV), young ovariectomized supplemented with a minimal dose of 17β-estradiol (OvxE), senile (SenV), and senile supplemented with the same minimal 17β-estradiol dose (SenE).

Methodology and Results

The young animals were ovariectomized (Ovx, n = 20) with xylazine/ketamine anesthesia (13 mg/kg xylazine and 40 mg/kg ketamine) to minimize pain and discomfort, using aseptic procedures. An incision was made in the abdominal zone to visualize the ovaries. A clip was placed 1 cm below the ovaries, which were then completely removed. A two-week recovery period was provided before hormone supplementation. Then, one of the young ovariectomized (OvxE) and one of the senile (SenE) groups were given hormone supplementation (10 μg of 17-β - estradiol in 0.2 ml oil solution). Two other groups (OvxV and SenV) received vehicle (0.2 ml of oil). The supplementation was administered subcutaneously every 24 h for 3 consecutive days. After the treatments, the animals were sacrificed, and the brains of the animals (in all groups) were extracted and distributed randomly (6 hemi-brains per assay) for different measurements. Quantification of lipid peroxidation and determination of its final products were performed using the technique of Triggs & Willmore (1984). The complete hippocampus of each of the 6 hemi-brains per group was carefully removed and homogenized in 3 ml of saline solution (0.9% NaCl in buffer); an aliquot of 1 ml of this homogenate was mixed with 4 ml of chloroform/methanol (2:1 v/v) and then left on ice for 30 min to allow phase separation; fluorescence of the chloroform phase was masured in a Perkin Elmer L5500B spectrophotometer (luminescence: excitation at 370 nm and emission at 430 nm). The spectrophotometer sensitivity was adjusted to 330 U of fluorescence with a standard solution of quinine (0.1μg/ml). The results were expressed in fluorescence units per gram of tissue. ANOVA tests showed significant differences in the levels of lipid peroxidation; they were similar in the young female rats in proestrus (Pro) and after treatment (OvxE). Moreover, supplementation with a low dose of 17β-estradiol produced a decrease in lipid peroxidation levels in senile females (SenE) as well as in young OvxE, as shown in Figure 1.

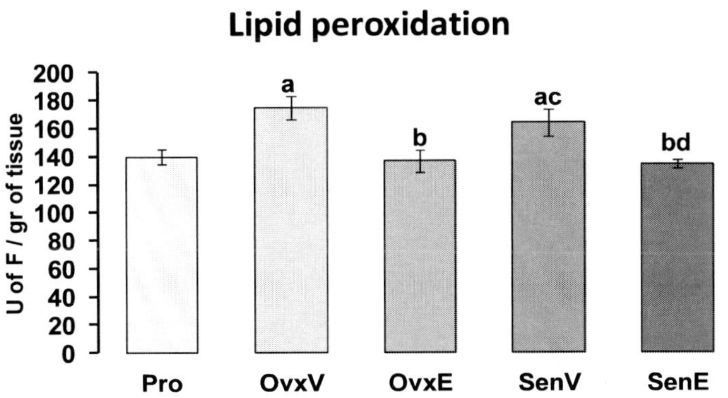

Figure 1. Mean ± SEM of fluorescence units (U of F) per gram of tissue and the significant differences ($p < 0.05$) between groups: a - vs Pro; b - vs OvxV; c - vs OvxE; d - vs SenV. Modified from Beltrán-Campos et al. (2011).

2. Estrogen Supplementation Effects on Spine Density

Structural synaptic changes are believed to be responsible for stabilizing the activity patterns in neuronal ensembles during memory consolidation (Hebb, 1949). Following learning, structural remodeling of synapses has been studied in different brain regions after varied learning experiences in several animal species (Bailey et al., 2008; Butz et al., 2009). In hippocampal CA1 pyramidal neurons, the number of dendritic spine increases when rats experience, for several days, a complex environment that promotes spatial learning (Moser et al., 1994). Also, training rats in the MWM spatial task induces changes in the distribution of dendritic spines in CA1 neurons, as observed using electron microscopy (Rusakov et al., 1997). Trace eyeblink conditioning training, which is an associative learning task dependent on the integrity of the hippocampus (Solomon et al., 1986), increases spine density in CA1 neurons as observed with Golgi staining 24 h after learning (Leuner et al., 2003). This staining method has also revealed that spatial water maze training increases the number of some, but not all, spine types in CA1 neurons (Diamond et al., 2006). Interestingly, the dendritic spine number in CA1 neurons can also be modulated by extrinsic factors such as circulating gonadal steroids (Brusco et al., 2008; González-Burgos, 2005). Dendritic spines have a highly plastic capacity and can modify their structure in response to hormonal influences (Murakami et al., 2006; Sato et al., 2007). For example, it is well established that ovariectomy in young animals reduces their dendritic spine number in CA1 hippocampal pyramidal neurons, and this effect is reversed by estradiol and progesterone replacement (Gould et al., 1990). We studied this effect in the same CA1 hippocampal pyramidal neurons by administering 17β-estradiol not only in ovariectomized young, but also in senile females, in order to know if these spines retain their plastic capacity as a result of estradiol influence. Moreover, we evaluated if the spine number recovered to levels similar to those observed in animals at proestrus, which are the highest of the estrous cycle.

Methodology and Results

The dorsal hippocampus (Bregma -2.8 to - 4.2; Paxinos & Watson, 1998) of each hemi-brain (10 per group) was carefully removed, immediately fixed in a 10% buffered formalin solution, and divided into 4mm-thick blocks after 4 h with the aid of a stereoscopic microscope. Each block was impregnated using the rapid Golgi technique following the modification of Díaz-Cintra et al. (1994). After 12 days, each block was transferred to a solution of 0.75% silver nitrate in double distilled water for 12 h, washed in 50% alcohol, embedded in low-viscosity nitrocellulose, and cut along the frontal plane at a thickness of 120 μm. Each section was collected in 70% alcohol, dehydrated, and mounted in Entellan® medium. Each slide had 16 sections of the dorsal hippocampus and was assigned a random number to ensure that observers were blind to experimental conditions. Morphometric analysis was made in six complete and well-impregnated CA1 dorsal hippocampus neurons chosen randomly from each of the 6 animals per group and was analyzed using an Optiphot-2 Nikon microscope. A 20x Plan® objective (0.5 NA) with an optically calibrated reticule and a 100× Plan-Apochromat® objective (1.3 NA) were used for the analysis. An image of the selected pyramidal cell was captured with the 20x objective by carefully identifying the optical plane in which the whole apical dendrite was visible. This image was then used as the reference image. This study was performed only in those CA1 Golgi-impregnated pyramidal neurons whose dendrites reached the *stratum lacunosum molecular (slm)*, as shown in Figure 2. Using the reference image, the apical dendrite segments were designated according to the following criteria: The proximal segment was considered as the first 100 μm closer to the soma. The distal segment was considered to start at the *slm*, where the apical dendrite folds. Finally, the medial segment was considered the whole section between the proximal and distal segments. The spine density analysis was performed on one secondary dendritic branch attached to the main apical dendrite of each segment. In each selected branch, a 25 μm length was chosen randomly for spine classification and density analysis. We analyzed secondary branches rather than the main dendritic shaft, because the proximal segment of the main apical dendrite is devoid of spines within the first 100 μm from the soma (Megías et al., 2001). Golgi-stained neurons were classified and analyzed for spine density by direct microscopic observation. Dendritic spine density was calculated as the number of spines divided by 125 microns (sum of these three segments) in the apical dendrite in hippocampal CA1 neurons, and analyzed by one-way ANOVA comparing groups (Pro, OvxV, OvxE, SenV and SenE). Significant differences ($P < 0.0001$) were found, and a subsequent *post hoc* Fisher´s test indicated significant reductions ($P < 0.0001$) in the OvxV and the SenV groups compared to the Pro group, as shown in Figure 2. These results show that the young animals tested during the proestrus stage had 1.7 spines per linear μm, but a decrease of more than 50% in Ovx animals was found. After the 10-μg dose of 17-β estradiol, spine density recovered and was similar to that in young animals at proestrus. Also, the spine density of the senile groups showed equivalent pruning and recovery effects, Figure 2.

3. Effect of 17β-Estradiol on Plasticity of Hippocampal MF

Studies testing the hippocampal plasticity show an increased propensity of MF synapses to reorganize in the inner molecular layer following seizures (Lin et al., 2011). Estrogen deprivation increases the vulnerability to injury of granule cells in the adult hippocampus and may predispose to neurological diseases and an increased incidence of memory deficits after menopause (Liu et al., 2001; Sherwin, 2012). In hippocampal pyramidal cells, estrogen has also been shown to enhance long-term potentiation and potentiate acute excitatory transmission, a cellular correlate of learning and memory (Woolley, 2007; Smejkalova & Wooley, 2010). It is well accepted that estrogen increases synaptic function and induces neurogenesis in the adult (Gould et al., 2000). Neurogenesis and less apoptosis in hippocampal dentate gyrus during proestrus and in rats with estrogenic supplementation have been reported (Tanapat et al., 2005). The MF system is highly plastic in the adult brain and is influenced by multiple factors including learning and memory. In addition, zinc plays an important modulatory role in hippocampal neuronal signal transduction (Sindreu & Storm, 2011) and in memory formation and stress. Since the relation between MF plasticity and zinc content in the whole hippocampus throughout the estrous cycle remains unknown, we designed this study in order to test estrogen (17ß-estradiol) modulation and zinc content of the hippocampus over the course of the female estrous cycle. Thus, ovariectomized female rats without (Ovx) or with estrogen supplement (OvxE) were compared with control rats at three stages of the estrous cycle: diestrus, proestrus, and estrus.

Methodology and Results

Subjects, their ovariectomy surgery, and estrogenic supplementation were described earlier in this chapter. In order to detect normal cycles, daily vaginal smears were taken for three days from 36 female rats that were euthanized at proestrus (P), estrus (Es), or diestrus (D) stages (12 rats per stage). Groups of six rats were used either for Timm staining or zinc measurement. For estrogen deprivation and replacement, 24 female rats were ovariectomized (Ovx), half of which were supplemented with E (OvxE). Four, six-rat groups were formed and studied either by Timm staining or zinc measurement. Additionally, 20 female rats were ovariectomized (Ovx), and ten of them supplemented with E (OvxE) and subjected to behavioral testing in the MWM (Section 4, Effects of ovariectomy on the performance of a spatial task).

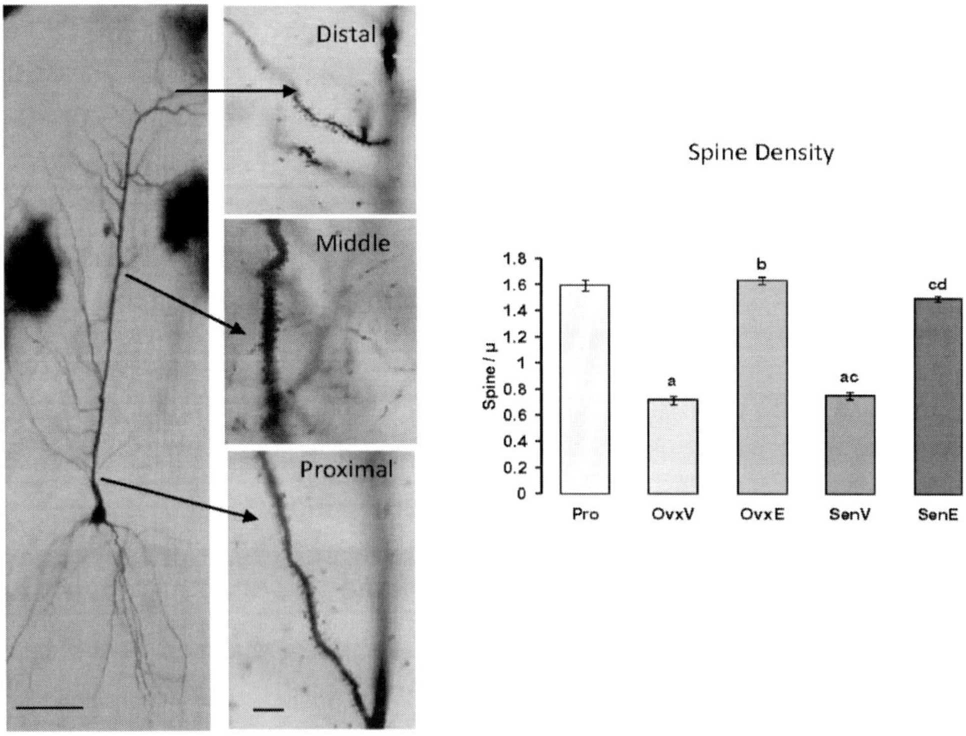

Figure 2. Example of a CA1 pyramidal cell stained with the rapid Golgi technique and enlargements of its dendritic segments (distal, middle, and proximal). Scale bars: 100 and 10 μm, on left and right, respectively. Graphs show the mean ± SEM spine density (spine / μ) in the five groups analyzed; significant ($p < 0.05$) reductions in OvxV and SenV groups and recovery with estrogen supplementation were found (OvxE and SenE groups); a - vs Pro; b - vs OvxV; c - vs OvxE; d - vs SenV. Modified from Beltrán-Campos et al. (2011).

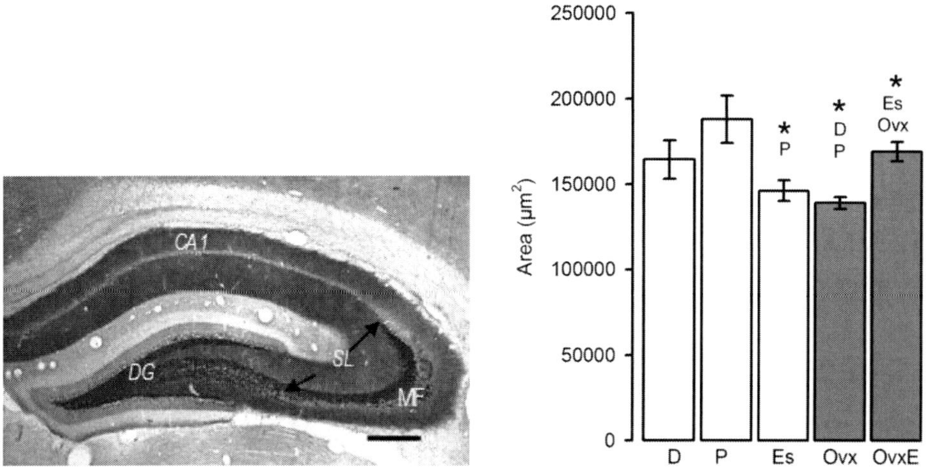

Figure 3. Example of hippocampal coronal section used to estimate the volume of the mossy fiber (MF) limit with arrows and to estimate areas: dentate gyrus (*DG*), *CA1,* and stratum lucidum (*SL*); bar, 300 μm. The graph shows the mean ±SEM of the MF *stratum lucidum* area in five groups: gonadally intact divided into: diestrus (D), proestrus (P), and estrus (Es) from cycling young female rats, and two ovariectomized (Ovx) without supplementation and with a 10-μg dose of 17β-estradiol (OvxE). Note the significant decreases in the Es ($p = 0.001$) and Ovx ($p = 0.01$) groups relative to the P group and a significant ($p = 0.001$) increase in OvxE with respect to the Ovx and Es groups. Modified from Padilla-Gómez et al. (2012).

Tissue collection. A total of 30 animals (P, Es, D, Ovx and OvxE), 6 per group, were studied with the histological Timm technique (Padilla-Gómez et al., 2011). Sections were serially mounted and processed using a modification of Timm's sulfide silver technique as described elsewhere (Granados et al., 2002). A coronal section from the hippocampal formation was obtained immediately after perfusion. These sections were used to estimate the area of the suprapyramidal bundle of the MF system. Every fifth section was selected from a random starting position within the first five serially mounted sections. Each slide was assigned a random number to ensure that the observer was unaware of the experimental conditions. The area of the MF system (expressed in μm^2) was measured in the suprapyramidal bundle, which broadly corresponds to the *stratum lucidum (SL),* and in the sections selected from the dorsal hippocampus (Figure 3A). The results are shown in Figure 3, with the mean area ±SEM of the MF system and *SL* in five groups: cycling female rats (D, P, Es) and Ovx alone or with 17β-estradiol supplement (OvxE). ANOVA testing showed significant ($p = 0.006$) differences among groups and Fisher´s *post hoc* test showed a significant ($p = 0.003$) area reduction in the Es and Ovx ($p=0.0007$) groups relative to P group. The zinc determination was made in six animals at each stage of the estrous cycle (D, P, Es), and in Ovx and OvxE. Hippocampal tissue was dissected out from the skull as rapidly as possible and placed in tubes previously washed with 30% nitric acid solution to avoid external contamination. All the hippocampus weights were recorded, and 1 ml of redistilled nitric acid was added to the samples. Tubes were then capped and placed on a shaking bath at 60°C for 30 min. The resulting solution was assayed for zinc content in an atomic absorption spectrophotometer equipped with a graphite furnace and Zeeman background correction (Analyst 600, Perkin Elmer). Results are expressed as μg of zinc per gram of wet tissue as shown in Figure 3b. This data showed that estrogen modulates the plasticity and maintenance of MF in hippocampal CA3 during proestrus because the MF area is reduced in Ovx animals and recovers to normal when they are supplemented with a physiological dose of 10 μg of 17β-estradiol. Estradiol supplementation had similar effects on the hippocampal zinc content in the same five experimental groups: cycling female rats (D, P, Es) and Ovx with or without E (OvxE) (Figure 4).

4. Effects of Ovariectomy on the Performance of a Spatial Task

Ovariectomy produces deficits in the performance of hippocampus-dependent learning tasks (Wallace et al., 2006); these deficits are ameliorated by estradiol administration (Xu & Zhang, 2006), demonstrating that they are due to inadequate levels of circulating estradiol. Some studies have found that ovariectomy may improve hippocampus-dependent learning (Bimonte-Nelson et al., 2003); however, this effect was observed 1.5–6 months after ovariectomy, when the endocrine system of the animal had already adapted to the lack of ovaries, and estrogens might be released from other sources, such as adipose tissue (for reviews see Mendelson & Simpson, 1987; Nelson & Bulun, 2001). Moreover, it has also been observed that low estrogen levels during the estrous cycle inhibit the acquisition of spatial tasks (Frye & Sturgis, 1995; Sarkaki et al., 2008), which is consistent with the detrimental effect of ovariectomy on hippocampus-dependent spatial-memory tasks. In order to demonstrate the effect of hormone replacement, we studied learning and memory in Ovx and OvxE groups using a MWM.

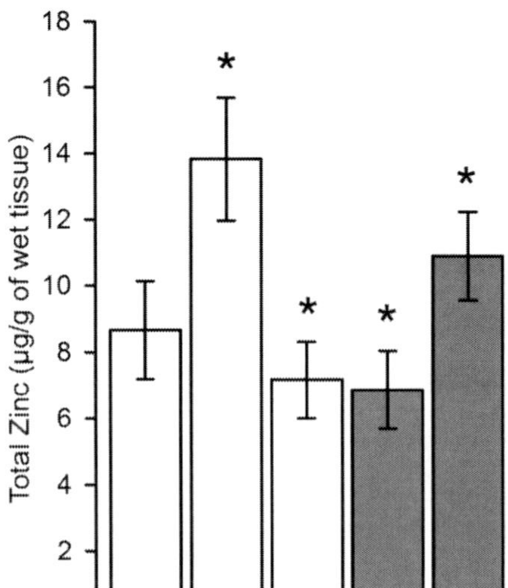

Figure 4. Zinc content (mean ± SEM) in five groups: gonadally intact: diestrus (D), proestrus (P), and estrus (E) from cycling female rats, Ovx and OvxE. Note the significant decreases in the E, D, and Ovx groups in relation to the P group and a significant increase in the OvxE compared to the Ovx group. Modified from Padilla-Gómez et al. (2012).

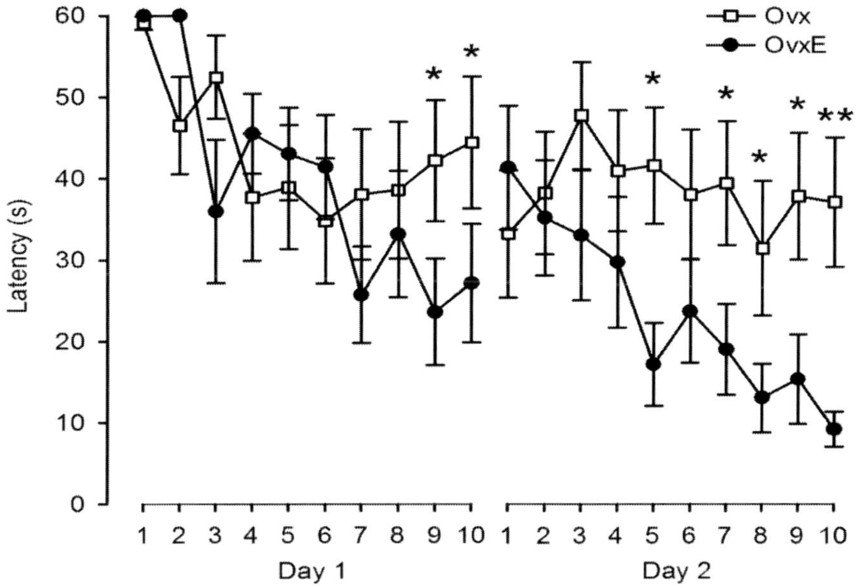

Figure 5. Mean ± SEM of acquisition performance of animals subjected to 2 days of training. Points represent the latency to reach the target platform on consecutive trials. Repeated measures ANOVA showed significant differences (*) between the Ovx and OvxE groups on trials 9 and 10 on day 1; and on trials 5, 7, 8, 9, and 10 on day 2. Also, between trials 1 to 10, only the OvxE group showed significantly reduced latency; the Ovx group did not reach the latency threshold (30 s) that would indicate learning. Modified from Padilla-Gómez et al. (2012).

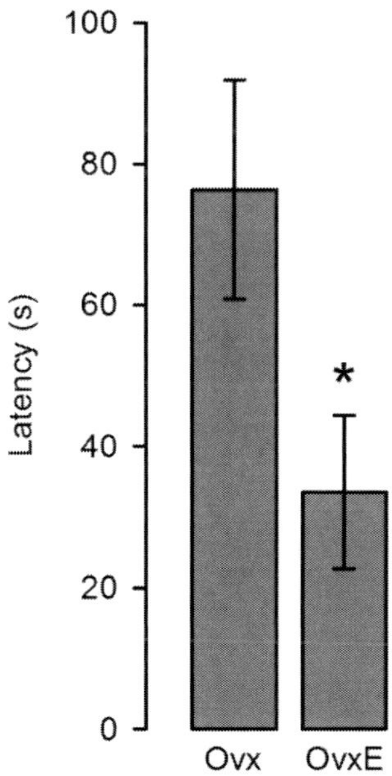

Figure 6. Mean ± SEM of water maze performance during the memory test after two days of learning. Latency in seconds spent by the Ovx and OvxE groups to locate the platform area. The Student's t-test showed significant differences (*) between groups. Modified from Padilla-Gómez et al. (2012).

Methodology and Results

We trained young Ovx and OvxE animals in the MWM spatial training task (Subjects described in Methodology for Section 3). The training consisted of one session of 10 trials. The animal was introduced into the pool at a different starting point for each trial up to a total of 10 trials (Ramírez-Amaya et al., 2001). The animal was allowed to swim for a maximum of 60 s or until it located the platform, and it was allowed to stand on the platform for 30 s. Escape latency was measured for each trial. Figure 5 shows that Ovx rats had higher latencies, indicating poorer performance in the MWM. Learning was evaluated in two sessions of 10 trials each, and memory was tested 24 h later. The OvxE group performed significantly better in both learning (trials 5, 8, 9, 10 on day 1, and trials 5, 9, 10 on, day 2) and in memory (Figure 6).

Concluding Remarks and Future Directions

We have reported that ovariectomy produces an increase in oxidative stress and spine pruning in CA1 pyramidal cells (Beltrán-Campos et al., 2010); other effects found are reduction in the MF area in the CA3 and a decrease in the level of total hippocampal zinc (Padilla-Gómez et al., 2011). Animals trated with a minimal dose of 17β-estradiol, showed a reversal of these latter effects and had MF areas and zinc levels similar to those observed during the proestrus stage of the estrous cycle. In addition, the OvxE group acquired and remembered the spatial task, suggesting the important role of estrogen for maintaining hippocampal plasticity and zinc level in MF-CA3 synapses during proestrus, parameters associated with better performance in learning and memory. While suggestive, these data are not sufficient to infer changes in synaptic connectivity; therefore, another approach to the problem will be to use electron microscopy to look for ultrastructural modifications at postsynaptic sites through the estrous cycle of rats.

The findings concerning spine density support the idea that gonadal activity is required for some structural changes in spines underlying hippocampus-dependent cognition in female animals (Gould et al., 1990; Woolley et al., 1993; 1997). We have reported (Beltrán-Campos et al., 2010) that the different dendritic spine types (stubby, thin, and mushroom) had different density distributions across the apical dendrite from CA1 pyramidal neurons, because the input sites are altered differentially. Ovariectomy (Ovx) produced spine pruning in all the dendritic segments. It is necessary to know the differential effects of estrogen supplementation on oxidative stress (protective), on hippocampal plasticity (maintenance) and on the density of spines (recovery), which have high plastic capacity to modify their structure in relation with estrogen levels.

Acknowledgments

This study was supported by PDCB, DGAPA-UNAM, and CONACYT fellowships (173299, 17276, 210873) and CB2012-178841, UNAM-PAPIIT IN-201613. The authors wish to thank A. Aguilar Vázquez, T. Martínez, L. Palma, N. Hernández, N. Serafin and M. García for technical assistance. We are grateful to Dr. D. Pless for proofreading.

References

Barron, A. M. & Pike, Ch. J. (2012). Sex hormones, aging, and Alzheimer's disease. *Front Biosci. 4*, 976–997.

Behl, Ch., Shutella, T., Lezoualc'h, F., Post, A., Widmann, M., Newton, ChJ. & Holsboer, F. (1997). Neuroprotection against Oxidative Stress by Estrogens: Structure-Activity Relationship. *Molec. Pharmacol. 51*, 535–541.

Behl, Ch. (2003). Estrogen can protect neurons, modes of action. *J Ster Biochemist. Molec. Biolog. 83*, 195–197.

Beltrán-Campos, V., Prado-Alcalá, R. A., León-Jacinto, U., Aguilar Vázquez, A., Quirarte, G. L., Ramírez-Amaya, V. & Díaz-Cintra, S. (2011). Increase of mushroom spine density in CA1 apical dendrites produced by water maze training is prevented by ovariectomy. *Brain Res, 1369*, 119-130.

Bailey, C. H. & Kandel, E. (2008). Synaptic remodeling, synaptic growth and the storage of long-term memory in Aplysia. *Prog. Brain Res. 169*, 179–198.

Bimonte-Nelson, H. A., Singleton, R. S., Hunter, C. L., Price, K. L., Moore, A. B. & Granholm, A. C. (2003). Ovarian hormones and cognition in the aged female rat, I. Long-term, but not short-term, ovariectomy enhances spatial performance. *Behav Neurosci. 117*, 1395-1406.

Brake, W. G., Alves, S. E., Dunlop, J. C., Lee, S. J., Bulloch, K., Allen, P. B., Greengard, P. & McEwen, B. S. (2001). Novel target sites for estrogen action in the dorsal hippocampus, an examination of synaptic proteins. *Endocrinology. 142*, 1284-1289.

Brusco, J., Wittmann, R., de Azevedo, M. S., Lucion, A. B., Franci, C. R., Giovenardi, M. & Rasia-Filho, A. A. (2008). Plasma hormonal profiles and dendritic spine density and morphology in the hippocampal CA1 stratum radiatum, evidenced by light microscopy, of virgin and postpartum female rats. *Neurosci Lett. 438*, 346-50.

Butz, M., Worgotter, F. & van Ooyen, A. (2009). Activity-dependent structural plasticity. *Brain Res. Rev. 60*, 287–305.

Caballero, B. & Coto-Montes, A. (2012). An insight into the role of autophagy in cell responses in the aging and neurodegenerative brain. *Histol Histopathol. 27*, 263-275.

Diamond, D. M., Campbell, A. M., Park, C. R., Woodson, J. C., Conrad, C. D., Bachstetter, A. D. & Mervis, R. F. (2006). Influence of predator stress *Hippocampus. 16*, 571-576.

Díaz-Cintra, S., Cintra, L., Galván, A., Aguilar, T., Kemper, Morgane, P. J. (1991). Effects of prenatal protein deprivation on the posnatal development of granule cell neurons in the fascia dentata. *J. Comp Neur. 310*, 356-364

Díaz-Cintra, S., García-Ruiz, M., Corkidi, G. & Cintra, L. (1994). Effects of prenatal malnutrition and posnatal nutritional rehabilitation on CA3 hippocampal pyramidal cells in rats of four ages. *Brain Res. 662*, 117-126.

Díaz-Cintra, S., González Maciel, A., Aguilar Vázquez, A. R., Morales, M. A., Cintra, L. & Prado-Alcalá, R. A. (2007). Protein malnutition differentially alters glutamic acid decarboxilase-67-Positive hippocampus interneurons. *Exp Neurol. 208*, 47-53

Feng, Z. & Zhang, J. T. (2005). Long-term melatonin or 17beta-estradiol supplementation alleviates oxidative stress in ovariectomized adult rats. *Free Radic Biol Med. 39*, 195-204.

Foy, R. (2010). Ovarian Hormones, Aging and Stress on Hippocampal Synaptic Plasticity Michael R. *Neurobiol Learn Mem. 95*, 134–144.

Frye, C. A. & Sturgis, J. D. (1995). Neurosteroids affect spatial/reference, working, and long-term memory of female rats. *Neurobiol Learn Mem. 64*, 83-96.

Garcia-Segura, L. M., Azcoitia, I. & donCarlos, L. L. (2001). Neuroprotection by estradiol. *Prog. Neurobiol. 63*, 29-60.

González-Burgos, I., Alejandre-Gomez, M. & Cervantes, M. (2005). Spine-type densities of hippocampal CA1 neurons vary in proestrus and estrus rats. *Neurosci. Lett. 379*, 52-54.

Gould, E., Tanapat, P., Rydel, T. & Hastings, N. (2000). Regulation of hippocampal neurogenesis in adulthood. *Biol Psychiatry. 48*, 715-720.

Gould, E., Woolley, C., Frankfurt, M. & McEwen, B. (1990). Gonadal steroids regulate dendritic spine density in hippocampal pyramidal cells in adulthood. *J. Neurosci. 10*, 1286-1291.

Granados-Rojas, L., Aguilar, A. & Díaz-Cintra, S. (2004). The mossy fiber system of the hippocampal formation is decreased by chronic and postnatal but not by prenatal protein malnutrition in rats. *Nutr Neurosci, 7*, 301-308.

Green, P. S. & Simpkins, J. W. (2000). Neuroprotective effects of estrogens. Potential mechanisms of action. *Int J Dev Neurosci. 18*, 347-358.

Hebb, D. O. (1945). The Organization of Behavior, *A Neuropsychological Theory*. John Wiley & Sons.

Janicki Sarah, C. & Nicole Schupf. (2010). Hormonal Influences on Cognition and Risk for Alzheimer Disease Curr Neurol Neurosci Rep. Author manuscript; available in PMC. *Curr Neurol Neurosci Rep. 10*, 359–366.

Koyama, R. & Ikegaya, Y. (2004). Mossy fiber sprouting as a potential therapeutic target for epilepsy. *Curr Neurovasc Res. 1*, 3-10.

Lee, S. J. & McEwen, B. S. (2001). Neurotrophic and neuroprotective actions of estrogens and their therapeutic implications. *Annu Rev Pharmacol Toxicol. 41*, 569-591.

Leuner, B., Falduto, J. & Shors, T. J. (2003). Associative Memory Formation Increases the Observation of Dendritic Spines in the Hippocampus *The Journal of Neuroscience. 23*, 659–665.

Lin, H., Huang, Y., Wang, Y. & Jia, J. (2011). Spatiotemporal profile of N-cadherin expression in the mossy fiber sprouting and synaptic plasticity following seizures. *Mol Cell Biochem. 358*, 201-205.

Liu, Z., Gastard, M., Verina, T., Bora, S., Mouton, P. R. & Koliatsos, V. E. (2001). Estrogens modulate experimentally induced apoptosis of granule cells in the adult hippocampus. *J Comp Neurol. 441*, 1-8.

Maggi, A., Ciana, P., Belcredito, S. & Vegeto, E. (2004). Estrogens in the nervous system, Mechanisms and nonreproductive functions. *Annu. Rev. Physiol. 66*, 291-313.

Megías, M., Emri, Z., Freund, T. F. & Gulyas, A. I. (2001). Total number and distribution of inhibitory and excitatory synapses on hippocampal CA1 pyramidal cells. *Neuroscience. 102*, 527-540.

Mendelson, C. R. & Simpson, E. R. (1987). Regulation of estrogen biosynthesis by human adipose cells in vitro. *Mol Cell Endocrinol. 52*, 169-176.

Moser, M. B., Trommald, M. & Andersen, P. (1994). An increase in dendritic spine density on hippocampal Cal pyramidal cells following spatial learning in adult rats suggests the formation of new synapses. *Proc. Natl. Acad. Sci. USA. 91*, 12673-12675.

Murakami, G., Tsurugizawa, T., Hatanaka, Y., Komatsuzaki, Y., Tanabe, N., Mukai, H., Hojo, Y., Kominινami, S., Yamazaki, T. & Kawato, S. (2006). Comparison between basal and apical dendritic spines in estrogen-induced rapid spinogenesis of CA1 principal neurons in the adult hippocampus. *Biochem. Biophys Res. Communic. 351*, 553-558.

Nelson, L. R. & Bulun, S. E. (2001). Estrogen production and action Source. *J Am Acad Dermatol. 45*, S116-124.

Nilsen, J. (2008). Estradiol and neurodegenerative oxidative stress. *Front Neuroendocrinol. 29*, 463-475.

Padilla-Gómez, E., Beltrán-Campos, V., Montes, S., Díaz-Ruíz, A., Quirarte, G., Ríos, C. & Diaz-Cintra, S. (2012). Effect of 17ß-estradiol on zinc content of hippocampal mossy fibers in ovariectomized adult rats. *Biometals. 25*, 1129-1139.

Palmiter, R. D., Cole, T. B., Quaife, C. J. & Findley, S. D. (1996). ZnT-3, a putative transporter of zinc into synaptic vesicles. *Proc Natl Acad Sci U S A. 93*, 14934-14939.

Paxinos, G. & Watson, C. (1998). The rat brain in stereotaxic coordinates. *Academic Press*, New York.

Poon, H. F., Calabrese, V., Calvani, M. & Butterfield, D. A. (2006). Proteomics analyses of specific protein oxidation and protein expression in aged rat brain and its modulation by l-acetylcarnitine, insights into the mechanisms of action of this proposed therapeutic agent for cns disorders associated with oxidative stress. *Antioxid. Redox. Signal. 8*, 381–394.

Prange-Kiel, J., Fester, L., Zhou, L., Lauke, H., Carretero, J. & Rune, G. M. (2006). Inhibition of hippocampal estrogen synthesis causes region-specific downregulation of synaptic protein expression in hippocampal neurons. *Hippocampus.16*, 464-471.

Ramírez-Amaya, V., Balderas, I., Sandoval, J., Escobar, M. L. & Bermúdez-Rattoni, F. (2001). Spatial long-term memory is related to mossy fiber synaptogenesis. *J. Neurosci. 21*, 7340-7348.

Ramírez-Amaya, V., Escobar, M. L., Chao, V. & Bermúdez-Rattoni, F. (1999). Synaptogenesis of mossy fibers induced by spatial water maze overtraining. *Hippocampus. 9*, 631-636

Richwine, A. F., Godbout, J. P., Berg, B. M., Chen, J., Escobar, J., Millard, D. K. & Johnson, R. W. (2005). Improved psychomotor performance in aged mice fed diet high in antioxidants is associated with reduced ex vivo brain interleukin-6 production. *Brain Behav Immun. 19*, 512–520.

Rusakov, D. A., Davies, H. A., Harrison, E., Diana, G., Richter-Levin, G., Bliss, T. V, & Stewart, M. G. (1997). Ultrastructural synaptic correlates of spatial learning *Neuroscience. 80*, 69-77.

Sarkaki, A., Amani, R., Badavi, M., Safahani, M. & Aligholi, H. (2008). Effect of ovariectomy on reference memory version of Morris water maze in young adult rats. *Iran. Biomed. J.* 12, 123-128.

Sato, K., Akaishi, T., Matsuki, N., Ohno, Y. & Nakazawa, K. (2007). Beta-Estradiol induces synaptogenesis in the hippocampus by enhancing. brain-derived neurotrophic factor release from dentate gyrus granule cells. *Brain Res. 1150*, 108-120.

Sherwin, B. B. (2012). Estrogen and cognitive functioning in women, lessons we have learned. *Behav Neurosci. 126*, 123-127.

Smejkalova, T. & Woolley, C. S. (2010). Estradiol acutely potentiates hippocampal excitatory synaptic transmission through a presynaptic mechanism. *J Neurosci. 30*, 16137-16148.

Solomon, P. R., Vander Schaaf, E. R., Thompson, R. F. & Weisz, D. J. (1986). Hippocampus and trace conditioning of the rabbit's classically conditioned nictitating membrane response. *Behav Neurosci, 100*, 729–744.

Spencer-Segal Joanna, L., Mumeko, C., Tsuda, Larissa Mattei, Waters, Elizabeth M., Romeo, Russell D., Milner, Teresa A., McEwen, Bruce S. & Sonoko Ogawa. (2012). Estradiol acts via estrogen receptors alpha and beta on pathways important for synaptic plasticity in the mouse hippocampal formation. *Neuroscience. Neuroscience. 202*, 131–146.

Srivastava, D. P. (2012). Two-Step Wiring Plasticity - A mechanism for estrogen-induced rewiring of cortical circuits. *J Steroid Biochem Mol Biol. 131*, 17-23.

Tanapat, P., Hastings, N. B. & Gould, E. (2005). Adult female rat in a dose- and time-dependent manner. *J Comp Neurol, 481*, 252-265.

Triggs, W. J. & Willmore, L. J. (1984). In vivo lipid peroxidation in rat brain following intracortical Fe2+ injection. *J. Neurochem. 42*, 976-980.

Wallace, M., Luine, V., Arellanos, A. & Frankfurt, M. (2006). Ovariectomized rats show decreased recognition memory and spine density in the hippocampus and prefrontal cortex. *Brain Res. 1126*, 176–182.

Woolley, C. S. (2007). Acute effects of estrogen on neuronal physiology. *Annu. Rev. Pharmacol. Toxicol. 47*, 657–680.

Woolley, C. S. & McEwen, B. S. (1993). Roles of estradiol and progesterone in regulation of hippocampal dendritic spine density during the estrous cycle in the rat. *J. Comp. Neurol. 336*, 293-306.

Xu, X. & Zhang, Z. (2006). Effects of estradiol benzoate on learning-memory behavior and synaptic structure in ovariectomized mice. *Life Sci. 79*, 1553-1560.

Yao, J., Chen, S., Cadenas, E. & Diaz Brinton, R. (2011). Estrogen Protection Against Mitochondrial Toxin-Induced Cell Death In Hippocampal Neurons, Antagonism by Progesterone. *Brain Res.1379*, 2–10.

Zhu, Y., Carvey, P. M. & Ling, Z. (2006). Age-related changes in glutathione and glutathione-related enzymes in rat brain. *Brain Res. 1090*, 35–44.

Index

A

B

D

E

G

H

I

J

K

L

M

N

O

P

Q

T

U

V